DRUGS IN OBSTETRICS AND GYNECOLOGY

DRUGS IN OBSTETRICS AND GYNECOLOGY

Editors

Ashok Kumar
MD PhD FAMS FICOG FICMCH
Director-Professor
Department of Obstetrics and Gynecology
Maulana Azad Medical College and
Lok Nayak Jai Prakash Narayan Hospital
New Delhi, India

Krishna Agarwal MS
Professor
Department of Obstetrics and Gynecology
Maulana Azad Medical College and
Lok Nayak Jai Prakash Narayan Hospital
New Delhi, India

Sudha Prasad MS
Director-Professor and Head
Department of Obstetrics and Gynecology
Maulana Azad Medical College and
Lok Nayak Jai Prakash Narayan Hospital
New Delhi, India

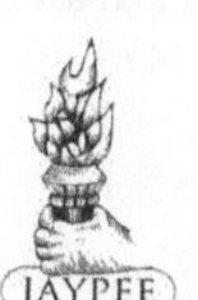

JAYPEE *The Health Sciences Publisher*
New Delhi | London | Philadelphia | Panama

Jaypee Brothers Medical Publishers (P) Ltd.

Headquarters
Jaypee Brothers Medical Publishers (P) Ltd.
4838/24, Ansari Road, Daryaganj
New Delhi 110 002, India
Phone: +91-11-43574357
Fax: +91-11-43574314
E-mail: jaypee@jaypeebrothers.com

Overseas Offices

J.P. Medical Ltd.
83, Victoria Street, London
SW1H 0HW (UK)
Phone: +44-20 3170 8910
Fax: +44(0) 20 3008 6180
E-mail: info@jpmedpub.com

Jaypee Medical Inc.
325, Chestnut Street
Suite 412
Philadelphia, PA 19106, USA
Phone: +1 267-519-9789
E-mail: jpmed.us@gmail.com

Jaypee Brothers Medical Publishers (P) Ltd.
Bhotahity, Kathmandu, Nepal
Phone: +977-9741283608
E-mail: kathmandu@jaypeebrothers.com

Jaypee-Highlights Medical Publishers Inc.
City of Knowledge, Bld. 237, Clayton
Panama City, Panama
Phone: +1 507-301-0496
Fax: +1 507-301-0499
E-mail: cservice@jphmedical.com

Jaypee Brothers Medical Publishers (P) Ltd.
17/1-B, Babar Road, Block-B, Shaymali
Mohammadpur, Dhaka-1207
Bangladesh
Mobile: +08801912003485
E-mail: jaypeedhaka@gmail.com

Website: www.jaypeebrothers.com
Website: www.jaypeedigital.com

Inquiries for bulk sales may be solicited at: jaypee@jaypeebrothers.com

Drugs in Obstetrics and Gynecology

First Edition: 2016, Reprint: **2025**

ISBN: 978-93-5250-168-7

Printed in India

Dedicated to

All patients who provide us
the opportunities to learn

Contributors

Anjali Tempe
Director-Professor
Department of Obstetrics and Gynecology
Maulana Azad Medical College and
Lok Nayak Jai Prakash Narayan Hospital
New Delhi, India

Anju Bhalotra
Professor
Department of Anesthesiology
Maulana Azad Medical College and
Lok Nayak Jai Prakash Narayan Hospital
New Delhi, India

Ankita Pal
Senior Resident
Department of Obstetrics and Gynecology
Maulana Azad Medical College and
Lok Nayak Jai Prakash Narayan Hospital
New Delhi, India

Anoosha K Ravi
Resident
Department of Obstetrics and Gynecology
Maulana Azad Medical College and
Lok Nayak Jai Prakash Narayan Hospital
New Delhi, India

Ashok Kumar
Director-Professor
Department of Obstetrics and Gynecology
Maulana Azad Medical College and
Lok Nayak Jai Prakash Narayan Hospital
New Delhi, India

Ashwani Khanna
State TB Officer
Delhi, India

Asmita M Rathore
Director-Professor
Department of Obstetrics and Gynecology
Maulana Azad Medical College and
Lok Nayak Jai Prakash Narayan Hospital
New Delhi, India

Asmita Patil
Assistant Professor
Department of Physiology
All India Institute of Medical Sciences (AIIMS)
New Delhi, India

Aswathy Kumaran
FNB Resident
Department of Obstetrics and Gynecology
Maulana Azad Medical College and
Lok Nayak Jai Prakash Narayan Hospital
New Delhi, India

B Nisha
Specialist
Department of Obstetrics and Gynecology
Maulana Azad Medical College and
Lok Nayak Jai Prakash Narayan Hospital
New Delhi, India

Bhoomika Tantuway
Senior Resident
Department of Obstetrics and Gynecology
Maulana Azad Medical College and
Lok Nayak Jai Prakash Narayan Hospital
New Delhi, India

Bidisha Singha
Specialist
Department of Obstetrics and Gynecology
Maulana Azad Medical College and
Lok Nayak Jai Prakash Narayan Hospital
New Delhi, India

Binni Makkar
Senior Resident
Department of Obstetrics and Gynecology
Maulana Azad Medical College and
Lok Nayak Jai Prakash Narayan Hospital
New Delhi, India

Chandan Dubey
Assistant Professor
Department of Obstetrics and Gynecology
Maulana Azad Medical College and
Lok Nayak Jai Prakash Narayan Hospital
New Delhi, India

Chetna Arvind Sethi
Specialist
Department of Obstetrics and Gynecology
Maulana Azad Medical College and
Lok Nayak Jai Prakash Narayan Hospital
New Delhi, India

Deepika S Sharma
Resident
Department of Obstetrics and Gynecology
Maulana Azad Medical College and
Lok Nayak Jai Prakash Narayan Hospital
New Delhi, India

Deepti Goswami
Professor
Department of Obstetrics and Gynecology
Maulana Azad Medical College and
Lok Nayak Jai Prakash Narayan Hospital
New Delhi, India

Devender Kumar
Professor
Department of Obstetrics and Gynecology
Maulana Azad Medical College and
Lok Nayak Jai Prakash Narayan Hospital
New Delhi, India

Gauri Gandhi
Director-Professor
Department of Obstetrics and Gynecology
Maulana Azad Medical College and
Lok Nayak Jai Prakash Narayan Hospital
New Delhi, India

Gunjan Bhatnagar
Senior Resident
Department of Obstetrics and Gynecology
Maulana Azad Medical College and
Lok Nayak Jai Prakash Narayan Hospital
New Delhi, India

Komal Rastogi
Resident
Department of Obstetrics and Gynecology
Maulana Azad Medical College and
Lok Nayak Jai Prakash Narayan Hospital
New Delhi, India

Krishna Agarwal
Professor
Department of Obstetrics and Gynecology
Maulana Azad Medical College and
Lok Nayak Jai Prakash Narayan Hospital
New Delhi, India

Latika Sahu
Professor
Department of Obstetrics and Gynecology
Maulana Azad Medical College and
Lok Nayak Jai Prakash Narayan Hospital
New Delhi, India

Madhavi M Gupta
Professor
Department of Obstetrics and Gynecology
Maulana Azad Medical College and
Lok Nayak Jai Prakash Narayan Hospital
New Delhi, India

Madhur Kumar
Resident
Department of Surgery
Government Medical College
Amritsar, Punjab, India

Meenoo S
Resident
Department of Obstetrics and Gynecology
Maulana Azad Medical College and
Lok Nayak Jai Prakash Narayan Hospital
New Delhi, India

Mridul Daga
Director-Professor
Department of Medicine
Maulana Azad Medical College and
Lok Nayak Jai Prakash Narayan Hospital
New Delhi, India

Nalini Bala
Medical Officer
Department of Obstetrics and Gynecology
Maulana Azad Medical College and
Lok Nayak Jai Prakash Narayan Hospital
New Delhi, India

Poonam Kashyap
Specialist
Department of Obstetrics and Gynecology
Maulana Azad Medical College and
Lok Nayak Jai Prakash Narayan Hospital
New Delhi, India

Poonam Sachdeva
Specialist
Department of Obstetrics and Gynecology
Maulana Azad Medical College and
Lok Nayak Jai Prakash Narayan Hospital
New Delhi, India

Preeti Singh
Assistant Professor
Department of Obstetrics and Gynecology
Maulana Azad Medical College and
Lok Nayak Jai Prakash Narayan Hospital
New Delhi, India

Purnima Gupta
Resident
Department of Obstetrics and Gynecology
Maulana Azad Medical College and
Lok Nayak Jai Prakash Narayan Hospital
New Delhi, India

Pushpa Mishra
Senior Medical Officer
Department of Obstetrics and Gynecology
Maulana Azad Medical College and
Lok Nayak Jai Prakash Narayan Hospital
New Delhi, India

Rachna Sharma
Specialist
Department of Obstetrics and Gynecology
Maulana Azad Medical College and
Lok Nayak Jai Prakash Narayan Hospital
New Delhi, India

Reena Rani
Senior Resident
Department of Obstetrics and Gynecology
Maulana Azad Medical College and
Lok Nayak Jai Prakash Narayan Hospital
New Delhi, India

Renu Tanwar
Professor
Department of Obstetrics and Gynecology
Maulana Azad Medical College and
Lok Nayak Jai Prakash Narayan Hospital
New Delhi, India

Reva Tripathi
Director-Professor
Department of Obstetrics and Gynecology
Maulana Azad Medical College and
Lok Nayak Jai Prakash Narayan Hospital
New Delhi, India

Sangeeta Bhasin
Chief Medical Officer
Department of Obstetrics and Gynecology
Maulana Azad Medical College and
Lok Nayak Jai Prakash Narayan Hospital
New Delhi, India

Sangeeta Gupta
Professor
Department of Obstetrics and Gynecology
Maulana Azad Medical College and
Lok Nayak Jai Prakash Narayan Hospital
New Delhi, India

Shailja Singh
FNB Resident
Department of Obstetrics and Gynecology
Maulana Azad Medical College and
Lok Nayak Jai Prakash Narayan Hospital
New Delhi, India

Shailja Verma
Senior Resident
Department of Obstetrics and Gynecology
Maulana Azad Medical College and
Lok Nayak Jai Prakash Narayan Hospital
New Delhi, India

Shakun Tyagi
Assistant Professor
Department of Obstetrics and Gynecology
Maulana Azad Medical College and
Lok Nayak Jai Prakash Narayan Hospital
New Delhi, India

Shweta Tahlan
Senior Resident
Department of Obstetrics and Gynecology
Maulana Azad Medical College and
Lok Nayak Jai Prakash Narayan Hospital
New Delhi, India

Snigdha Pathak
Resident
Department of Obstetrics and Gynecology
Maulana Azad Medical College and
Lok Nayak Jai Prakash Narayan Hospital
New Delhi, India

Sudha Prasad
Director-Professor and Head
Department of Obstetrics and Gynecology
Maulana Azad Medical College and
Lok Nayak Jai Prakash Narayan Hospital
New Delhi, India

Supriya Hajela
Senior Resident
Department of Obstetrics and Gynecology
Maulana Azad Medical College and
Lok Nayak Jai Prakash Narayan Hospital
New Delhi, India

Swati Kumari
Resident
Department of Obstetrics and Gynecology
Maulana Azad Medical College and
Lok Nayak Jai Prakash Narayan Hospital
New Delhi, India

Swati Priya
Senior Resident
Department of Obstetrics and Gynecology
Maulana Azad Medical College and
Lok Nayak Jai Prakash Narayan Hospital
New Delhi, India

Tanvi Raj
Senior Resident
Department of Obstetrics and Gynecology
Maulana Azad Medical College and
Lok Nayak Jai Prakash Narayan Hospital
New Delhi, India

Vaishali Paliwal
Resident
Department of Obstetrics and Gynecology
Maulana Azad Medical College and
Lok Nayak Jai Prakash Narayan Hospital
New Delhi, India

YM Mala
Professor
Department of Obstetrics and Gynecology
Maulana Azad Medical College and
Lok Nayak Jai Prakash Narayan Hospital
New Delhi, India

Preface

Drugs are the integral part of medicine. The rational use of drugs has saved enumerable lives, prevented epidemics and promoted health in general. Accessibility to essential medicines is an essential element of a health system. However, to accrue the optimum benefits, the drugs have to be used optimally—the right indication, right drug, right dose, right duration, minimal toxicity, and at the lowest cost, denoted as "rational drug therapy".

Unfortunately, despite knowing the benefits of rational drug therapy, irrationality in the use of drugs is rather rampant to the extent that it has been identified as a major public health problem. Apart from causing harm to the health of people, it is responsible for high cost of health care impoverishing people and communities. As per a recent estimate, over 53 million people get impoverished due to health care cost and cost of drugs constitutes a major part of it. Irrational use of antimicrobial drugs resulting in high level of antimicrobial resistance has almost pushed us to preantibiotics era.

The specialty of obstetrics and gynecology is different from other specialties of medicine in many different ways. A practitioner of this specialty has to have artistic skills of a surgeon as well as wisdom of a physician. Unfortunately, this does not happen in reality and we tend to falter on the very basic principles of pharmacotherapy. Despite being a physician for a significant part of our routines, we keep getting confused when confronted with names of drugs—new or old, as well as pharmacological terms associated with it. One of the reasons is the unavailability of 'resource book' that is concise yet provides optimum amount of details to help us make well-informed decisions about the use of drugs.

We have attempted to fill this void through this modest attempt. The book includes description of commonly used drugs in obstetrics and gynecology. In the beginning of a chapter, common-related drugs are given in a table for quick-reference followed by other required details in the text. There are a total of 35 chapters, each one being concise enough to be read over a short time. We have tried to maintain uniformity throughout the book to make it more predictive and easy to understand. Enough number of tables are provided on essential information. The section on antimicrobials provides optimum choice of antibiotics in different clinical conditions. A table has been provided on classification of commonly used antibiotics, which will help the reader in choosing the right agent in different situations.

We hope that the book would serve its purpose and help practicing physicians as well as postgraduate students to practice rational drug therapy in their day-to-day practice. It was a great learning experience for us to go through the nuances of the subject. Despite of observing due diligence, we are sure that there would be mistakes and errors, which we hope that the generous readers would overlook and provide us feedback for improvement in the future editions.

We thank the contributors for painstakingly compiling their chapters. Mr Jai Mohan deserves special thanks for coordinating with the contributors and the publisher. We also thank M/s Jaypee Brothers Medical Publishers, New Delhi, India, for bringing out this work wonderfully.

Ashok Kumar
Krishna Agarwal
Sudha Prasad

Contents

SECTION IX Anticancer Drugs

SECTION X Miscellaneous

FDA PREGNANCY DRUG CATEGORIES

FDA Category	*Type of Studies Available*
A	Adequate, well-controlled studies in pregnant women have not shown an increased risk of fetal abnormalities in any trimester of pregnancy
B	Well-controlled studies in animals have revealed no evidence of harm to the fetus
C	No animal studies or the one's reported have shown an adverse effect on the fetus and there are no adequate and well-controlled studies in pregnant women
D	Risk to the fetus demonstrated in well-controlled or observational studies in pregnant women, however, the benefits of therapy could outweigh the potential risk. Acceptable for use in a life-threatening situation only
X	Positive evidence of harm to the fetus seen in well-controlled or observational studies in both animals and pregnant women. The use of the drug is contraindicated in women who are or might become pregnant
N	Not classified by FDA

LACTATION DRUG CATEGORIES

Category	*Safety*	*Type of Studies Available*
L1	Safest	Controlled studies in breastfeeding women have not shown any risk to the breastfeeding infant and possibility of harm is remote
L2	Safer	Drugs which have been studied in limited number of breastfeeding women without any increase in adverse effects in the breastfeeding infant
L3	Moderately safe	There are no controlled studies, but risk of untoward effects on breast-fed infant is possible OR Controlled studies show minimal nonlife-threatening adverse effects. These drugs are given when potential benefit outweighs potential risk to the mother
L4	Possibly hazardous	There is evidence of risk to the breastfed infant or to the breast milk production. But these drugs can be used in life-threatening situation and when safer drugs cannot be used
L5	Contraindicated	Human studies showed significant risk to the infant, the risk of using drug clearly outweighs any possible benefit from breastfeeding. The drug is contraindicated during lactation

Section I

PRINCIPLES OF DRUG THERAPY

CHAPTER

CHAPTER 1

Rational Drug Therapy

Krishna Agarwal

INTRODUCTION

'Rational drug therapy' literally means using a right drug in right dose and for right duration. The irrational use of drugs is not only dangerous in short-term but is on its way to cause long-term destructive consequences.

The concept of rational drug use is age old. Reference about 'rational drug use' has been made as early as 300 BC by an Alexandrian physician Herophilus who stated that "medicines are nothing by themselves but are the very hands of god if employed with reason and prudence".

Definition

WHO defines rational drug use as "rational use of drug requires that patient receives medication appropriate to their clinical needs in doses that meet their own individual requirements for an adequate period of time, at the lowest cost to them and their community.[1]

This definition requires following criteria (*IA-PIM*) to be fulfilled:

- *Appropriate indication*: It is based on the medical rationale that the drug is effective and safe in a particular clinical situation.
- *Appropriate agent*: Selection of drug is based on the efficacy, safety and cost of the therapy.
- *Appropriate patient*: Drug is acceptable to the patient, no contraindications and the possibility of adverse drug reaction is minimum.
- *Appropriate information*: Patient should be given information regarding the disease and medicines which are prescribed.
- *Appropriate monitoring*: Any unexpected effects of drug should be monitored and appropriate measures taken.

However, more often than not, prescriptions do not follow the steps and are irrational with respect to one or more reasons.

Epidemiology

Magnitude of Irrational Drug Use

Unfortunately, irrational use of drugs is rampant all over the globe including India. It is estimated that half of the prescriptions are irrational.

Various studies from developing and developed world have revealed the pattern of irrationality such as drug not related to diagnosis, use of costlier drugs when the cheaper and effective drugs are available, polypharmacy (defined as prescription, administration, or use of more medications than are clinically indicated, or when a medical regimen includes at least one unnecessary medication), improper use of antibiotics, irrational self-medication and inadequate dose of medications.[2]

Studies from Canada, USA, Australia have revealed that the irrational drug use is quite prevalent even in the developed world. A Canadian study from a teaching hospital revealed 50% of the prescriptions of antibiotics in gynecologic patients were irrational and of these 86.8% irrational prescriptions were used for prophylaxis.[3] Study from USA revealed 41% cases with inappropriately used antibiotics in hospital patients.[4]

A study from a teaching hospital in South Africa showed 54% irrational drug use in gynecology in patients.[5] A study from university care center from Croatia highlighted high prescription rate of antibiotics, concomitant use of antibiotics with a similar spectrum of activity.[6]

A study on the use of antimicrobials in obstetrics and gynecology in a tertiary care unit of India revealed that antibiotic use was to the tune of 95%. Out of these only 12% (42/340) prescriptions were rational, 33% (112/340) were semirational and 40% (136/340) were irrational.[7] Study from city of Jammu showed that drugs used were inappropriate in 33% cases and large number of prescriptions did not confirm to ideal patterns.[8]

Impact on Morbidities, Mortality, Economic Burden and Hospital Stay

Irrational drug use may lead to increase in morbidity and sometimes even mortality tA recent review by Institute of Medicine, USA has estimated that 1 out of 131 outpatients and 1 out of 854 inpatients die due to medication error.[9]

A few studies from India reveal that antibiotics are being misused which increases the cost of therapy several times resulting in economic burden on already compromised health system. In an Indian study it was estimated that this irrational use had led to 75% extra cost of the treatment.[7]

In a study from Pakistan, it was seen that after use of antibiotics according to ACOG guidelines, the cost of antibiotics per patient was reduced by 90%. Decrease in the length of hospital stay and workload on nursing staff was also observed.[10]

Common Forms of Irrationality in Drug Use

Antimicrobials, analgesics and supplements are the most commonly used but sadly the most commonly misused drugs.

The Antimicrobials

Widespread irrational use of antibiotics is a vivid example of irrationality which has started showing off its devastation in form of immerging antimicrobial resistance (AMR).

It has been known that antibiotics affect healthy gut flora and diarrhea is a common side effect of some of the antibiotics. Diarrhea is common with the use of amoxicillin and clavulanic acid. Fluoroquinolone, a commonly used antibiotic, is known to affect the microbiome. Frequent and irrational use of antibiotics has been linked to a change in human microbiome and many diseases. The human microbiome constitutes healthy microorganisms residing in our body—skin, gastrointestinal tract, respiratory tract, genital tract, surface of eyes and others. Recently, this change in microbiome has been even linked with the diabetes, hypertension, asthma and even obesity.[11,12]

Irrational use of antibiotics is common in obstetrics and gynecology **(Table 1.1)**. We need to base our prescriptions of antibiotics after carefully considering the clinical evidence, sensitivity pattern of the causative agent for a particular condition, local or national guidelines and choosing as far as possible from the essential drug list (prescribed by the hospital, country or World Health Organization).

Use of antimicrobials can be rationalized if the individual hospitals develop their own guidelines based on the national and international guidelines.

Table 1.1: Antimicrobials in obstetrics and gynecology

S. No.	*Clinical situation*	*Common irrationality*	*Rational use*
1.	Normal vaginal delivery with or without episiotomy	Oral antibiotics such as ampicillin, metrogyl, amoxicillin—clavulanic acid and cephalexin are commonly used for 5–7 days	No prophylactic antibiotic is required. Maintaining proper asepsis is what is sufficient[13,14]
2.	Elective cesarean section	Injectable antibiotics—ampicillin, gentamicin, metronidazole, cephalosporins, amoxicillin-clavulanic acid given for 5–7 days	Cefazolin 1–2 g IV or Clindamycin 600 mg IV or Erythromycin 300 mg IV 15–60 minutes before the incision[13,14]
3.	Emergency cesarean section	Fixed drug combinations—ceftazidime, gentamicin and metronidazole for 7–10 days	Same as above However, if the procedure extends beyond 3 hours or bleeding more than 1500 mL, one more dose needs to be given[13,14]
4.	Preterm premature rupture of membrances (PPROM)	Ampicillin + gentamicin + metronidazole for 10–14 days Ceftazidime + gentamicin + metronidazole for 10–14 days	Erythromycin 250 mg 6 hourly for 10 days
5.	Preterm labor with intact membranes	Ampicillin + gentamicin + metronidazole for 10–14 days Ceftazidime + gentamicin + metronidazole for 10–14 days	No antibiotics
6.	Elective total abdominal hysterectomy	Ampicillin + gentamicin + metronidazole for 10–14 days Ceftazidime + gentamicin + metronidazole for 10–14	Single dose of injection cefazolin 1–2 g IV Or Clindamycin 600 mg IV or Erythromycin 300 mg IV, 15–60 minutes before the incision[15]
7.	Infertility	Rampant use of ATT on positive polymerase chain reaction (PCR) for tuberculosis (TB) in blood	PCR for TB based on detection of DNA and RNA of tubercular bacillus is a nonspecific test. In a meta-analysis, sensitivity and specificity of PCR for TB ranged from 9% to 100% and from 25% to 100%, respectively. ATT should be started on only a strong suspicion and in consultation with a DOTS center[16]
8.	Upper respiratory infection (URI) and viral fevers	Levofloxacin, ceftazidime, Amoxicillin and clavulanic acid combination for variable duration	No antibiotics required

Analgesics

Use of analgesics is another example of dug misuse (**Table 1.2**). Analgesics are being given for relief of pain without finding out the cause which may lead to prolongation of disease. Giving long-term analgesics could cause addiction or even have bad effect on the important organs like liver and kidney.

Supplements

During pregnancy, supplementation of only iron and folic acid is recommended by World Health Organization and the Government of India. Rest all supplements are of no proven benefit. However, the prescriptions in antenatal patients are replete with all micronutrients and protein powder. These all drastically increase the cost of therapy with possible side effects or harmful effects (**Table 1.3**).

Hormones

Use of various progestogens during pregnancy is quite common (**Table 1.4**). It is prescribed even to the pregnant women with no high risk factors. This practice of prescribing progestogen thinking that "even if there no benefit it would not cause any harm to the woman," should be stopped.

Table 1.2: Analgesic use in obstetrics and gynecology

S. No.	*Clinical situation*	*Common irrationality*	*Rational use*
1.	Chronic pelvic pain	Long-term use of NSAIDs (diclofenac) and opioids (tramadol)	Find out the cause of pain (endometriosis), evaluate for depression or sexual abuse and treat the cause
2.	Postoperative pain	Round the clock injectable diclofenac or tramadol for up to 7–10 days	After 48 hours analgesics could be given on demand

Table 1.3: Supplements use during pregnancy

S. No.	*Clinical situation*	*Common irrationality*	*Rational use*
1.	Low risk and high risk pregnancies	Multivitamin commonly prescribed	No proven role and should not be prescribed[16]
2.	Low risk and high risk pregnancies	Micronutrients which include zinc, copper, magnesium, selenium	No proven role and should not be prescribed[17]
3.	Pregnancies at risk of pre-eclampsia-history of pre-eclampsia in previous pregnancy or current gestational hypertension	Antioxidants	Role in pre-eclampsia is proposed but not yet proven, should not be prescribed.[18]

Table 1.4: Progestogen use during pregnancy

S. No.	*Common prescribed*	*Common irrationality*	*Rational use*
1.	Micronized progestogen or hydroxyprogesteron injections in treatment and prophylaxis of threatened miscarriage	No proven role	Should not be prescribed.[19,20]

Drugs Used in Pre-eclampsia and Eclampsia

Pre-eclampsia and eclampsia, which are one of three leading causes of maternal deaths, if not treated properly could lead to maternal mortality. Administration of magnesium sulfate as anticonvulsant and hydralazine or labetalol as antihypertensive is the first drug of choice. Use of diazepam for control of convulsion or frusemide for control of hypertension could result in maternal death **(Table 1.5)**.

Drugs During Labor

A woman in labor mostly requires monitoring and no medications. Induction of labor is being performed without any indication. Woman in latent phase or active phase of labor are being started oxytocin infusion and given antispasmodics for pain relief. These medications have no role and may sometimes harm the patient **(Table 1.6)**.

Antenatal Steroids

Antenatal steroids are used in women at risk of preterm vaginal delivery. However, multiple courses and its use beyond 34 completed weeks is common **(Table 1.7)**.

Drugs Used for Ovulation-induction

As the incidence of infertility is on the rise, there is increase in the rate of complications due to misuse of drugs used for its treatment **(Table 1.8)**.

Measures for Promoting Rational Drug Use

To fulfill the IA-PIM criteria for rational drug prescription (WHO), process of prescribing would require stepwise approach in following manner:

- Defining patient's problem (diagnosis)
- Defining effective and safe treatment (drugs and nondrugs)

Table 1.5: Use of anticonvulsants and diuretics in pre-eclampsia and eclampsia

S. No.	*Clinical situation*	*Common irrationality*	*Rational use*
1.	Eclampsia	Intravenous diazepam for control of convulsions	Could lead to respiratory depression and death. IV loading dose of magnesium sulfate should be given
2.	Pre-eclampsia, eclampsia	Injectable furosemide for control of blood pressure	Could lead to shock and death. For control of BP, IV labetalol or nitroglycerine infusion can be used

Table 1.6: Commonly used drugs during labor

S. No.	*Clinical situation*	*Common irrationality*	*Rational use*
1.	Woman admitted in labor	Use of enema	Increases incidence of neonatal infection. Should not be used
2.	Woman admitted with labor pains	Augmentation of labor with oxytocin infusion	No need for augmentation in a low risk woman, it increases incidence of fetal distress, rate of cesarean section and increased risk of birth asphyxia
3.	For relief of pain in labor	Use of antispasmodics like hyoscine bromide	No proven role[21]
4.	In advanced labor to increase softness and dilatability of cervix	Use of valethamate bromide	No proven role[21]

Table 1.7: Use of steroids during pregnancy

S. No.	Clinical situation	Common irrationality	Rational use
1.	Pregnancy before 34 weeks of pregnancy	Repeated doses of dexamethasone or betamethasone	Can cause fetal growth restriction, not indicated
2.	Preterm labor beyond 34 completed weeks	Antenatal steroids	No benefit

Table 1.8: Ovulation inducing agents for treatment of infertility

S. No.	Clinical situation	Common irrationality	Rational use
1.	Infertility	Use of clomiphene without ruling out all causes of infertility	Establish that the couple is infertile and that anovulation is the cause of infertility and all other causes have been ruled out
2.	Infertility	Use of latrozole	Should not be used, banned by DCGI because of suspicion that it increases risk of congenital malformations

- Selecting appropriate drug/drugs, dose, and duration
- Writing the prescription
- Providing adequate information to the patient
- Planning for evaluation of treatment response.

Defining Patient's Problem

This is the basic requirement for drug prescription. The physician must confirm the diagnosis before prescribing the medicine.

Like in a case of chronic pelvic pain, cause of pain should be established before prescribing her the medicine. Before starting ovulation induction, ensure that the cause for infertility is defective ovulation and all other causes of infertility have been ruled out.

Defining Effective and Safe Treatment (Drugs and Nondrugs)

Once diagnosis is established, next step is to know what would be the effective as well as safe treatment for the patient. Use of a drug should be based on the clinical guidelines which may be hospital based, national or international guidelines. In the absence of any such guidelines, the treatment may be based on the evidences which may be in the form of meta-analysis, systematic reviews, well conducted randomized controlled trials or sometimes the cohort studies.

Selecting Appropriate Drug(s), Dose and Duration

The knowledge regarding the available drugs for a particular condition and choosing amongst them the first drug of choice after excluding the contraindications for that drug would constitute the rational use.

Use of hospital drug formulary, national drug formulary or even choosing from the WHO essential drug list would take care of this aspect of rational drug therapy. WHO essential drug list enlists the most suitable drugs to be used in common clinical conditions of different specialties. Sometimes if the guidelines are not available or the drug is not included in the essential drug list then, drug treatment should be based on the clinical evidences.

Writing the Prescription

This step in drug therapy is very important. Literature is full of untoward incidences due dispensing of wrong drugs because the prescription was not written clearly. Even MCI has given directions to practitioners to use capital letters while writing the names of the drugs. The MCI directs to write generic names. It has been proven that when generic names are used, it has helped in rationalizing the drug use by directly linking the disease and the drug.[22]

The prescription should be written on a proper drug slip meant for writing a prescription. For a private practitioner, the prescription slip carries name, address and phone numbers of the prescriber.

Patient's name, age, address and date should be written. Symbol Rx is written before writing the drug name. This is an abbreviation for a Latin phrase that means "take thou." Dose of the drug, frequency, route of administration and duration of the drug intake should be clearly mentioned. In the end the prescriber should sign the prescription. Every aspect of prescription writing is important and the clinician must master the art of prescription writing during their training.

Providing Adequate Information to the Patient

Patient is provided with the information about what would be the effect of drug , how to take the medicine and for how much duration. The patient should be warned about the side effects of a particular drug and what to do if patient has some side effects.

Planning for Evaluation of Treatment Response

This step should always be a part of drug therapy and evaluation may be planned in a way which is convenient to the patient. Quality improvement (QI) initiatives at national and hospital level could provide guidance on the rationality of drug use. A QI in a tertiary care hospital in Pakistan has proved to effectively decrease the use of irrational antibiotics. This study revealed that use of antibiotics according to ACOG guidelines led to decrease in the use of antibiotics from 97% to 8% and surgical site infections rates came down to less than 5%.[11]

Regulatory Body for Promotion of Rational Use

There is a national regulatory body in India that guides us about the use of drugs and provides some safeguard in case of an untoward adverse drug reaction.

Central Drug Standard Control Organization (CDSCO)

It is the national regulatory agency for Indian pharmaceuticals and medical devices. It serves same function in India as the Food and Drug Administration (FDA) in United States.

It is headed by Drug Controller General of India (DCGI). DCGI is responsible for approval of new drugs, conduct of clinical trials in the country, laying down standards for drugs, controls the quality of imported drugs, coordination of the activities of State Drug Control Organizations and provision of expert opinion about the enforcement of Drugs and Cosmetics Act. The office of CDSCO is located at FDA Bhawan, Kotla Road, New Delhi 110002 and functions under the Directorate General of Health Services.

The Central Government has established four zonal offices of the Central Drug Standard Control Organization at Mumbai, Kolkata, Chennai, and Ghaziabad. The zonal offices work in close collaboration with the State Drug Control Administration and assist them in securing uniform enforcement of the Drug Act and other connected legislations, on all India basis.

Pharmacovigilance

This is a relatively new concept for enhancing the rational drug use.[23]

WHO defines pharmacovigilance (PV) as the science and activities relating to the detection, assessment, understanding and prevention of adverse effects or any other drug-related problem. It established its International pharmacovigilance program after the Thalidomide disaster detected in 1961. It promotes PV at country level and by the end of 2010, 134 countries including India were part of WHO PV program.

The Pharmacovigilance Program of India (PVPI) was started in India in July 2010 by CDSCO under the aegis of Ministry of Health and Family Welfare. At present the national coordinating center for PVPI is Indian Phamacopoeia Commisssion (IPC), Ghaziabad, UP. Any adverse drug reaction should be informed to the office of PvPI on following address:

Secretary-cum-Scientific Director
Indian Pharmacopoeia Commission
Ministry of Health & Family Welfare
Government of India
Sector-23, Raj Nagar, Ghaziabad-201 002
Telephone: 0120-2783400, 2783401, 2783392,
FAX: 0120-2783311
E-mail: ipclab@vsnl.net

REFERENCES

1. Promoting rationale use of medicines: core components. WHO policy perspectives on medicines, 2002.
2. Hogerzeil HV. Promoting rational prescribing: an international perspective. British Journal of Clinical Pharmacology. 1995;39(1):1-6.
3. Achong MR, Hauser BA, Krusky JL. Rational and irrational use of antibiotics in a Canadian teaching hospital. Can Med Assoc J. 1977; 116(3): 256-9.
4. Maki DG, Schuna AA. A study of antimicrobial misuse in a university hospital. Am J Med Soc 1978; 275:271-82.
5. Till B, Williams L, Oliver SP, Pillans PI. A survey of inpatient antibiotic use in a teaching hospital. S Afr Med J. 1991;80:7-10.
6. Erdeljić V, Francetić I, Macolić Sarinić V, Bilusić M, Huić M, Merćep I, Makar-Ausperger K. [Evaluation of justification for antibiotic use at the Internal Medicine Clinic of the Clinical Hospital in Zagreb. Acta Med Croatica. 2004;58(4):293-9.
7. Amane H, Kop P. Prescription analysis to evaluate rational use of antimicrobials. Int J of Pharma & Bioscience. 2011:2;314-9.
8. Sharma P, Kapoor B. Study of prescribing patterns for rationale drug therapy. JK Science. 2003;5:107-9.
9. Wittich CM, Burkle CM, Lanier WL. Medication errors: an overview for clinicians. Mayo Clin Proc. 2014;89(8):1116-25.
10. Nausheen S1, Hammad R, Khan A. Rational use of antibiotics—a quality improvement initiative in hospital setting. J Pak Med Assoc. 2013;63(1):60-4.
11. De Lastours V, Fantin B. Impact of fluoroquinolones on human microbiota. Focus on the emergence of antibiotic resistance. Future Microbiol. 2015;29:1-15.
12. Nobel YR, Cox LM, Kirigin FF, Bokulich NA, Yamanishi S, Teitler I, Chung J, Sohn J, et al. Metabolic and metagenomic outcomes from early-life pulsed antibiotic treatment. Nat Commun. 2015;6:7486.
13. Antibiotic prophylaxis in Obstetrics. SOGC clinical practice guidelines, 2010.
14. Prophylactic antibiotics in Obstetrics and Gynaecology. C-Gen 17. The Royal Australian and New Zealand College of Obstetricians and Gynaecologists.
15. ACOG guidelines for antibiotic prophylaxis for gynecological procedures. Am Fam Physician, 2007;75(7):1094-6.
16. Sarmiento OL, Weigle KA, Alexander J, Weber DJ, Miller WC. Assessment by meta-analysis of PCR for diagnosis of smear-negative pulmonary tuberculosis. J Clin Microbiol. 2003;41(7):3233-40.
17. Kawai K, Spiegelman D, Shankar AH, Fawzi WW. Maternal multiple micronutrient supplementation and pregnancy outcomes in developing countries: meta-analysis and meta-regression. Bull World Health Organ. 2011;89(6):402-411B.
18. Salles AM, Galvao TF, Silva MT, Motta LC, Pereira MG. Antioxidants for preventing preeclampsia: a systematic review. Scientific World Journal. 2012;243-476.

19. Oates-Whitehead RM, Haas DM, Carrier JA. Progestogen for preventing miscarriage. Cochrane Database Syst Rev. 2003;(4):CD003511. Review. Update in: Cochrane Database Syst Rev. 2008;(2):CD003511.
20. Wahabi HA, Abed Althagafi NF, Elawad M, Al Zeidan RA. Progestogen for treating threatened miscarriage. Cochrane Database Syst Rev. 2011;(3):CD005943.
21. Rohwer AC, Khondowe O, Young T. Antispasmodics for labour. Cochrane Database Syst Rev. 2012;8:CD009243.
22. URL http://ipc.nic.in/index2.asp?slid=43&sub linkid=8&lang=1&EncHid=Acessed on 6th July 2015.
23. URL http://www.indiamedicaltimes.com/2013/01/23/mci-directs-doctors-to prescribe-drugs-with-generic-names/Acessed on 6th July 2015.

Section II

EMERGENCY DRUGS

CHAPTER

CHAPTER 2

Drugs Used in Medical Emergencies

Shakun Tyagi, Swati Kumari

INTRODUCTION

Most of the obstetric and gynecological emergencies require a combination of medical and surgical management. Medical emergencies such as shock, congestive heart failure, convulsions, electrolyte imbalance, hypocalcemia, bradycardia and anaphylactic shock are common medical emergencies which are encountered in obstetric and gynecological practice. This chapter will describe the drugs and their usage in these medical emergencies **(Table 2.1)**.

Table 2.1: Drugs used in commonly encountered medical emergencies

Emergency	*Drug(s)*
Shock	Adrenaline, noradrenaline, dopamine, dobutamine
Convulsions	Diazepam, phenytoin, midazolam
Electrolyte imbalance, acidosis	Potassium chloride, sodium bicarbonate
Hypocalcemia	Calcium gluconate
Bradycardia	Atropine
Anaphylactic shock	Hydrocortisone, adrenaline, chlorpheniramine, pheniramine

Drugs Used in Shock

Adrenaline (Epinephrine)

Pharmacology: It is a sympathomimetic catecholamine.

Indications of use: During emergency, it is used in following conditions:

- Hypotension and bradycardia
- Anaphylaxis
- Asystole, ventricular fibrillation (VF) and pulseless electrical activity (PEA).

Contraindications: It is given in life saving emergencies.

Dosage

- Bradycardia and hypotensive states, as IV infusion at an initial rate of 2–10 μg/min and increased stepwise gradually until the desired heart rate is achieved.[1]
- *Anaphylaxis:* 0.3–0.5 mg of undiluted adrenaline (1:1000) administered intramuscularly or subcutaneously in anterolateral aspect of thigh, repeated every 5–10 minutes as necessary.[2]
- In asystole, ventricular fibrillation (VF) and pulseless electrical activity, it is used in 1:10,000 dilutions in dose of 1.0 mg IV bolus dose.

Preparation: Adrenaline is available in 1 mL ampoule with concentration of 1 mg/mL.

Preparation of IV Infusion: Dilute 1 mg in 250 mL of 5% dextrose or NS, this will make the concentration of adrenaline as 4 µg/mL. This fluid is then infused initially at the rate of 1 µg/min (15 macrodrops or 60 micro- drops per minute) and increase to desired dose.

1:1000 adrenaline concentration is:

- One ampoule of 1:1000 adrenaline in 1 mL volume
- This equals 1 mg in 1 mL
- This equals 1000 µg/mL.

If one ampoule is diluted to 10 mL:

- This equals 0.1 mg/mL
- This equals 100 µg/mL
- This equals 1:10,000 adrenaline concentration.

Adverse drug reaction: Anxiety, apprehensiveness, tremors, palpitations, headache, arrhythmias.

Drug interaction: Monoamine oxidase inhibitors, antidepressants imipramine or triptyline group of drugs.

Monitoring: Pulse rate, blood pressure, ECG, symptomatic improvement.

Safety during pregnancy: It is used as life saving drug for the mother in case of emergency.

It is FDA Category B.

Noradrenaline (Norepinephrine)

Pharmacology: It is a sympathomimetic catecholamine. Its action on alpha-1 adrenergic receptors results in peripheral vasoconstriction and ionotropic action on heart, whereas its action on beta adrenergic receptors leads to dilatation of coronary arteries.

Indications of use: Noradrenaline is used in hypotension to preserve cardiac and cerebral blood flow along with volume replacement. During shock volume replacement and treatment of the underlying cause are the mainstay.

Contraindications: It should not be used in hypovolemia without concurrent volume replacement; it is contraindicated in cases of chronic mesenteric or peripheral vasoconstriction unless as a lifesaving procedure.

Dosage: The infusion fluid is prepared by adding 2 mg of norepinephrine to 500 mL of 5% dextrose. Each milliliter of this solution contains 4 µg of noradrenaline. Initial dose is 2–3 mL (8–12 µg) of the diluted drug per minute. The rate is adjusted to maintain 100–120 mm Hg of systolic blood pressure. Average maintenance dose ranges from 0.5 mL to 1.0 mL (2 mcg to 4 mcg) per minute.[3]

Intravenous infusion is prepared in dextrose or dextrose normal saline as dextrose solution prevents loss of potency due to oxidation. *It is never diluted in saline.*

Adverse drug reaction: Tissue hypoxia, lactic acidosis and ischemic injury may occur if norepinephrine is given without plasma volume correction.

Bradycardia as a reflex result of rise in blood pressure and arrhythmias.

Drug interaction: Monoamine oxidase inhibitors, antidepressants imipramine or triptyline group of drugs. Norepinephrine injection use is contraindicated with anesthetic drugs like halothane or with cyclopropane as it can result in ventricular tachycardia or fibrillation.

Monitoring: Pulse rate, blood pressure, ECG, symptomatic improvement.

Preparation: Norepinephrine (Generic preparation)—available as 4 mL ampoule containing 1 mg per mL.

Safety during pregnancy: It is used as lifesaving drug for the mother.

It is FDA Category C.

Dopamine

Pharmacology: The action of dopamine differs according to the concentration at which it is used.

- It acts as strong beta-1 adrenergic when given at rate of 2–10 mcg/kg/min
- It has alpha-adrenergic and dopaminergic effects at rate of more than 10 mcg/kg/min
- It has dopaminergic effect at rate of 0.5–2 mcg/kg/min.

Indications of use

- Used as an adjunct to other measures for treatment of hypotension
- In low cardiac output and poor perfusion of vital organs
- To increase mean arterial pressure in patients with septic shock which is refractory to volume expansion.

Contraindications: Pheochromocytoma, uncorrected tachyarrhythmia, ventricular fibrillation, allergy to corn or corn products, occlusive vascular diseases, patient using monoamine oxidases.

Dosage

- To increase renal blood flow and urine output: 1–5 mcg/kg/min IV infusion.
- To increase cardiac output, heart rate, cardiac contractility: 5–15 mcg/kg/min IV
- Increase in blood pressure but with vasoconstriction, may increase risk of tachyarrhythmias: 20–50 mcg/kg/min.

Increase in dosage may be at the rate of 1–4 mcg/kg/min at 10–30 minutes interval for desired response.

Simple formula for preparing the solution for IV infusion and calculating infusion rate in mL per hour.[4]

$$\frac{\text{Ordered amount of drug (mcg/kg/min)} \times \text{patient's weight (kg)} \times 60}{\text{Drug concentration (mcg/mL)}} = \text{IV infusion rate (mL/hour)}$$

So, if ordered amount of drug = 5 mcg/kg/min IV infusion

Weight of patient = 60 kg

Drug concentration = 3200 mcg/mL prepared by dissolving 1600 mg in 500 mL normal saline

$$\frac{5 \times 60 \times 60}{3200} = 5.6 \text{ mL per hour}$$

If infusion pump is not available then it can be given by microdrip set at rate of 20-25 microdrops per minute (1 mL equals 60 microdrops).

Adverse drug reaction: It may cause ventricular arrhythmia, hypertension or angina at higher doses. It can cause gangrene of extremities if high doses are administered for prolonged periods, which can occur even at low doses in patients with occlusive vascular disease.

It may rarely cause anaphylaxis.

Drug interaction: Monoamine oxidase inhibitors.

If used with phenytoin it can cause hypotension and bradycardia.

Oxytocic agents may cause severe hypertension when given with dopamine.

Monitoring: Pulse rate, blood pressure, ECG, input/output, symptomatic improvement.

Preparation: Dopamine (Generic drug)—available as 5 mL ampoule containing 40 mg/mL.

Safety during pregnancy: It is FDA Category C.

Dobutamine

Pharmacology: It has inotropic action through direct effect on the beta adrenergic receptors on heart. It has onset of action within two minutes but peak action occurs after 10 minutes.[5]

Indications of use: It is used in patients of cardiac decompensation and low cardiac output states.

Contraindications: Dobutamine should not be used in cases of cardiac decompensation due to mechanical obstruction of ventricular filling and/or of outflow, such as pericardial tamponade, constrictive pericarditis, hypertrophic obstructive cardiomyopathy, idiopathic hypertrophic subortic stenosis. Some patients may have hypersensitivity to this drug.[3]

Dosage

Cardiac decompensation: 0.5–1 mcg/kg/min continuous infusion initially, then 2–20 mcg/kg/min, maximum dose 40 mcg/kg/min.

Low cardiac output: 2–20 mcg/kg/min IV, not exceeding 40 mcg/kg/min (this use is off label).

For preparing solution and calculating drip rate please refer to formula described in dopamine section, page 17.

Adverse drug reaction: The common side effects are nausea, headache, hypertension, tachycardia, premature, and ventricular ectopic. Rarely can it cause hypotension.

Drug interaction: This might be ineffective when used with beta blocking drugs. Side effects may be increased when it is used with cimetidine or methyl dopa. Do not add to injection sodium bicarbonate as chemically incompatible.

Monitoring: Pulse rate, blood pressure, ECG, input/output, symptomatic improvement.

Preparation: Generic drug available as 20 mL ampoule containing 12.5 mg/mL.

Safety during pregnancy: It is FDA Category B.

Drugs Used in Treatment of Convulsions

Diazepam

Pharmacology: It belongs to benzodiazepam group of drugs and acts on limbic, thalamus and hypothalamus.

Indications of use

- For acute control of seizure
- Premedication before anesthesia.

Contraindications: Hypersensitivity, glaucoma.

Dosage

- For acute control of seizure— 5-10 mg IV slowly over 2 minutes.
- Premedication before anesthesia—10 mg IM.

Adverse drug reaction: Drowsiness, confusion or depression, respiratory depression.

Drug interaction: Phenothiazines, narcotics, barbiturates, monoamine oxidase (MAO) inhibitors.

Monitoring: Patient should be monitored for cardiorespiratory depression. If any evidence of respiratory depression, antidote flumazenil should be used after measures to secure the airway, ventilation and intravenous access are taken.

Preparation

Diazepam (Generic drug): Available as 10 mL ampoule containing 5 mg/mL.

Safety during pregnancy: It is FDA Category C.

Increased risk of congenital malformations with use in first trimester.

Phenytoin

Pharmacology: It acts by preventing repetitive detonation of normal brain cells during depolarization shift that occurs in epileptic patients and consists of synchronous and large depolarization over which action potentials are superimposed. Its half-life is 12–24 hours and it gets metabolized in liver by hydroxylation and glucuronide conjugation.

Indications of use

- It is used as first-line drug in cases of generalized tonic-clonic seizures (GTCS).
- It is also used in cases of simple and complex partial seizure and status epilepticus occasionally.
- As an alternative in eclampsia when magnesium sulfate is contraindicated.

Contraindications: Hypersensitivity, sinus bradycardia, sinoatrial block, second and third degree A-V block, Adams-Stokes syndrome.

Dosage: Initially a loading dose of 10–15 mg/kg is given over two to three minutes then infusion is given by diluting the desired dose in 100–250 mL normal saline over 35 minutes. It must not be diluted in glucose solution.[3]

It should be delivered via large gauge cannula in a large vein. Line must be flushed with saline before and after administration.

The rate must not exceed 50 mg/min.

Adverse drug reaction: Extravasation of drug can cause severe thrombophlebitis. Sometimes it may cause hypotension, arrhythmias, or respiratory depression.

Drug interaction: Chloramphenicol, isoniazid, cimetidine and warfarin inhibit phenytoin metabolism and can precipitate its toxicity.

Monitoring: Heart rate, blood pressure, respiratory rate, and ECG monitoring should be done throughout when the loading dose is being given. Inspection of delivery site is important to look for any evidence of extravasation.

Preparation: Dilantin-5 mL ampoule containing 50 mg/mL.

Safety during pregnancy: Prenatal exposure to fetus increases risk of fetal malformations and other adverse developmental outcomes.

It is FDA Category D drug.

Midazolam

Pharmacology: Midazolam is a short acting benzodiazepine and act as central nervous system depressant. It primarily act by facilitating inhibitory GABAergic transmission.

After intramuscular injection, the onset of action is after 15 minutes with peak action at 30–60 minutes. It is faster acting, shorter acting and 3 times more potent than diazepam. It is used via intravenous route for induction of anesthesia.

It is metabolized in liver by hydroxylation; the metabolites get conjugated and excreted in urine.

Indications of use: Sedation, anxiolysis, amnesia during for short surgical procedures.

Preanesthetic agent for induction of anesthesia.

Contraindications: Hypersensitivity, open angle glaucoma.

Dosage

Intravenous dose: 1 mg slowly over two minutes, then response is assessed, not more than 2.5 mg is given, maintenance dose is usually 25% of the dose required to achieve adequate sedation.[3]

Adverse drug reaction: Cardiorespiratory depression, sedation, light headedness, psychomotor and cognitive impairment, vertigo.

Drug interaction: Its sedative action is accentuated by morphine, fentanyl, etc.

Caution exhibited with drugs that inhibit P450-3A4 enzyme system (erythromycin, diltiazem, verapamil, ketoconazole).

Monitoring: For IV use, response is assessed with respect to responsiveness, speech, facial expression and eyes status.

Close cardiorespiratory monitoring by measuring SpO_2, pulse rate, blood pressure and respiratory rate.

Preparation: Midazolam (Generic drug)—available as 2 mL ampoule containing 1 mg/mL.

Safety during pregnancy: Increased risk of congenital malformations.

It is FDA Category D.

Drugs Used is Electrolyte Imbalance

Potassium Chloride

Pharmacology: It directly corrects the ionic concentration and the onset of action is immediate.

Indications of use: It is used in conditions which cause hypokalemia like excessive vomiting and diarrhea, with diuretic drugs, diabetic ketoacidosis, adrenal gland disorder, etc. It is given if serum potassium levels fall below 2.5 mEq/L.

Contraindications: Renal failure, Addison's disease, severe burns, etc.

Dosage: Potassium chloride solution is prepared in concentration 20–40 in 500 mL of NS or 5% dextrose solution. It is transfused at rate not exceeding 10 mEq/hour and in 24 hours the dose should not exceed 200 meq.

If serum potassium level is less than 2.0 mEq/L with ECG changes it can be infused at the rate of 40 mEq/hour with maximum of 400 mEq in 24 hours.

Adverse drug reaction: These are muscle weakness, limp feeling, severe stomach pain, numbness or tingling in hands, feet and mouth, cardiac arrhythmias, heart blocker even cardiac arrest may occur.

Drug interaction: Hyperkalemia can occur with potassium sparing diuretics.

Monitoring: Pulse rate, BP, ECG monitoring.

Preparation: Potassium hydrochloride—available as ampoules containing 20 mEq/50 mL.

Safety during pregnancy: Usually used in life-threatening conditions.

It is FDA Category C.

Sodium Bicarbonate

Pharmacology: It is used as intravenous bolus or infusion for correction of acid-base imbalance.[6]

Indications of use: It is used in metabolic acidosis as in circulatory insufficiency due to shock or severe dehydration, severe renal disease, uncontrolled diabetes, etc.

Contraindications: Metabolic and respiratory alkalosis, hypocalcemia, etc.

Dosage: Depends on the indication and weight of the patient according to arterial blood gas (ABG) findings.

Requirement of sodium bicarbonate (mEq) can be calculated by following formula:

- 0.2 × weight of the patient (kg) × base deficit Or
- 0.5 × weight (kg) × [24-serum HCO_3 (mEq/L)].

Solution for IV infusion is prepared by dissolving required amount of sodium bicarbonate in 500 L of normal saline. Initially an infusion of 2–5 mEq/kg body weight is transfused over a period of 4–8 hours. This will produce a measurable improvement in the abnormal acid-base status of the blood. Then further dose is calculated based on patient's response and base deficit on ABG.

Adverse drug reaction: Infection at site of injection, phlebitis, suppression of respiratory drive, hypernatremia resulting in.

Drug interaction: None.

Monitoring: ABG is to be repeated to know pH of blood.

Preparation: 50 mL single dose vial containing 8.4% sodium bicarbonate which is equal to 1 mEq per mL (84 mg sodium bicarbonate equal to 1 mEq sodium bicarbonate).

Safety during pregnancy: Used for life-threatening emergencies.

It is FDA Category C.

Drugs Used in Hypocalcemia

Calcium Gluconate

Pharmacology: Calcium is an important body constituent and essential for maintenance of physiology of nervous, muscular, skeletal systems, cell membranes, coagulation and capillary permeability.

Onset of action occurs in 5 minutes.

Indications of use: Hypocalcemic tetany, hypocalcemia related to hypoparathyroidism, magnesium sulfate toxicity.

Contraindications: Hypercalcemia, ventricular fibrillation, digitalis use.

Dosage: Dose depends on the requirement of the individual patient.

In case of severe hypocalcemia (ionized serum calcium less than 1 mmol per liter).

- Without seizure or tetany—0.5 mg/kg/hour IV infusion with maximum dose of 3-4 g IV over 4 hours
- In hypocalcemic tetany—2 g calcium gluconate given IV over 5-10 minutes, followed by continuous IV infusion at 0.5 mg/kg/hour.

Infusion fluid is prepared by dissolving calcium gluconate in 500 mL of normal saline. The number of ampoules depends on the concentration required.

Adverse drug reaction: Local reaction occurs if drug gets extravasated. There is sense of warmth on intravenous injection. Rapid injection may cause vasodilatation, hypotension, bradycardia, cardiac arrhythmias, syncope and cardiac arrest.[3]

Drug interaction: It is contraindicated in digitalized patient.

Monitoring: Pulse rate, blood pressure, respiratory rate, ECG and serum calcium levels every 6 hours.

Preparation: Calcium gluconate (Generic drug)—10 mL ampoule containing 100 mg per mL of calcium gluconate.

Safety during pregnancy: It is used during possibly life-threatening disorders.

It is FDA Category C.

Drug Used in Bradycardia

Atropine

Pharmacology: Atropine acts by inhibiting the muscarinic actions of acetylcholine. This action occurs at post ganglionic parasympathetic neuro-effector sites like smooth muscles, secretory glands and CNS sites. The action is dose related. It is rapidly absorbed and the half-life is 3-4 hours. It is metabolized in liver and excreted in the urine.[5,6]

Indications of use

- Sinus bradycardia with hypotension
- As anesthetic premedication
- Organophosphorus poisoning.

Contraindications: Absolute contraindicated are narrow iridocorneal angle, myasthenia gravis, obstructive GI diseases, e.g. pyloric stenosis.

Dosage: For sinus bradycardia with hypotension—0.5-1 mg IV every five minutes not more than 3 mg.[3]

Adverse drug reaction

Anticholinergic side effects: Patient may experience dry mouth; difficulty in talking swallowing; dry, flushed and hot skin; fever; difficulty in micturition; dilated pupil, photophobia and blurring of near vision; palpitation, excitement, ataxia and delirium. Overdosage may lead to hypotention, thready pulse or cardiovascular collapse.

Drug interaction: It delays absorption of most of drugs as it slows gastric emptying. It has additive effect with antihistaminic, tricyclic antidepressants and pethidine.

Monitoring: Cardiovasular monitoring.

Preparation: Atropine sulfate (generic preparation)—10 mL vial containing 0.1 mg/mL.

Safety during pregnancy: Safe.

Category B Drug: It is used for maternal life-threatening conditions.

Drugs Used in Anaphylactic Shock

Hydrocortisone Sodium Succinate

Pharmacology: It is a short-acting synthetic steroid with both glucocorticoid and mineralocorticoid action. It increases absorption of sodium in distal convoluted tubules of loop of Henle in kidney and increase excretion of potassium and hydrogen. It has anti-inflammatory action.[7]

It has half-life of 1.5 hours. It gets metabolized primarily by hepatic microsomal enzymes reduction, hydroxylation and oxidation and then gets conjugated with glucuronic acid or sulfate. It is excreted in urine, excretion is complete in 12 hours therefore 4-6 hourly dose is required.

Indications of use

- Shock unresponsive to conventional therapy
- Adrenocortical insufficiency
- Status asthmaticus
- Tubercular meningitis
- Acute exacerbation of various autoimmune and allergic disorders like systemic lupus erythematosus (SLE).

Dosage

- In shock and status asthmaticus—1-2 mg/kg slow IV for 24 hours followed by maintenance dose of 0.5-1 mg/kg slow IV every 6 hourly
- Acute adrenal insufficiency—100 mg IV bolus followed by 100 mg 8 hourly IV slowly over 30 seconds.

Adverse drug reaction: It can lead to fluid retention, hypertension, hypokalemia, alkalosis, and hyperglycemia, aggravates peptic ulcers. Congestive heart failure in susceptible patient, increased intraocular pressure.

Drug interaction: Phenobarbiturates and phenytoin the induce metabolism.

Monitoring: No short-term side effects. Long-term use can cause suppression of Hypothalamo pituitary adrenal axis.

Preparation: 100 mg vial containing 100 mg hydrocortisone sodium succinate in powder form to be reconstituted by adding 2 mL of water for injection.

Safety during pregnancy: It should be given when benefit clearly outweighs the risk.

It is FDA Category C.

Chlorpheniramine Maleate and Pheniramine Maleate

Pharmacology: They are selective antagonist for H1 histaminic receptors. Onset of action is within half an hour and duration of action is 4-6 hours. It is metabolized in liver and gets excreted in urine.

Indications of use: Allergic reaction to blood or plasma products, anaphylaxis and for treatment of allergic symptoms like bronchoconstriction, urticaria, and itching.

Contraindications: Narrow angle glaucoma, hypersensitivity.

Dosage: In the above conditions, chlorpheniramine is used in dose of 10-20 mg by IV, IM, or as SC injection single dose, maximum dose is 40 mg.

Injection pheniramine given in dose of 22.75 mg IV or IM.

Adverse drug reaction: Adverse effects such as sedation, diminution in alertness and concentration, light headedness, motor incoordination, fatigue, tendency to sleep, dryness of mouth, alteration in bowel habit, urinary hesitancy and blurring of vision is due to its anticholinergic action, epigastric discomfort, acute overdose can produce central excitation tremors, hallucination, convulsions, hypotension, fever.

Drug interaction: Monoamine oxidase inhibitors, phenytoin, drugs causing sedation.

Monitoring

- Monitoring is not required for IM dose.
- Pulse rate, blood pressure, ECG for IV use.

Preparation: Chlorpheniramine maleate (generic drug)—1 mL ampoule for injection containing 10 mg/mL.

Injection avil-available as vial containing 22.75 mg/mL.

Safety during pregnancy: Nonteratogenic.

It is FDA Category B.

REFERENCES

1. Anantharaman V, Gunasegaran K. Advanced Cardiac Life Support guidelines, 2011. Singapore Med J. 2011; 52(8): 548-55.
2. Simons FE. Anaphylaxis: Recent advances in assessment and treatment. J Allergy Clin. Immunol. 2009;124(4):625-36.
3. United State Food and Drug Administration website "Drugs@FDA". *http://www.accessdata.*

fda.gov/scripts/cder/drugsatfda accessed on September 10, 2015.
4. Ira Gene Reynolds. Calculating IV. Drip rates with confidence. American Nurse Today;2006. pp.62-5.
5. Cheung WK, Chau LS, Mak II, et al. Clinical management for patients admitted to a critical care Unit with severe sepsis or septic shock. Intensive Crit Care Nurs. 2015;17:S0964-3397.
6. Wilkman E, Kaukonen KM, Pettilä V, Kuitunen A, Varpula M. Association between inotrope treatment and 90-day mortality in patients with septic shock. Acta Anaesthesiol Scand. 2013;57(4):431-42.
7. Yeager MP, Rassias AJ, Pioli PA, et al. Pretreatment with stress cortisol enhances the human systemic inflammatory response to bacterial endotoxin. Crit Care Med. 2009;37(10):2727-32.

Section III

ANTIMICROBIALS USED IN DIFFERENT CLINICAL CONDITIONS

CHAPTERS

CHAPTER 3

Antibiotic Classification

Krishna Agarwal

Antibiotic use is rampant in obstetrics and gynecology, both rational and irrational. This is most of the time empirical and not based on the spectrum of microorganisms responsible for infection. **Table 3.1** provides working information of all the important antibiotics which are used in different clinical conditions in obstetrics and gynecology. This table also provides salient features of these antibiotics, their spectrum of coverage and the adverse effects.

Table 3.1 Classification and important features of common antibiotics used in obstetrics and gynecology practice (This is not an exclusive but a working list of antibiotics with emphasis on those available in Indian market and are commonly prescribed by physicians)

S. no.	*Antibiotics class/ subclass/name*	*Antibacterial spectrum*				*Special precautions Common side effects*
		Gram-positive	*Gram-negative*	*Anaerobes*	*Others*	
1.	Beta lactams					
	1.1. Penicillins					
	• Penicillin G • Benzathine and procaine salts provide repository forms for IM injections (susceptible to hydrolysis by beta lactamases therefore not effective against bacteria producing them)	Gram-positive organisms	Gram-negative cocci Not active against gram-negative rods	nonbeta lactamase producing anaerobes		Remarkably safe; hypersensitivity, autoimmune reactions, skin rashes especially when give in viral infections
	• Antistaphylococcal penicillins such as methicillin, nafcillin, cloxacillin (susceptible to hydrolysis by beta lactamases therefore not effective against bacteria producing them)	Staphylococci, streptococci and pneumococci not active against enterococci, *Listeria*, MRSA	Not active	Not active		
	• *Extended spectrum*: Ampicillin, amoxicillin (have better stability; better oral absorption)	Same as penicillin G Penicillin resistant pneumococci Ampicillin active against penicillin sensitive enterococci, and *Listeria*	Better coverage than penicillin G Ampicillin (not amoxicillin) effective in shigellosis, *E. coli*, *Salmonella*, H. influenzae Ampicillin not active against *Klebsiella*, *Enterobacter*, *Pseudomonas*, *Citrobacter*, *Serratia*, indole positive *Proteus*	Yes Not active against gram-negative anaerobes		

Contd...

Contd...

S. no.	*Antibiotics class/ subclass/name*	*Antibacterial spectrum*				*Special precautions Common side effects*
		Gram-positive	*Gram-negative*	*Anaerobes*	*Others*	
	• *Antipseudomonal*: Piperacillin (used in combination with aminoglycoside or fluoroquinolone)	Same as penicillin G	Gram-negative cocci *Pseudomonas, Klebsiella* and other gram-negative rods	Yes- *Clostridium difficile,* and *Bacteroides fragilis*		
	1.2. *Cephalosporins*: Similar to penicillins but more stable to beta-lactamases and have broader spectrum activities; not active against enterococci and *Listeria monocytogenes*					
	• *1st generation*: Cephalexin, cefazolin, cefadroxil—these are oral preparations	Very active against gram-positive cocci (Staphylococci, streptococci and pneumococci) not active against MRSA, enterococci	Gram-positive rods such as *E. coli, Klebsiella, Proteus* Not active against *P. aeruginosa*, indole positive Proteus, *Serratia marcescens*, enterobacter, *Citrobacter* and *Acinetobacter*	Anaerobic cocci (*Peptococcus* and *Peptostreptococcus*) not active against Bacteroides fragilis		As of penicillins
	• *2nd generation*: Cefaclor, cefuroxime, cefoxitin, cefazolin—they have marked individual differences in activity, pharmacokinetics and toxicity. Cefazolin is drug of choice for surgical prophylaxis	Same as 1st generation	Extended activity against gram-negative bacteria not active against *P. aeruginosa*	Active		
	• *3rd generation*: Cefoperazone, cefotaxime, ceftazidime, ceftizoxime, ceftriaxone, cefixime, cefpodoxime	Reduced activity against gram-positive organisms; not active against MRSA	Expanded gram-negative cover, also active against citrobacter, *S. marcescens, Providencia* Ceftazidime and cefoperazone effective against *P. aeruginosa*	Ceftriaxone active against B. fragilis		

Contd...

Contd...

S. no.	*Antibiotics class/ subclass/name*	*Antibacterial spectrum*				*Special precautions Common side effects*
		Gram-positive	*Gram-negative*	*Anaerobes*	*Others*	
	• *4th generation*: Cefepime	Good activity against *Staphylococcus aureus, Pneumococcus*	Good activity against *Pseudomonas, Enterobacteriaceae, H. influenzae, Neisseria* resistant to hydrolysis by chromosomal beta-lactamases	No		
	1.3. *Monobactams*: Aztreonam	No activity	Similar to third generation cephalosporins, *P. aeruginosa*	No activity		
	1.4. *Carbapenems*: Doripenem, ertapenem, imipenem, meropenem (Not inactivated by most beta-lactamases except metallo-beta-lactamases; Imipenem is inactivated by dehydropeptidases in renal tubules, resulting in low urinary concentration, it is therefore given in combination with cilastatin for clinical use. Meropenem and doripenem do not require concomitant administration of cilastatin)	Gram-positive organisms not active against MRSA and *E. faecium* Imipenem has higher activity against gram-positives than mero or doripenem	Gram-negative including *P. aeruginosa*, those producing ESBL not active against Burkholderia cepacia, *Stenotrophomonas maltophilia* Mero or doripenem has higher activity against gram-negatives than imipenem	Yes Not active against Clostridium difficile		As of penicillins
2.	*Tetracyclines*: Tetracycline, doxycyclines and minocyclines and tigecycline Tigecycline effective against bacteria resistant to other tetracyclines	Gram-positive	Gram-negative	Yes	Chlamydiae, rickettsiae, mycoplasma, amoeba	Skin sensitivity, GI upset, abdominal pain, headache

Contd...

Contd...

S. no.	Antibiotics class/ subclass/name	Antibacterial spectrum				Special precautions Common side effects
		Gram-positive	Gram-negative	Anaerobes	Others	
3.	*Macrolides*: Erythromycin, azithromycin, clarithromycin All of them have similar activities Erythromycin is destroyed by stomach acidity-must be given as enteric coated tablets Food interferes with absorption-give empty stomach Azithromycin has long half-life and can be given in OD doses	Gram-positive (Strept, Staph and *Corynebacterium*, *Campylobacter jejuni*	Neisseria, Bordetella and Bartonella		Chlamydiae, helicobacter, *Listeria*, *Treponema pallidum*, rickettsiae, *Mycoplasma*, amoeba	QT prolongation, myopathy, GI upset, cholestasis
4.	Clindamycin	Stept, Staph, Penumo *Enterococccus* is resistant	Not active	Yes		GI upset, joint pains, vaginal itching, heart burn
5.	Oxazolidinones Linezolid	Gram-positive cocci including Staph, MRSA, Strept, vancomycin resistant enterococci, cornybacteria and Listeria	Not active	No		Chills, confusion, dizziness, tachycardia, fever blood in stool, urine, convulsion
6.	*Aminoglycosides*: Genta, amika, neo, kana, tobra, netil	Some gram-positive bacteria including MRSA but not active against most gram-positive bacteria Synergistic effect with beta lactum and vancomycin	Gram-negative enteric pathogens	Facultative anaerobic bacilli		Hearing loss, tinnitus, fullness in ears, nephrotoxicity, skin rash, weakness, drowsiness, dizziness

Contd...

Contd...

S. no.	*Antibiotics class/ subclass/name*	*Antibacterial spectrum*				*Special precautions Common side effects*
		Gram-positive	*Gram-negative*	*Anaerobes*	*Others*	
7.	Sulfonamides, trimethoprim	Gram-positive	Gram-negative	No	Nocardia, chlamydiae, and rickettsiae not inhibited	Hypersensitivity, dizziness, fever, rash, GI upset
8.	*Quinolones*: Norfloxacin, Nalidixic acid, ciprofloxacin, levofloxacin	Newer agent have improved activity	Good activity	No		GI upset, headache, insomnia, exacerbation of neurological disorder, arthropathy in children
9.	Glycopeptides					
	Vancomycin (IV)	Gram-positive bacteria including MRSA	None	None		Rash, infusion related reactions (red man syndrome), nephrotoxicity and ototoxicity
	Teicoplanin (IV and IM)	Similar to vancomycin	None	None		Fever, itching, pain, Red ness of the skin, skin rash
10.	Nitrofurantoin Highly stable to development of bacterial resistance due to multiplicity of mechanisms of action; selectively concentrated in urinary tract and GI tract	*Staphylococcus aureus*, streptococci, *Corynebacterium* and enterococci	*E. coli, Enterobacter, Neisseria, Salmonella, Shigella* not active against *Pseudomonas* and *Proteus spp.*	No		ECG changes, pseudotumor cerebri, confusion, depression, headache, alopecia, erythema multiforme, hyperphosphatemia, brown color urine, hypersensitivity, arthralgia

Beta lactamases (BL) are the enzymes produced by different bacteria (gram-positive as well as gram-negative) that destroys beta lactam antibiotics. There are many different types of BL. The capability to produce BLs is developed in bacteria on exposure to antibiotics and then this capability is transmitted from one to other bacteria. There many varieties of BLs and include the ones capable of destroying penicillins (penicillinase), cephalosporins (cephalosporinases) and even monobactam and carbapenems (carbapenemases). The BLs capable of destroying third generation cephalosporins (cefotaxime, ceftazidime, ceftriaxone) and monobactums (aztreonum) are known as extended spectrum BLs (ESBLs). The ESBL positive bacteria can be treated by carbapenems.

CHAPTER 4

Antibiotic Prophylaxis in Obstetrics and Gynecology

Preeti Singh

INTRODUCTION

Inpatients that are undergoing any operative procedure, risk of infection is a real challenge. In addition to adopting aseptic practices, antibiotic prophylaxis is important for achieving best results. However, it should be judiciously used as indiscriminate antibiotic use can lead to antibiotic resistance. Presence of antibiotics in tissues at the time of surgery prevents endogenous pathogens from gaining foothold and helps in prevention of infection. During gynecological and obstetric surgical procedures the common pathogens are from the patient's own skin and vagina.

Hence prophylactic antibiotics have a role in prevention of postoperative morbidity in terms of an abdominal wound infection, wound discharge or abscess, pelvic inflammatory disease, pelvic cellulitis, pelvic abscess, and septicemia.[1-5]

Before deciding the antibiotic to be used in prophylaxis before surgery. It is important to know about these microorganisms. The endogenous flora which have potential to cause infection are enlisted in **Table 4.1**.

Table 4.1 Endogenous flora in human body

Organ	*Microbial flora*
Skin	*Staphylococcus aureus* and epidermis *Micrococcus* species Nonpathogenic *neisseria* species Hemolytic and nonhemolytic streptococci *Propionobacterium* species *Peptostreptococcus* species
Vagina	Group B Streptococci Anaerobic streptococci Alpha hemolytic streptococci *Streptococcus* viridans *Prevotella* *Clostridia* *Gardnerella vaginalis* Aerobic and anaerobic lactobacilli
Urethra	Staphylo epidermidis *Streptococcus faecalis* Diphtheroid *Staphylococcus saprophyticus*
Intestine	*About 96–99% are anaerobes* • *Bacteroides* species B fragilis • *Fusobacterium* species • Anaerobic lactobacilli–bifido bacteria • *Clostridium perfringens* • Anaerobic gram-positive cocci *About 1–4% facultative anaerobes* • Gram-negative coliform • Enterococci • Small number of Protei • *Pseudomonas* • Lacto bacilli • *Candida*

Principles of Antibiotic Prophylaxis

The antibiotic chosen for prophylaxis of infection should be effective against the likely organism which may be responsible for postoperative or postprocedure infection. The

Table 4.2: Classification of surgical wound by center for disease control and prevention[6]

Class of wound	*Characteristics of the wound*
Class I—clean	When the operative wound is uninfected and the respiratory, alimentary, genital or urinary tract is not entered
Class II—clean contaminated	If during surgery the respiratory, alimentary, genital, or urinary tracts are entered but under controlled conditions and there is no unusual contamination
Class III—contaminated	If during surgery there is major breaks in sterile technique or there is gross spillage from the gastrointestinal tract or incisions in which nonpurulent inflammation is encountered
Class IV—dirty, infected	When there is old traumatic wound with retained devitalized tissue and that involves existing clinical infection or perforated viscera

antibiotic should be administered just prior to or at the start of surgery or procedure so as to cover the time during which microbial inoculation of the surgical wound may occur. The antibiotic chosen must be effective, safe and the dose should be such that the tissue concentration remains in the therapeutic range throughout the surgery and for few hours later.[6-8] **Table 4.2** provides classification of surgical wound by Center for Disease Control and Prevention (CDCP). It helps in planning antibiotic for prophylaxis and treatment before surgery.

Use of Antibiotic Prophylaxis in Obstetrics

Cesarean Section

It is well proven fact that cesarean delivery carries 5-20 times higher risk of maternal infection as compared to vaginal birth and this is the most important risk factor for puerperal sepsis.[9] Incidence of wound infection and associated serious complications may be increased to 25%.[10]

A Cochrane review (2002) assessed the effect of prophylactic antibiotics versus placebo or no treatment on prevention of infection after elective as well as emergency cesarean section. There were 2000 women in each arm. The meta-analysis revealed that the risk of endometritis and wound infection was significantly reduced in both elective and emergency cesarean section.[11]

Most of the guidelines recommend use of cefazolin as the first line antibiotic for prophylaxis before cesarean section. Patients who are obese have higher risk of infection after cesarean section therefore double the normal dose is given in these patients with BMI more than 35.[11]

Second line antibiotics, clindamycin and erythromycin, can be used in patients allergic to cefazolin **(Table 4.3)**.

Cefazolin

Pharmacology: It belongs to the first generation cephalosporin category. It has broad spectrum antibacterial cover and provides good cover for gram-positive bacteria and modest cover for gram-negative microbes.

Indications of use: For prophylaxis of infection before most surgical procedures **(Tables 4.4 and 4.5)**.

Contraindications: Allergy.

Dosage: 1-2 g, IV within 30 minutes of skin incision. Additional dose is given if blood loss is in excess of 1500 mL or in case of prolonged surgery for more than 4 hours. In patients with BMI more than 35, double the dose is administered for prophylaxis.

Adverse drug reaction: Local phlebitis, seizures, pruritus, skin rash, nausea vomiting, diarrhea, leukopenia, thrombocytopenia, anaphylaxis, renal failure, increased creatinine, fever etc.

Table 4.3 Antibiotics used for prophylaxis before cesarean section

Antibiotic	*Dosage*
Cefazolin (drug of choice)	1–2 g, IV within 30 minutes of skin incision. Additional dose is given if blood loss is in excess of 1500 mL or in case of prolonged surgery for more than 4 hours. In patients with BMI more than 35, double the dose is administered for prophylaxis
Clindamycin	600 mg IV if allergic to cefazolin
Erythromycin	500 IV is third line antibiotic

Table 4.4 Prophylactic antibiotic recommendations for obstetrical procedures[12-19]

Procedure	*Antibiotic*	*Dosage*
Cesarean section (elective and emergency) If allergic then	Cefazolin Clindamycin or Erythromycin	1–2 g IV, 15–60 minutes before skin incision 600 mg IV single dose 500 mg IV single dose
Repair third or fourth degree perineal laceration	Cefoxitin or Cefotetan	1 g IV 1 g IV
Operative vaginal delivery	Not recommended	NA
Manual removal placenta	Not recommended	N/A
Postpartum dilatation and curettage	Not recommended	N/A
Cerclage	Not recommended	N/A

Table 4.5 Prophylactic antibiotic recommendations for gynecological procedures[31]

Procedure	*Antibiotic*	*Dosage*
Vaginal and abdominal hysterectomy If allergic then	Cefazolin Clindamycin or Erythromycin	1–2 g IV, 15–60 minutes before skin incision 600 mg IV 500 mg IV
Laparoscopic hysterectomy	Same as above	Same as above
Pelvic organ prolapse and stress incontinence surgery	Same as above	Same as above
Hysteroscopy	Not recommended	
Surgical abortion	Doxycycline	100 mg orally before the procedure and 200 mg orally after the procedure
IUD insertion	None recommended	
Endometrial biopsy	None recommended	
Hysterosalpingogram	If STI treat accordingly if tubed dilated, give doxycycline	

Drug interaction: It may increase effect of phenytoin and warfarin.

Probenecid may increase concentration of cefazolin.

Monitoring: CBC, kidney function tests and liver function. Its dose needs to be modified in patients with deranged kidney functions.

Preparations: Azolin, cefazolin, ozolin, prezolin-500 mg and 1 g injection.

Safety during pregnancy: FDA category B drug and safe during lactation (American Academy of Pediatrics).[17]

Clindamycin

Pharmacology: Clindamycin is a potent lincosamide antibiotic. It is completely absorbed after oral administration and the t½ is 2.9 hours. It is largely metabolized and metabolites are excreted in the urine and bile. Hence dose adjustments are required in severe hepatic failure.

Antimicrobial spectrum: It inhibits protein synthesis by binding to 50s bacterial ribosome. It is effective against gram-positive cocci and especially against the toxin producing strains of *Staphylococcus* and *Streptococcus*. However, gram-negative organisms like pseudomonas, enterocbacter and acinetobacter spp are resistant to clindamycin because the cellular wall is impermeable to the drug. It is not effective against MRSA but highly effective against anaerobes especially bacteroides.

Contraindications: Allergy.

Dosage

Oral dose: 150–300 mg four times a day, maximum up to 600 mg 6 hourly.

IV dose: 600–900 mg 8 hourly, maximum 4800 mg per day.

Adverse effects: Rashes, urticaria and abdominal pain. But the major problem is diarrhea and pseudomembranous enterocolitis due to toxin by organism clostridium difficile.

Drug interactions: It should not be combined with macrolides because both have same mechanism of action. It should not be used in patients on neuromuscular blocking agents because it has neuromuscular blocking properties.

Monitoring: KFT and LFT should be monitored and watch for occurrence of side effects especially diarrhea.

Preparations: Dalcinex 300 mg per 2 mL and 600 mg per 4 mL injection.

Safety during pregnancy and lactation: The drug crosses placenta achieving maximum cord serum levels of 50% of the maternal serum levels, however there are no reports linking the use of clindamycin with congenital defects. The American Academy of Pediatrics classifies clindamycin compatible with breastfeeding. It is FDA category B drug.

Erythromycin

Pharmacology: Belongs to macrolide group.

Indications of use

- Treatment of infections caused by *Streptococcus, Staphylococcus, Chlamydia* and *Gonococcus.*
- Surgical prophylaxis.

Contraindications: Hypersensitivity.

Dosage

- Oral 250–500 mg 6–12 hourly, maximum 4 g daily.
- Intravenous 500–1 g 6 hourly, maximum 4 g daily.

Adverse drug reaction: Anorexia nausea abdominal pain, pruritus jaundice, weakness allergy.

Drug interaction: Budesonide, calcium channel blockers, domperidone, ergot derivatives, fluconazole, ulipristal, zafirlukast.

Preparation

Erythrocin—100, 250 mg tablets
Erythrokem—250 mg tablets

Erythromycin lactobionate powder for injection —500 mg and 1 g.

Safety during Pregnancy: It is category B drug.

Cefoxitine

Pharmacology: It is a parenteral semi synthetic cephalosporin antibiotic. Cefoxitin is more active than any other first or second generation cephalosporin against anaerobes specially Bacteroides fragilis.

Cefoxitin has special role for treatment of mixed aerobic and certain anaerobic infections.

Indications of use: For prophylaxis in major gynecological surgeries.

Contraindications: Hypersensitivity

Dosage: In PID (CDC2010): 2 g IV every 6 hourly with doxycycline for 24 hours after the clinical improvement followed by doxycycline to complete 14 days.

For perioperative prophylaxis—2 g IV, 30-60 minutes before incision, then 2 g every 6 hours for not more than 24 hours after the procedure.

Adverse drug reaction: Most common is diarrhea. Rarely can cause anaphylaxis, bone marrow depression, fever, nephrotoxicity, skin reactions, nausea and vomiting.

Drug interaction: It enhances nephrotoxicity of aminoglycosides, should not be used with it. It enhances anticoagulant effects, e.g. of warfarin.

Monitoring: CBC, KFT and LFTs.

Preparation: Acifox, zepax, foxitin, geoxin—available as powder for 1 g injection.

Safety during pregnancy lactation: It crosses placenta but is FDA category B drug. Very small amount of drug is excreted in the breast milk but should be cautiously used.

The transplacental passage of cefoxitin has been reported but no apparent adverse effect was noted in any of the new. borns.[28,29] It is secreted into breast milk in low concentrations. American Academy of Pediatrics classifies Cefoxitin as compatible with breast feeding.[12-29]

Use of Antibiotic Prophylaxis in Gynecological Surgeries

Hysterectomy

Hysterectomy is associated with opening of vaginal into the peritoneal cavity therefore it belongs to class II or clean contaminated wound. However, route of hysterectomy affects the risk of postoperative infection.[30] The antibiotic prophylaxis after vaginal, abdominal and laparoscopic hysterectomy is summarized in **Table 4.5.**[31,32]

Surgical Abortion (Induced and Therapeutic Abortion)

Risk of infection after surgical abortion before 16 weeks is shown to be significantly reduced with prophylactic antibiotics as compared to placebo. This was shown in a meta-analysis which included 12 randomized controlled trials (RCTs). Importantly this benefit was seen in both the subjects who were considered to be low and high risk for infection. Therefore the study recommended use of antibiotic prophylaxis in all cases of surgical abortion. However, the choice of antibiotics is only based on the results of a trial which revealed statistically significant reduction in infection rate with the use of 100 mg oral doxycycline before the procedure and 200 mg after the procedure **(*See* Table 4.5)**.

REFERENCES

1. Allen JL, Rimpone JF, Wheeless CR. Use of Prophylactic antibiotic in elective major gynecological operations. Obstet & Gynecol. 1972;39:218.
2. Berger SA, Nagar H, Gordin M. Antimicrobial Prophylaxis in Obst Gyane Surgery: a critical review. J Reprod Med. 1980;24:185.
3. Hemsell DL, Cunninghem FG, Kappas S, et al. Cefoxitin for prophylaxis in premenopausal women undergoing vaginal hysterectomy. Obstet & Gynecol. 1980;56:629.

4. Meckal A, Curole D, Levis C. Cefoxitin sodium: double blind vaginal hysterectomy prophylaxis in premenopausal patients. Obstet Gynecol. 1980;56:222.
5. Cresmen WT, Hill GA, Weed JC Jr, et al. A trial of prophylactic cefamandole in extended gynecologic surgery. Obstet Gynecol. 1982;59:303.
6. Mangam AJ, Horen TC, Peason ML, Silver LC, Jaevis WRJ Guideline for prevention of surgical site infection, 1999. Centre for Disease Control and Prevention (CDC) Hospital Infection Control Practices Advisory Committee. AMJ Infect Control. 1999;27:97-134.
7. Burke JF. The effective period of preventive antibiotic action in experimental incisions and dermal lesions. Surgery. 1961;50:161-8.
8. Classen DC, Evans RS, Pestonik SL, Horn SD, Menlove RL, Burke JP. The timing of prophylactic administration of antibiotics and the risk of surgical wound infection. N Engl J Med. 1992;326:281-6.
9. Gibbs RS. Clinical risk factors for puerperal infections Obstet & Gynecol. 1980;55(Suppl): 185-1845.
10. Henderson E, Love EJ. Incidence of hospital acquired infections associated with caesarean sectum. J Hosp Infect. 1995:29:245-55.
11. Smaill F, Hofmeyr GJ. Antibiotic prophylaxis for caesarean section. Cochrane Database Syst Rev 2002 ;(3) CD00093
12. Gordon SM. Antibiotic prophylaxis against postoperative wound infections. Cleve Clin J Med. 2006;73(Suppl 1):S42-5.
13. Sullivan SA, Smith T, Chang E, Hulsey T, Vondersten JP, Soper D. Administration of Cafazolin prior to skin incision is superior to Cefazolin at cord clamping in preventing post ceaserean infections morbidity: a randomised, controlled trial. Am J Obstet Gynecol. 2007;196:455 e1-5.
14. Dekel A, Elean l, Gibor Y, Goldman JA. Transplanted passage of Cefazolin in the first trimester of pregnancy. Eur J Obst Gynecol Reprod Biol. 1980;10:303-7.
15. Bernard B, Barton L, Abate M, Bellard CA, Maternal fetal transfer of Cafezolin in the first twenty weeks of pregnancy. J Infect Dis. 1977;136: 377-82.
16. Cho N, HOT, Secto T, et al. Clinical studies in Cefazolin in the field of Obstetrics and Gynecology. Chemotherapy. 1970;18:770-7.
17. Brown CEL, Christmas JJ, Bowdon RE. Placental transfer of Cefazolin and piperacillin in pregnancies remote from term completed by Rh iso immunisation. AM J Obst Gynecology. 1990;163:938-43.
18. Committee in drugs. American Academy of Pediatrics. The transfer of drugs & other chemicals into human milk. Pediatrics. 2001:108:776-89.
19. Heslehurst N, Simpson H, Ells LJ, Rankin J, Wilkinson J, Lang R, et al. The impact of maternal BMI status on pregnancy outcomes with immediate short-term obstetric resource implications: a meta-analysis. Obes Rev. 2008;9635-83.
20. Lee CE, Zembower TR, Fotis MA, Postelnick MJ, Greenberger PA, Peterson LR, et al. The incidence of antimicrobial allergies in hospitalized patients: implications regarding prescribing patterns and emerging bacterial resistance. Arch Intern Med. 2000;160:2819-22.
21. Sogn DD, Evans R 3rd, Shepherd GM, Casale TB, Condemi J, Greenberger PA, et al. Results of the National Institute of Allergy and Infectious Diseases collaborative clinical trial to test the predictive value of skin testing with major and minor penicillin derivatives in hospitalized adults. Arch Intern Med. 1992;152:1025.
22. Real GA, Rose ME, Ramirez-Atamoros MT, Hammel J, Gordon SM, Arroliga AC, Arroliga ME. Penicillin skin testing in patients with a history of beta-lactam allergy. Ann Allergy Asthma Immunol. 2007;98:355-9.
23. International Rheumatic Fever Study Group. Allergic reactions to long-term benzathine penicillin propylaxis for rheumatic fever. Lancet. 1991;337(8753):1308-10.
24. Dash, CH. Penicillin allergy and the cephalosporins. J Antimicrob Chemother. 1975;1:107.
25. Daulat S, Solensky R, Earl HS, Casey W, Gruchalla RS. Safety of cephalosporin administration to patients with histories of penicillin allergy. J Allergy Clin Immunol. 2004;113:1220.
26. Fonacier L, Hirschberg R, Gerson S. Adverse drug reactions to a cephalosporins in hospitalized patients with a history of penicillin allergy. Allergy Asthma Proc. 2005;26:135.
27. Philipson A, Sabath LD, Challeso. Transplacental passage of Azithromycin and Clindamycin. N England Journal Med. 1973;288:19-21.
28. Wenstein AJ, Gibbs RS, Gallaghen M. Placental transfer of Clindamycin and Gentamycin I term

pregnancy. American Journal Obstet Gynaecol. 1976;124:688-91.

29. Committee on Drugs. American Academy of Pediatrics. De transfer of drugs and other chemicals into human milk. Pediatrics. 2001; 108:776-89.
30. Bergogne Berezin B, Morel O, Kafe H, Bethelot G, Bernard Y, Lambert Zeechevsky N, Rouvillos JL. Pharmacokinetic study of cefoxitin in man: diffusion into bronchi and transfer across placenta. Threrapie. 1979;34:345-54.
31. Roex AJM, Van Loenen AC, Puyenbroek JI, Arts NFT. Secretion of cefoxitin in breast milk following short term prophylactic administration in caesrean section. Eur J Obstet Gynecol Reprod Biol. 1987;25:299-302.
32. Schalkwyk VJ, EYK, VN. Antibiotic prophylaxis in obstetrical procedures JOGC, September 2010. No. 247;879-85.

CHAPTER 5

Preterm Premature Rupture of Membranes and Chorioamnionitis

Krishna Agarwal, Shailja Verma

INTRODUCTION

Preterm premature rupture of membranes (PPROM) is spontaneous rupture of membranes prior 37 weeks of gestation. Therefore we often need to continue pregnancy with conservative management till the fetal lung maturity is obtained.

Amniotic fluid is normally sterile but when there is prolong rupture of membranes there are chances of ascending infection from vagina which can infect the decidua and lead to chorioamnionitis.[1]

Chorioamnionitis is notoriously difficult to diagnosis. It comprises mainly of maternal pyrexia (>38° C); and atleast two of either of the following:[2]

- Maternal tachycardia with pulse rate more than 100 beats per minute
- Fetal tachycardia with fetal heart rate more than 160 beats per minute
- Uterine tenderness
- Offensive vaginal discharge
- Raised C-reactive proteins
- Raised maternal total leukocyte count.

In women with PPROM, timely initiation of antibiotics prevents development of chorioamnionitis, a dreadful clinical event. Also when PPROM is at less than 34 weeks period of gestation, corticosteroids are required for fetal lung maturity prior to termination.

When chorioamnionitis is clinically suspected pregnancy has to be terminated. Simultaneouly, woman is started on antibiotics and the choice of antibiotics is usually in line with postpartum endometritis as both are caused by ascending infection and spectrum of causative organisms in both the conditions are same.

WHAT STUDIES HAVE TO SAY?

ORACLE trial was the first acceptable study to demonstrate a role for oral erythromycin in PPROM regimens. This was large randomized controlled trial which included 4826 women with PPROM. In singleton pregnancies, erythromycin alone was associated with a significant reduction (from 14.4–11.2%) in neonatal mortality and major morbidity whereas coamoxiclav was associated with significant rise in cases of necrotizing enterocolitis. ORACLE II trial has laid guidelines on the use of broad spectrum antibiotics for spontaneous preterm labor.[3,4]

Though there is no good trial to guide about the best place for management of PPROM but as it is recognized that 48–72 hours is the critical time during which many women will go in labor or develop clinical chorioamnionitis, it is recommended to manage them as indoor patients. During this stay intravenous antibiotics are used for atleast for 48 hours followed by oral antibiotics.

Antenatal steroid are associated with a significant reduction in rates of neonatal deaths, respiratory distress syndrome (RDS) and intraventricular hemorrhage especially with a single course given between 26 and 34 weeks gestation and is safe for the mother also.[5] They are most effective in reducing RDS in pregnancies that deliver 24 hours after and up to 7 days after administration of the second dose of antenatal corticosteroids.[5]

ANTIBIOTIC TREATMENT IN PPROM AND CHORIOAMNIONITIS

Role of antibiotics in PPROM is to prolong pregnancy, prevent puerperal sepsis and neonatal sepsis.[1,2,6,7] The choice of antibiotics in these two clinical conditions is given in **Table 5.1**.

Table 5.1: Antibiotics recommended in PPROM and chorioamnionitis[8-10]

Choice of antibiotic	*Antibiotic*	*Dosage*
Preterm premature rupture of membranes (PPROM)		
Drug of choice	Erythromycin: It is effective against most gram-positive and few gram-negative organisms, highly effective against *Streptococcus, Pneumococcus, Gonorrhea, Chlamydia* and *Mycoplasma*	250–500 mg erythromycin IV 6 hourly for 48 hours, 250 mg orally 6 hourly for total 10 days
Additional therapy	If vaginal swab grows group B streptococcus-ampicillin or any penicillin can be added except for coamoxiclav (increased incidence of necrotizing enterocolitis in newborns) Ampicillin and sulbacin is another alternative	Ampicillin 0.5–2 g IV every 6 hours for 48 hours and then 0.5–2 g orally 6 hourly for 10 days
Second-line	If patient is sensitive to penicillin	Clindamycin 600–900 mg IV 8 hourly for 48 hours followed by 150–300 mg four times a day for total 10 days
Chorioamnionitis*		
Drug of choice	Ampicillin, gentamicin and metronidazole The combination provides broad spectrum antibiotic coverage for gram-positive and negative organisms and anaerobes	Ampicillin 1–2 g IV 6 hourly, gentamicin 1.5 mg per kg body weight IV 8 hourly and metronidazole 500 mg IV 8 hourly
Second-line	If allergic to penicillin	Cefotaxime 1–2 g IV or IM 8 hourly OR ceftriaxone 1–2 g IV or IM 8–12 hourly OR cefuroxime 1.5 IV or IM mg 8 hourly PLUS metronidazole 500 mg IV 8 hourly
	If patient does not respond to above regimen	Imipenem plus cilastatin OR Piperacillin plus tazobactam
	If MRSA suspected	Vancomycin OR Teicoplanin OR linezolid

* The treatment is continued till 24 hours after the patient becomes afebrile

REFERENCES

1. Preterm prelabor rupture of membrane. Green-top Guideline 44, 2010.
2. Bacterial Sepsis in Pregnancy. Green-top Guideline no. 64a. 2012.
3. Kenyon S, Taylor DJ, Tarnow-Mordi WO, ORACLE Collaborative Group. ORACLE-antibiotics for preterm prelabour rupture of the membranes: Short-term and long-term outcomes. Acta Paediatr Suppl. 2002;91(437):12-5.
4. Kenyon SL, Taylor DJ, Tarnow-Mordi W, et al. Broad-spectrum antibiotics for spontaneous preterm labour: The ORACLE II randomised trial. The Lancet. 2001;357(9261):989-94.
5. Antenatal Corticosteroids to Reduce Neonatal Morbidity and Mortality, Royal College of Obstetricians and Gynecologists. Green-top Guidline no.7, 2010.
6. Cousens S, Blencowe H, Gravett M, et al. Antibiotics for preterm prelabour rupture of membranes: Prevention of neonatal deaths due to complications of preterm birth and infection. Int J Epidemiol. 2010;39 (Suppl 1):134-43.
7. Prevention of Early Onset Neonatal Group B Streptococcal Disease, Royal College of Obstetricians and Gynaecologists. Green-top Guideline no. 36, 2012.
8. Chapman E, Reveiz L, Ellanes E, et al. Antibiotic regimens for management of intra-amniotic Infection. Cochrane Database Syst Rev. 2014;12:CD010976.
9. Mercer BM, Miodovnik M, Thurnau GR, et al. Antibiotic therapy for reduction of infant morbidity after preterm premature rupture of the membranes. A randomized controlled trial. National Institute of Child Health and Human Development Maternal-Fetal Medicine Units Network. JAMA. 199;278(12):989-95.
10. Kenyon S, Boulvain M, Neilson J. Antibiotics for preterm premature rupture of membranes. Cochrane Database Syst Rev. 2001;(4):CD001058. Review. Update in: Cochrane Database Syst Rev. 2003;(2):CD001058.

CHAPTER 6

Puerperal Infection

Poonam Kashyap

Bacterial infection of genital tract after child birth is generally referred to as puerperal infections or sepsis. This is one of the most common causes of preventable maternal morbidity and mortality not only in the developing countries but in developed countries. It is the most common cause of puerperal pyrexia.[1]

Puerperal sepsis was defined using the WHO criteria as the infection of the genital tract occurring anytime between the rupture of membranes or labor and the 42nd day postpartum in which two or more of the following were present: pelvic pains, fever, i.e. oral temperature of 38°C or more, abnormal vaginal discharge, abnormal smell or foul odor of discharge and delay in the rate of uterine involution (less than 2 cm per day in the first 8 days).[2]

Mostly puerperal infection after vaginal or cesarean delivery presents as metritis and pelvic cellulitis. These patients respond to antibiotics in more than 90% cases. In the remaining following complications may arise:

- Wound infection, dehiscence or necrotizing fasciitis
- Peritonitis
- Parametrial phlegmon
- Ovarian or pelvic abscess
- Septic pelvic thrombophlebitis
- Infection of perineum, vagina and cervix
- Toxic shock syndrome.

The transmissions of infecting organisms are typically categorized into nosocomial, exogenous, and endogenous. Nosocomial infections are acquired in hospitals or other health facilities and may come from the hospital environment or from the patient's own flora. Exogenous infections come from external contamination, especially when deliveries take place under unhygienic conditions. Endogenous organisms, consists of mixed flora colonizing the woman's own genital tract.

Mostly the source of infection in puerperal sepsis is endogenous infection. Aseptic precautions, advances in investigative tools and the use of antibiotics have played a major role in reducing the incidence of puerperal infections.

Selection of antibiotics should be based on the understanding of the multibacterial dimensions of pelvic infections, the pattern of sensitivity to the antibiotics and presence of antimicrobial resistance. Infection of genital tract is mostly caused by bacteria which are normally present in the female genital tract. The major pathogens responsible for genital tract infection are given in **Table 6.1**.

Antibiotic therapy for any infection should ideally be based on the culture and gram staining reports of any swab, aspirate or biopsy specimen. However, in practice the patient is usually sick and broad spectrum antibiotics

Table 6.1 Common bacteria responsible for puerperal sepsis[2]

Class	*Species of bacteria*
Gram-positive bacteria	*Streptococcus pyogenes* (also known as group A *Streptococcus* or GAS), *Streptococcus pneumoniae, Staphylococcus aureus*, methicillin resistant *Staphylococcus aureus* (MRSA)
Gram-negative bacteria	*E. coli, Klebsiella, Neisseria gonorrhoeae*, Chlamydia, *Enterobacter, Proteus, Pseudomonas, Haemophilus influenzae*
Anaerobes	*Clostridium, Bacteroides, Listeria monocytogenes*

Table 6.2 Antibiotic choice in treatment of puerperal sepsis[4]

Line of treatment	*Drug regimen*
First-line treatment	Clindamycin 900 mg IV plus 1.5 mg per kg of body weight plus gentamicin 8 hourly Add injection ampicillin 1 gm IV 6 hourly if does not respond within 48 hours or enterococcal infection is suspected
	If patient has renal insufficiency, replace gentamicin with aztreonam
Second-line treatment	Amoxicillin plus clavulanic acid plus gentamicin plus metronidazole OR Ampicillin plus sulbactam plus gentamicin plus metronidazole
	If patient is sensitive to penicillins, give cefotaxime OR cefuroxime plus metronidazole
If patient does not respond to above regimen	Imipenem plus cilastatin OR Piperacillin plus tazobactam
If MRSA suspected	Vancomycin OR Teicoplanin OR Linezolid

should be immediately started based on the knowledge of commonly responsible pathogens. In case of suspicion of severe sepsis, intravenous broad-spectrum antibiotics should be started within 1 hour **(Table 6.2)**.

Mostly after vaginal delivery, genital tract infection is mild and responds to combination of ampicillin and gentamicin. However after cesarean section and in cases of severe peripartum sepsis where group A *Streptococcus* and *Staphylococcus* have potential to cause toxic shock syndrome, injectable clindamycin is recommended.[3] This should be combined with gentamicin to cover for gram-negative bacteria. Clindamycin is effective against most gram-positive aerobes and anaerobes except enterococcus. For gram-negative coverage gentamicin is added. Ninety five percent times patients respond to this treatment. In some cases if patient does not respond in 48 hours, ampicillin is added in presumption to treat persisting *Enterococcus* infection which is not covered by clindamycin. In case of deranged kidney functions gentamicin should be replaced by aztreonam.

Beta lactam penicillins (amoxicillin, ampicillin, piperacillin) are usually safe except for allergy and are free from toxicity. In case of severe infection they can be used combined with beta-lactamase inhibitors (clavulanic acid, sulbactam and tazobactam). In patients who are allergic to penicillins, third generation cephalosporins (cefotaxime or cefuroxime) can be used. In addition to penicillin metronidazole for covering most anaerobes and an aminoglycoside for gram-negative organism should be combined. Whereas cephalosporins cover gram-positive and gram-negative bacteria and require coverage with metronidazole for anaerobic cover.

In patients not responding to above regimen then higher antibiotic imipenem is used. It has broad spectrum of coverage against most organism responsible for puerperal sepsis. Imipenem is combined with cilastatin because cilastatin prevents renal metabolism of imipenem by competitive inhibition of dehydropeptidase along the brush borders of renal tubules. Another alternative is piperacillin-tazobactam combination.

In case of MRSA, even higher antibiotics like vancomycin, teicoplanin or linezolid may have to be used.

REFERENCES

1. Bacterial sepsis following pregnancy. Green-top guideline No. 64b, 2012.
2. Managing puerperal sepsis. Education material for teachers of midwifery. Midwifery education modules-2nd edition. World Health Organization, 2008.
3. Dizerega G, Yonekura L, Roy S, et al. A comparison of clindamycin-gentamycin and penicillin gentamycin in treatment of post caesarean section endomyometritis. Am J Obstet Gynecol. 1979;134:238.
4. Cunningham, Leveno, Bloom, Hauth, Rouse, Spong. Puerperal infection. In Williams Obstetrics, 23rd edn. McGraw-Hill Publishers, 2010.pp.661-71.

CHAPTER 7

Human Immunodeficiency Virus During Pregnancy

YM Mala, Bhoomika Tantuway, Arushika Yedla

INTRODUCTION

The scenario of human immunodeficiency virus (HIV) in India has changed over the past years. There are an estimated 2.1 million people living with HIV in India, with national adult HIV prevalence of 0.27% (2011). Between 2004 and 2013, the number of pregnant women tested annually under the prevention of parent-to-child-transmission (PPTCT) program has increased from 0.8 million to 8.83 million.[1]

DRUGS FOR HIV POSITIVE PREGNANT WOMEN

Latest WHO guidelines for ART in pregnant women strongly recommend that all pregnant and breastfeeding women with HIV should initiate triple antiretrovirols (ARVs) antiretroviral therapy (ART), which should be maintained lifelong for all women or at least for women meeting treatment eligibility criteria.[2]

National AIDS Control Organisation (NACO) has also decided to provide lifelong ART for all pregnant and breastfeeding women living with HIV **(Table 7.1)**. Triple drug ART regimen, Tenofovir + Lamivudine + Efavirenz (**TDF + 3TC + EFV)** is recommended as first-line ART in pregnant and breastfeeding women and women of childbearing age regardless of CD4 count or WHO clinical stage[1] **(Table 7.2)**.

HIV infected pregnant women who have had previous exposure to Sd NVP (or EFV) for PPTCT prophylaxis in prior pregnancies, an NNRTI-based ART regimen such as TDF+3TC+EFV may not be fully effective due to persistence of

Table 7.1: Dose and duration of infant daily nevirapine (NVP) prophylaxis (NACO)

Birth weight	*NVP dose in mg*	*NVP dose in mL**	*Duration*
Infants with birth weight <2000 g	2 mg/kg once daily	0.2 mL/kg once daily	Up to 6 weeks irrespective of whether exclusively breastfeed or exclusively replacement feed may be extended to 12 weeks, if mother has not received ART for adequate duration, i.e. at least 24 weeks
Birth weight 2000–2500 g	10 mg once daily	1 mL once a day	
Birth weight more than 2500 g	15 mg once daily	1.5 mL once a day	

*1 mL suspension contains of 10 mg Nevirapine (NVP)

archived mutation to NNRTIs **(Table 7.3)**. Thus, these women will require a protease-inhibitor (Lopinavir/Ritonavir) based ART regimen viz.[1]

The nevirapine prophylaxin and ART in women with tuberculosis and hepatitis B infection have been given in **Tables 7.4** and **7.5** respectively.

Co-trimoxazole in Pregnancy

- Co-trimoxazole should be started if CD4 count is ≤250 cells/mm³ and continued through pregnancy, delivery and breast-feeding as per national guidelines (Dose: Double strength tablet – 1 tab daily). Dose

Table 7.2: ART regimens in pregnancy

ART for HIV positive pregnant women	***Preferred first line regimen***	***Alternative regimens***
	TDF (300 mg) + 3TC (300 mg) + EFV (600 mg)	AZT+ 3TC+EFV (600, 300, 600) AZT+3TC+NVP (600, 300, 200) TDF+ 3TC+NVP (300, 300, 200)

Table 7.3: ART in previous exposure of Sd NVP

ART for HIV positive pregnant women who have had previous exposure to Sd NVP (EFV)	***Preferred regimens***
	TDF (300 mg) + 3TC (300 mg) + LPV (200 mg)/r (50 mg), 2 tab BD

Table 7.4: ART in special circumstances:[2]

With tuberculosis	Start ART (TDF + 3TC + EFV) in all individuals with active TB disease regardless of CD4 cell count
Hepatitis B coinfection	Initiate in all individuals nonpregnant women with CD4 ≤500 cells/mm³ and in patients of severe chronic liver disease, ART should be started irrespective of CD4 count (TDF + 3TC + EFV)

Table 7.5: Classification of antiretroviral drugs

Entry inhibitors	***Maraviroc, Enfuvirtide***	
Reverse transcriptase inhibitors	NRTI	Lamivudine Abacavir Zidovudine Didanosine Emtricitabine Tenofovir
	NNRTI	Efavirenz Nevirapine
Integrase inhibitors	Raltegravir	
Protease inhibitors	Fosamprenavir Lopinavir/ritonavir (Ritonavir is used as a boosting agent) Saquinavir	
Multiclass combination products	2 or more classes in a single product	

of co-trimoxazole for adults is 800 mg sulfamethoxazole + 160 mg trimethoprim.

- Pregnant women should take their folate supplements regularly.

The drugs used in the treatment of HIV are classified into 5 groups.[3] Each class of drugs attacks virus at a different stage of the HIV life cycle. Therefore, drug classification is on the basis of their interference in the steps of HIV replication **(Table 7.5).**

1. *Entry inhibitors*: They interfere with the virus ability to bind the receptors on the outer surface of the cell.
2. *Reverse transcriptase inhibitors*: Inhibits a process known as reverse transcription by which, single stranded HIV RNA get converted into double stranded HIV DNA. There are two types of RT inhibitors:
   Nucleoside/nucleotide RT inhibitors (NRTIs) are faulty DNA building blocks. When one of these faulty building blocks is added to a growing HIV DNA chain, no further correct DNA building blocks can be added on, thus halts HIV DNA synthesis.
   - Lamivudine (3TC)
   - Abacavir
   - Zidovudine (AZT)
   - Didanosine (ddI)
   - Emtricitabine
   - Tenofovir (TDF)

   Non-nucleoside RT inhibitors (NNRTIs) acts by binding to RT, therefore prevents conversion of HIV RNA into HIV DNA
   - Efavirenz (EFV)
   - Nevirapine (NVP)
3. *Integrase inhibitors*: These drugs block the HIV enzyme integrase, by this enzyme virus inserts its genetic material into the infected cells DNA e.g. raltegravir.
4. *Protease inhibitors*: These drugs interfere with enzyme protease. Protease function is to cut long chains of HIV proteins.
   - Fosamprenavir
   - Lopinavir/ritonavir (Ritonavir is used as a boosting agent)
   - Saquinavir.
5. *Multiclass combination products*: HIV drugs from two or more classes combine into a single product.

Tenofovir Disoproxil Fumarate[4]

Pharmacology

- The oral bioavailability is approximately 25%
- Tenofovir disoproxil fumarate (TDF) gets eliminated by combination of glomerular filtration and active tubular secretion
- Following IV administration, approximately 70–80% of the dose is recovered in the urine.

Indications

- Used in HIV treatment regimen
- TDF is also an HBV reverse transcriptase inhibitor, therefore used to treat chronic HBV in adults and children of 12 years and above.

Contraindications: Tenofovir should be avoided with concurrent or recent use of nephrotoxic agent (e.g. high-dose or multiple nonsteroidal anti-inflammatory drugs).

Dosage: 300 mg once a day.

Adverse drug reactions: Side effects can be life-threatening, example lactic acidosis. Other side effects of tenofovir include:

- Headache, abdominal pain, fever
- Diarrhea, nausea, vomiting
- Lipodystrophy
- Arthralgia, myalgia
- Depression, insomnia, peripheral neuropathy
- Pneumonia
- Immune reconstitution inflammatory syndrome (IRIS), it occur when immune system begins to recover after treatment. As the immune system gets stronger, it may have an increased response to a previously hidden infection.

Precautions: Tenofovir should be withheld in patients of lactic acidosis or hepatotoxicity (which may include hepatomegaly and steatosis).

Patients with HBV who discontinue tenofovir should be closely monitored with both clinical and laboratory follow-up for at least several months after stopping treatment.

Preparations
Tavin, Tenof.
Pregnancy category: B.

Lamivudine (3TC)[5]

Pharmacology

- Absolute bioavailability 85–87%
- The majority of lamivudine is eliminated unchanged in urine.

Indication: Treatment of HIV infection in combination with other antiretroviral agents.

Contraindication: Previous history of clinically significant hypersensitivity reaction (e.g. anaphylaxis).

Dosage: 300 mg once a day.

Adverse drug reactions

- Lactic acidosis and severe hepatomegaly with steatosis
- Hepatic decompensation in patients co-infected with HIV-1 and hepatitis
- Pancreatitis
- Nausea, vomiting, abdominal pain, diarrhea, headache, hair loss, fever, joint pains, insomnia, rash, tiredness and hypersensitivity.

Preparation
Lambda.
Pregnancy category: C.

Efavirenz (EFV)[6]

Pharmacology

- Efavirenz is principally metabolized by the cytochrome P450 system to hydroxylated metabolites
- Efavirenz induces its own metabolism by inducing CYP enzymes
- Efavirenz is highly bound to human plasma proteins (approximately 99.5–99.75%), predominantly to albumin
- 14–34% of efavirenz was eliminated in the urine and 16–61% eliminated in the feces.

Indication
Treatment of HIV infection.

Contraindications: In patients with previously demonstrated clinically significant hypersensitivity (e.g. Stevens-Johnson syndrome, erythema multiforme, or toxic skin eruptions).

Dosage: 600 mg once a day.

Adverse drug reactions

- Psychiatric symptoms, severe depression, suicidal ideation, nonfatal suicide attempts, aggressive behavior, paranoid reactions, and manic reactions
- Rash
- *Hepatotoxicity*: Monitoring of liver enzymes before and during treatment is recommended for patients with underlying hepatic disease, including hepatitis B or C infection
- Convulsions have been observed in adult and pediatric patients receiving efavirenz, generally in the presence of known medical history of seizures.

Drug interaction: Plasma concentrations of the drug may be altered by substrates, inhibitors, or inducers of CYP3A.

Preparation
Efavir.

Pregnancy category: D.
Potential risk of neural tube birth defects (very low risk in humans). A recent meta-analysis found no overall increase in the incidence of birth defects for first-trimester EFV exposure compared with other ARV drugs.

Zidovudine (AZT)[7]

Pharmacology

- Oral bioavailability 65%
- After oral administration, zidovudine is rapidly absorbed and distributed and peak serum concentrations occur within 1 to 1.5 hours

- Zidovudine is primarily eliminated by hepatic metabolism.

Indications
- HIV infection treatment
- Prevention of mother to child transmission of HIV.

Contraindication: Contraindicated in patients who had a potentially life-threatening hypersensitivity reaction (e.g. anaphylaxis, Stevens-Johnson syndrome).

Dosage: 250 mg twice a day.

Adverse drug reactions
- Hematologic toxicity (neutropenia and anemia). Therefore, in patients with bone marrow compromise (granulocyte count less than 1,000 cells per mm^3 or hemoglobin less than 9.5 g per dL) zidovudine should be used cautiously
- Lactic acidosis and severe hepatomegaly with steatosis
- Hepatic decompensation in patients co-infected with HIV-1 and hepatitis C
- Nausea, vomiting, fatigue, headache, dizziness, weakness, muscle pain, loss of appetite, fever.

Drug interactions
- Exacerbation of anemia due to ribavirin has been reported when zidovudine is part of the HIV regimen. Hematological toxicity of zidovudine got increased when used along with ganciclovir, interferon alfa, ribavirin, and other bone marrow suppressive or cytotoxic agents.
- Concomitant use of zidovudine with stavudine should be avoided (antagonistic relationship has been demonstrated).

Preparation
Zidine.

Pregnancy category: C.

Nevirapine (NVP)[8]

Pharmacology
- Nevirapine is readily absorbed (greater than 90%) after oral administration
- Primary route of nevirapine biotransformation and elimination in humans is by cytochrome P450 metabolism, glucuronide conjugation, and urinary excretion of glucuronidated metabolites
- It induces hepatic cytochrome P450 (CYP) enzymes.

Indication
Treatment of HIV Infection.

Contraindications
- Contraindicated in patients with moderate or severe hepatic impairment
- Contraindicated for use as part of occupational and nonoccupational post-exposure prophylaxis (PEP) regimen.

Dosage: 200 mg once a day for 14 days, followed by 200 mg twice daily.

Adverse drug reactions
- The most common adverse reaction is rash
- The most serious adverse reactions are hepatic failure, hepatitis, hypersensitivity, Stevens-Johnson syndrome and toxic epidermal necrolysis reactions
- Fatigue, malaise, muscle or joint aches, oral lesions, blisters, conjunctivitis, facial edema, granulocytopenia, eosinophilia, lymphadenopathy, or renal dysfunction.

Preparations
Nev, Neve.

Pregnancy category: B.

Ritonavir (RTV)[9]

Pharmacology
- Food decreased the bioavailability of the ritonavir
- Ritonavir is metabolized by cytochrome P450 3A (CYP3A).

Indication
Treatment of HIV Infection.

Contraindications
- Along with other protease inhibitors
- Patients with known hypersensitivity (e.g. toxic epidermal necrolysis (TEN) or Stevens-Johnson syndrome)

- Coadministration of ritonavir with other classes of drugs (e.g. antiarrhythmics, ergot alkaloid preparations, sedative or hypnotics) as it may result in potentially serious adverse events due to effects of ritonavir on the hepatic metabolism.

Dosage

Lopinavir/Ritonavir 400 mg/100 mg twice daily.

Adverse drug reactions: Diarrhea, nausea, vomiting, abdominal pain, neurological disturbances, rash, and fatigue/asthenia. As monotherapy resistant virus emerges rapidly.

Drug interactions: Ritonavir is a CYP3A inhibitor, therefore it leads to increased, prolonged therapeutic or adverse effects, potentially leading to severe, life-threatening or fatal events along with concomitant medications.

Preparations

Empetus, Ritomax

Pregnancy category: B.

REFERENCES

1. Kumari G, Kanchar A, Rewari B, Sivalenka S, Rao R, Rani N. Prevention of Parent to Child Transmission (PPTCT) of HIV using Multi Drug Anti-retroviral Regimen in India. Ministry of Health and Family Welfare Department of AIDS Control Basic Services Division Chandralok Building, Janpath New Delhi; 2013.
2. World Health Organization. Consolidated guidelines on the use of Antiretroviral drugs for treating and preventing HIV infection, Recommendations for a public health approach [document on internet]. [Cited 2013 June]. Available from: *http://www.who.int/iris/bitstream/10665/85321/1/9789241505727_eng.pdf.*
3. Types of HIV/Retroviral drug [Internet] 2009 [updated September 13 2013]. Available from: *http://www.niaid.nih.gov/topics/HIVAIDS/Understanding/Treatment/pages/arvdrugclasses.aspx.*
4. AIDS info Drug Database [Internet] 2015 [updated June 2015]. Available from: *https://aidsinfo.nih.gov/drugs/290/tenofovir-disoproxil-fumarate/0/professional.*
5. AIDS info Drug Database [Internet] 2015 [updated March 2015]. Available from: *https://aidsinfo.nih.gov/drugs/126/lamivudine/0/professional.*
6. AIDS info Drug Database [Internet] 2015 [updated May 2014]. Available from: *https://aidsinfo.nih.gov/drugs/269/efavirenz/0/professional.*
7. AIDS info Drug Database [Internet] 2015 [updated December 2014]. Available from: *https://aidsinfo.nih.gov/drugs/4/zidovudine/0/professional.*
8. AIDS info Drug Database [Internet] 2015 [updated January 2015]. Available from: *https://aidsinfo.nih.gov/drugs/116/nevirapine/0/professional.*
9. AIDS info Drug Database [Internet] 2015 [updated February 2015]. Available from: *https://aidsinfo.nih.gov/drugs/244/ritonavir/33/professional.*

CHAPTER 8

Pelvic Inflammatory Disease

YM Mala, Bhoomika Tantuway

Inflammatory disorders of the upper female genital tract either endometritis or salpingitis or tubo-ovarian abscess or pelvic peritonitis or their combinations comprises pelvic inflammatory disease (PID).

According to centers for Disease Control and Prevention (CDC) 2015 guidelines,[1] presumptive treatment for PID should be started in sexually active young women and other women who are at risk for sexually transmitted diseases (STDs):

- If they are experiencing pelvic or lower abdominal pain
- If no cause for the illness other than PID can be identified
- If one or more of minimum clinical criteria are present on pelvic examination (**Table 8.1**).

TREATMENT FOR PELVIC INFLAMMATORY DISEASE

Treatment for mild-to-moderately severe acute PID intramuscular/oral therapy can be considered. Women not responding to IM/oral therapy within 72 hours should be re-evaluated and intravenous therapy should be administered. CDC 2015 guidelines are given in **Table 8.2.**

Metronidazole[2]

Pharmacology

- Oral metronidazole permeate into all tissues by simple diffusion
- Within 1–3 hours peak plasma concentrations are reached.

Table 8.1: Diagnosis of pelvic inflammatory disease (CDC, 2015)

Minimum clinical criteria	*Additional criteria**	*Specific criteria*
• Cervical motion tenderness or • Tenderness of uterus or • Adnexal tenderness	• Oral temperature >101°F (>38.3°C) • Abnormal cervical friability or mucopurulent discharge • Presence of abundant WBC on vaginal fluid saline microscopy • Elevated erythrocyte sedimentation rate and C-reactive protein • Laboratory documentation of cervical infection with gonorrhoeae or *C. trachomatis*	• Endometrial biopsy of endometritis on histopathological report • Transvaginal sonography or magnetic resonance imaging techniques showing thickened, fluid-filled tubes with or without free pelvic fluid or tubo-ovarian mass, or Doppler studies suggesting pelvic infection (e.g. tubal hyperemia) • Laparoscopic findings of PID

* Enhance the specificity of the minimum clinical criteria

Table 8.2: Treatment of PID (CDC, 2015)	
Parenteral regimens (transition to oral therapy can be initiated within 24–48 hours of clinical improvement)	*Intramuscular/Oral regimens*
• *Cefotetan* 2 g IV, every 12 hours plus *doxycycline* 100 mg orally or IV 12 hourly or • Cefoxitin 2 g IV every 6 hourly plus doxycycline 100 mg orally or IV every 12 hourly or • Clindamycin 900 mg IV every 8 hourly plus gentamicin loading dose IV or IM (2 mg/kg), followed by a maintenance dose (1.5 mg/kg) 8 hourly	• Ceftriaxone 250 mg IM single dose plus doxycycline 100 mg orally twice daily for 14 days with or without metronidazole 500 mg orally twice daily for 14 days or • Cefoxitin 2 g IM single dose and probenecid 1 g orally single dose plus doxycycline 100 mg orally twice daily for 14 days with or without metronidazole 500 mg orally twice daily for 14 days

- Plasma protein binding is low (10–20%)
- Metronidazole half-life—7.5 hours
- Metronidazole metabolites are excreted mainly in the urine
- Plasma clearance of metronidazole decreases in patients with impaired liver function.

Mechanism of Action

Metronidazole is nitroimidazole antiprotozoal drug also has potent antibacterial activity against anaerobes, metronidazole is selectively absorbed by anaerobic bacteria and sensitive protozoan. Inside bacteria and protozoan it is nonenzymatically reduced by reacting with reduced ferredoxin. Products formed after reduction are toxic to anaerobic cells. This process of reduction occurs only in anaerobic cells, while human cells or aerobic bacteria has relatively little effect.

Indications

- Trichomoniasis
- Treatment of asymptomatic sexual partners
- Amebiasis
- Giardiasis
- Anaerobic bacterial infections, intra-abdominal infections, intra-abdominal abscess, peritonitis, and liver abscess, caused by *Bacteroides* species
- Skin and skin structure infections caused by *Bacteroides* species
- Gynecologic infections, including endometritis, postsurgical vaginal cuff infection, tubo-ovarian abscess
- Central nervous system (CNS) infections, including brain abscess, meningitis
- Bone and joint infections.

Contraindications

- *Hypersensitivity*: Among patients with a prior history of hypersensitivity to metronidazole
- Metronidazole causes psychotic reaction with disulfiram therefore should not be administered to patients who have taken disulfiram within the last two weeks
- With alcohol use of oral metronidazole is associated with a disulfiram-like reaction, including abdominal cramps, nausea, vomiting, headaches, and flushing.

Adverse Drug Reactions

- Nausea, dry mouth, metallic taste, headache occurs commonly. Infrequent adverse effects include vomiting, diarrhea, dysuria, dark urine, insomnia, dizziness, weakness, thrush, rash, vertigo, paresthesias, and neutropenia
- Pancreatitis
- Severe central nervous system toxicity (seizures, encephalopathy, ataxia).

Preparations

Flagyl, Metro

Pregnancy category: B

REFERENCES

1. Kimberly A Workowski, Gail A Bolan. Sexually Transmitted Diseases Treatment Guidelines, 2015. US Department of Health and Human Services, Centers for Disease Control and Prevention.
2. Brtram G Katzung, Susan B Masters, Anthony J Trevor. Basic and clinical Pharmacology. New York City: LANGE; 2015.

CHAPTER 9

Vaginitis/Vulvitis

YM Mala, Bhoomika Tantuway

VAGINAL DISCHARGE

Among women of reproductive age group three common categories of altered vaginal discharge **(Table 9.1)**.[1]

Summary of signs and symptoms of infective causes of vaginal discharge **(Table 9.2)**.[2]

Bacterial Vaginosis

Bacterial vaginosis is a clinical syndrome characterized by replacement of the normal *Lactobacillus* spp. in the vagina with high concentrations of anaerobic bacteria, such as *G. vaginalis* and *Mycoplasma hominis*. The current recommendation is to treat symptomatic female. According to CDC 2015 guidelines recommended regimens are[3]

- Metronidazole 500 mg orally twice daily for 7 days

OR

- Metronidazole gel 0.75%, 5 g twice daily intravaginally for 5 days

OR

- Clindamycin vaginal cream 2%, 5 g at bedtime intravaginally for 7 days.

Alternative Regimen[1,3]

- Tinidazole 2 g orally once daily for 2 days

OR

- Tinidazole 1 g orally once daily for 5 days

OR

- Clindamycin, 300 mg orally twice daily for 7 days.

Follow-up

If symptoms persist patients should be advised to return as retreatment may be required. In case of recurrence, treatment with different

Table 9.1: Causes of vaginal discharge

Infective (Nonsexually transmitted)	*Infective (Sexually transmitted)*	*Noninfective*
• Bacterial vaginosis • Candida	• *Chlamydia trachomatis* • *Neisseria gonorrhoeae* • Herpes simplex virus • *Trichomonas vaginalis*	• Foreign bodies (e.g. retained tampons, condoms) • Cervical polyps and ectopy • Fistulae • Allergic reactions • Genital tract malignancy

Table 9.2: Diagnostic features of vaginitis

Signs and symptoms	*Bacterial vaginosis*	*Candidiasis*	*Trichomoniasis*
	Approximately 50% asymptomatic	10–20% asymptomatic	10–50% asymptomatic
Discharge	Thin	Thick curdy white	Scant to profuse
Odor	Offensive/fishy	Nonoffensive	Offensive
Itch	None	Vulval itch	Vulval itch
Other possible symptoms		Soreness Dysuria Superficial dyspareunia	Lower abdominal pain Dysuria
Visible signs	Discharge coating the vagina and vestibule No vulval inflammation	Normal findings Or Vulval erythema Edema Fissuring Satellite lesions	Frothy yellow discharge Vulvitis Vaginitis Cervicitis 'Strawberry cervix' (Ectocervix sometimes resembles surface of strawberry)
Vaginal pH	>4.5	≤4.5	>4.5

recommended regimen is justified. In women with multiple episode of recurrence, 0.75% metronidazole gel twice a week for duration of 4–6 months will decrease recurrence.

Management of Sexual Partner

Routinely treatment of sexual partners is not recommended.

Bacterial Vaginosis in Pregnancy

During pregnancy, bacterial vaginosis is associated with an increased incidence of adverse outcomes (e.g. premature rupture of membranes, preterm delivery). Symptomatic pregnant women should be treated, and screening of pregnant female with previous obstetric history of preterm delivery should be screened to detect asymptomatic infections. According to CDC 2015 guidelines either of the oral or vaginal regimens can be used to treat symptomatic pregnant women.

Candidiasis[1,3]

Classification of Vulvovaginal Candidiasis

Table 9.3 shows classification of vulvovaginal candidiasis (VVC).

Table 9.3: Classification of vulvovaginal candidiasis

Uncomplicated VVC	*Complicated VVC*
• Sporadic or infrequent vulvovaginal candidiasis • Mild-to-moderate in nature • Likely to be *C. albicans* • Nonimmunocompromised women	• Recurrent • Severe vulvovaginal candidiasis • Nonalbicans candidiasis • Usually seen in women with uncontrolled diabetes, debilitation, or immunosuppression

Recommended Regimens: Uncomplicated (CDC 2015)[3]

- Clotrimazole (1%) 5 g cream intravaginally for 7–14 days **or**
- Clotrimazole (2%) 5 g cream intravaginally for 3 days **or**
- Miconazole (2%) 5 g cream intravaginally for 7 days **or**
- Miconazole 200 mg intravaginally, once daily for 3 days **or**
- Miconazole 100 mg vaginal suppository, one suppository for 7 days **or**
- Fluconazole 150 mg orally, as a single dose.

Complicated Candidiasis (CDC 2015)[3]

- *Recurrent vulvovaginal candidiasis*: Defined as four or more episodes of symptomatic VVC in 1 year (<5%). Treatment is longer duration of initial therapy, i.e. 7–14 days of topical therapy. But first line of treatment is 100 mg or 150 mg or 200 mg oral fluconazole every third day, total 3 doses (day 1, 4, and 7). Maintenance doses of oral fluconazole (i.e. 100 mg or 150 mg or 200 mg dose) is given weekly for 6 months.
- *Severe VVC:* Extensive vulvar erythema, edema, excoriation, and fissure formation) is treated with either topical azole for 7–14 days or oral fluconazole 150 mg in two sequential doses (second dose 72 hours after first).
- *Nonalbicans VVC:* The optimal treatment remains unknown. Options include longer duration of therapy (7–14 days) with a nonfluconazole azole drug (oral or topical) as first-line therapy. In case of recurrence, 600 mg of boric acid in gelatin capsule vaginally once daily for 2 weeks.

Vulvovaginal Candidiasis in Pregnancy

Only topical azoles should be used to treat pregnant women as oral treatments are not safe or effective.

Management of Sexual Partners

Not recommended.

Trichomonas vaginalis Infection[1,3]

According to CDC 2015 guidelines.

Recommended Regimen

- Metronidazole, 2 g oral (single dose)

  or
- Tinidazole, 2 g oral (single dose).

Alternative Regimen

- Metronidazole, 400 mg oral, twice a day for 7 days.

Management of Sexual Partners

All sexual partners should be notified and treated, and advice against sexual intercourse should be given until both the index patient and the partner(s) are treated.

Other Sexually Transmitted Infections[3]

Treatment guidelines according to CDC 2015 **(Table 9.4)**.

Clindamycin[4]

Pharmacology

- The drug is about 90% protein bound
- Clindamycin is metabolized by the liver, and excreted in bile and urine
- The half-life is about 2.5 hours.

Mechanism of action: Inhibits protein synthesis by binding to 50S subunit of bacterial ribosomal.

Indications

- Infections originating in the female genital tract, e.g. pelvic inflammatory disease, septic abortion, pelvic abscesses.
- Clindamycin is indicated for treatment of skin and soft-tissue infections caused by streptococci and staphylococci.
- It is also active against community acquired strains of methicillin resistant *S. aureus* infections. Clindamycin is also indicated for treatment of anaerobic organism.

Table 9.4: Treatment of sexually transmitted infections (CDC guidelines 2015)

	Viral infections	
Genital herpes simplex: First clinical episode	Acyclovir 400 mg orally 3 times/day for 7–10 days **or** Acyclovir 200 mg orally 5 times/day for 7–10 days **or** Valacyclovir 1 g orally 2 times/day for 7–10 days	
For recurrent genital herpes: Episodic therapy	Acyclovir 400 mg orally 3 times/day for 5 days **or** Acyclovir 800 mg orally 2 times/day for 5 days **or** Valacyclovir 500 mg orally 2 times/day for 3 days **or** Famciclovir 125 mg orally 2 times/day for 5 days	
For recurrent genital herpes: Suppressive therapy	Acyclovir 500 mg orally once a day **or** Valacyclovir 400 mg orally 2 times/day **or** Famciclovir 250 mg oral 2 times a day	
Genital warts: (Human Papillomavirus) External genital and perianal warts	Imiquimod 3.75%/5% cream or solution or gel of Podofilox 0.5%	
	Bacterial	
Syphilis: Primary, secondary, or early latent <1 year	Benzathine penicillin G 2.4 million units IM (Single dose)	Doxycycline 100 mg 2 times daily for 14 days **or** Tetracycline 500 mg orally 4 times daily for 14 days
Latent >1 year, latent of unknown duration	Benzathine penicillin G 2.4 million units IM in 3 doses each at 1 week intervals (7.2 million units total)	Doxycycline 100 mg 2 times daily for 28 days **or** Tetracycline 500 mg orally 4 times daily for 28 days
Gonococcal infections: Uncomplicated gonococcal infections of the cervix, urethra, and rectum	Ceftriaxone 250 mg IM in a single dose **PLUS** Azithromycin 1 g orally in a single dose	If Ceftriaxone unavailable: Cefixime 400 mg orally, single dose **plus** Azithromycin 1 g orally, single dose
	Chlamydial	
Chlamydial infections: Adults and adolescents	Azithromycin 1 g oral single dose or doxycycline 100 mg oral 2 times a day for 7 days	Erythromycin base 500 mg oral 4 times a day for 7 days
Pregnancy	Azithromycin 1 g oral single dose	Amoxicillin 500 mg orally 3 times a day for 7 days or Erythromycin base 500 mg orally 4 times/day for 7 days
Lymphogranuloma venereum	Doxycycline 100 mg oral 2 times a day for 21 days	Erythromycin base 500 mg oral 4 times a day for 21 days
Persistent and recurrent NGU	Azithromycin 1 g orally in a single dose **or** doxycycline 100 mg orally 2 times/day for 7 days	Erythromycin base 500 mg orally 4 times/day for 7 days
	Parasitic	
Pediculosis pubis	Permethrin cream 1% apply to affected area, wash off after 10 minutes	Malathion 0.5% lotion, applied
Scabies	Permethrin cream 5% apply to all areas of body from neck, wash off after 8–14 hours **or** Ivermectin 200 µg/kg orally, repeated in 2 weeks	

- Clindamycin in combination with aminoglycoside or cephalosporin, is used to treat penetrating wounds of the gut and abdomen.
- Clindamycin is now recommended over erythromycin for prophylaxis of endocarditis in patients with valvular heart disease who are undergoing dental procedures and have penicillin allergies.
- Clindamycin plus primaquine is an effective alternative to trimethoprim-sulfamethoxazole for moderate to moderately severe *Pneumocystis jiroveci* pneumonia in AIDS patients.

Adverse drug reactions

- Nausea, diarrhea, and skin rashes
- Impaired liver function (with or without jaundice)
- Neutropenia
- Clindamycin is risk factor for colitis and diarrhea due to *C. difficile.*

Preparations

Climycin.

Pregnancy category: B

Benzathine Penicillin[4]

Pharmacology: Penicillin is mainly excreted by kidneys; small amounts are excreted by other routes. About 90% of renal excretion by tubular secretion and 10% is by glomerular filtration.

Half-life of penicillin G is approximately 30 minutes. In renal failure, it may be as long as 10 hours.

Mechanism of action: Penicillins contain a characteristic four-membered beta-lactam ring. Penicillin kills bacteria through binding of the beta-lactam ring to DD-transpeptidase, inhibiting its cross-linking activity and preventing new cell wall formation. Without a cell wall, a bacterial cell is vulnerable to outside water and molecular pressures, and quickly dies. Since human cells do not contain a cell wall, penicillin treatment results in bacterial cell death without affecting human cells.

Indications: Penicillin G is a drug of choice for infections caused by streptococci, meningococci, penicillin-susceptible pneumococci, non-β-lactamase-producing staphylococci, some enterococci, *Treponema pallidum, Clostridium* species, Actinomyces and certain other gram-positive rods, and non-β-lactamase-producing gram-negative anaerobic organisms.

Adverse drug reactions: Serious adverse effects are due to hypersensitivity. Test dose should always be given. Allergic reactions include anaphylactic shock (very rare—0.05%); serum sickness-type reactions (urticaria, fever, joint swelling, angioneurotic edema, intense pruritus, and respiratory compromise occurring 7–12 days after exposure); and a variety of skin rashes. Oral lesions, fever, interstitial nephritis (an autoimmune reaction to a penicillin-protein complex), hemolytic anemia, eosinophilia and other hematologic disturbances, and vasculitis may also occur.

Preparation

Bicillin CR

Pregnancy category: B

Azithromycin[4]

Pharmacology: The drug is slowly released from tissues (tissue half-life of 2–4 days) to produce an elimination half-life approaching 3 days. These unique properties permit once-daily dosing and shortening of the duration of treatment.

Mechanism of action: Inhibition of protein synthesis occur via binding to the 50S ribosomal RNA.

Active Against

Mycobacterium avium complex, *Mycobacterium leprae, Toxoplasma gondii, H. influenza* and *Chlamydia* species.

Adverse drug reactions: More common are diarrhea and loose stools, less common are blistering, crusting, irritation, itching, or reddening of the skin, cracked, dry or scaly skin.

Preparations
Zithromax, Zmax
Pregnancy category: B

Erythromycin[4]

Pharmacology

- Erythromycin base is destroyed by stomach acid therefore must be administered with enteric coating.
- Food interferes with its absorption.
- Large amounts of dose are excreted in the bile and lost in feces, and only 5% is excreted in the urine.

Mechanism of action: Bactericidal, inhibition of protein synthesis occurs via binding to the 50S ribosomal RNA.

Indications

- Erythromycin is a drug of choice in corynebacterial infections (diphtheria, corynebacterial sepsis and erythrasma)
- Used in respiratory, ocular, or genital chlamydial infections
- Treatment of community-acquired pneumonia because its spectrum of activity includes *Pneumococcus, M. pneumoniae.*
- Prophylaxis against endocarditis during dental procedures in individuals with valvular heart disease, although clindamycin, which is better tolerated, has replaced it.

Adverse drug reactions: Nausea, vomiting, diarrhea and anorexia are common. Most common reason for discontinuing is gastrointestinal intolerance, which is due to a direct stimulation of gut motility.

Preparations
Calthrox, Eltocin ER
Pregnancy category: B

Ceftriaxone[4]

Pharmacology

- Ceftriaxone (half-life 7–8 hours) can be injected once every 24. A single daily 1 g dose is sufficient for most serious infections
- Excretion of ceftriaxone is mainly through the biliary tract therefore no dosage adjustment is required in renal insufficiency.

Mechanism of action: Cephalosporins are *bactericidal.* Cephalosporins disrupt the synthesis of the *peptidoglycan* layer forming the bacterial *cell wall.* These drugs have expanded gram-negative coverage.

Active Against

Ceftriaxone are approved for treatment of meningitis, including meningitis caused by pneumococci, meningococci, *H influenzae,* and susceptible enteric gram-negative rods.

Ceftriaxone are the most active cephalosporins against penicillin nonsusceptible strains of gram-negative cocci. Other potential indications include empirical therapy of sepsis of unknown cause in both immunocompetent and immunocompromised patient.

Adverse drug reactions: Cephalosporins are sensitizing and may elicit a variety of hypersensitivity reactions that are identical to those of penicillins, including anaphylaxis, fever, skin rashes, nephritis, granulocytopenia, and hemolytic anemia.

After intramuscular injection local irritation can produce pain and after intravenous injection thrombophlebitis can occur.

Preparations
Aacef, Abicef
Pregnancy category: B

Doxycycline[4]

Pharmacology: Doxycycline is eliminated by nonrenal mechanisms, therefore do not accumulate significantly, and require no dosage adjustment in renal failure.

Mechanism of action: Tetracyclines are broad-spectrum bacteriostatic antibiotics that inhibit protein synthesis. It binds reversibly to the 30S subunit of the bacterial ribosome, blocking the binding of aminoacyl-tRNA to the acceptor site on the mRNA ribosome complex. This prevents addition of amino acids to the growing peptide.

Adverse drug reactions

Gastrointestinal: Nausea, vomiting, and diarrhea are the most common reasons for discontinuing.

Bony structures and teeth: Tetracyclines are readily bound to calcium deposited in newly formed bone or teeth in young children. When a tetracycline is given during pregnancy, it can be deposited in the fetal teeth, leading to fluorescence, discoloration, and enamel dysplasia. It can also be deposited in bone and it may lead to deformity or growth inhibition. Because of these effects, tetracyclines are contraindicated in pregnancy. If the drug is given for long periods to children younger than 8 years, similar changes can occur.

Preparations
Doxy 100, Vibramycin.
Pregnancy category: D

Fluconazole[4]

Pharmacology

- Fluconazole has the widest therapeutic index, therefore can be used in variety of fungal infections
- Fluconazole is highly water soluble and have good cerebrospinal fluid penetration
- Better gastrointestinal tolerance and fewer hepatic enzyme interactions.

Mechanism of action: Antifungal activity of azole results from the reduction of ergosterol synthesis by inhibition of fungal cytochrome P450 enzymes.

Indications

- Fluconazole most commonly used for treatment of mucocutaneous candidiasis
- Fluconazole is the azole of choice in the treatment and secondary prophylaxis of cryptococcal meningitis
- Intravenous fluconazole has been shown to be equivalent to amphotericin B in treatment of candidemia in ICU patients with normal white blood cell counts
- The spectrum of action of azole medications is broad, including many species of *Candida, C neoformans,* the endemic mycoses (blastomycosis, coccidioidomycosis, histoplasmosis), the dermatophytes.

Adverse drug reactions: The most common adverse reaction is relatively minor gastrointestinal upset

Abnormalities in liver enzymes and clinical hepatitis can also occur very rarely.

Preparations
Abcan, Flucan.

Pregnancy category: The pregnancy category for a single dose of fluconazole 150 mg to treat vaginal candidiasis is category C.

High doses (400–800 mg/day) may be associated with a rare and distinct set of birth defects (brachycephaly, abnormal facies, abnormal calvarial development, cleft palate, femoral bowing, thin ribs, long bones, arthrogryposis, and congenital heart disease) in infants whose mothers were treated with the drug during the first trimester of pregnancy: for this pregnancy category D.

Acyclovir[4]

Pharmacolgy: The bioavailability of oral acyclovir is low (15–20%) and it is not affected by food. An intravenous formulation is also available. Topical formulations produce high concentrations in herpetic lesions.

Acyclovir is cleared primarily by glomerular filtration and tubular secretion. The half-life is 2.5–3 hours in patients with normal renal function and it increases to 20 hours in patients with anuria.

Mechanism of action: Acyclovir triphosphate inhibits viral DNA synthesis.

Adverse drug reactions

- Nausea, diarrhea, and headache
- Intravenous infusion may be associated with reversible renal toxicity (i.e. interstitial nephritis or crystalline nephropathy) or

neurologic effects (e.g. seizures, tremors, delirium).

Preparations
Zovirex, Aclovir.
Pregnancy category: B

REFERENCES

1. England. Faculty of Sexual & Reproductive Health Care. Management of Vaginal Discharge in Non-Genitourinary Medicine Settings. Clinical Effectiveness Unit; February 2012.
2. Sherrard J, Donders G, White D. European Guideline on the Management of Vaginal Discharge. 2011.
3. Workowski KA, Bolan GA. Sexually Transmitted Diseases Treatment Guidelines. US Department of Health and Human Services, Centers for Disease Control and Prevention. 2015.
4. Katzung BG, Masters SB, Trevor AJ. Basic and Clinical Pharmacology. New York City: Lange. 2015.

CHAPTER 10

Tuberculosis

B Nisha, Ashwani Khanna

INTRODUCTION

Use of appropriate antitubercular drugs is the only way to stop spread of tuberculosis in the community. Irrational use of these lifesaving drugs has resulted in emergence of multidrug resistant tuberculosis. Here we would describe the salient features of antitubercular drugs and antitubercular therapy.

CLASSIFICATION OF CURRENTLY USED ANTITUBERCULAR DRUGS[1]

Antitubercular drugs are classified based on efficacy, toxicity and their use into follows:

- *First-line drugs*: They have high antitubercular efficacy as well as low toxicity and are used routinely. These are isoniazid, rifampicin, pyrazinamide, ethambutol and streptomycin.
- *Second-line drugs*: These drugs have either low antitubercular efficacy or high toxicity or both and are used in special circumstances only **(Table 10.1)**.
- The alternative classification classifies antitubercular drugs into 5 groups based on the mode of administration (oral or injection), if they belong to the fluoroquinolones group and unclear efficacy **(Table 10.2)**.

First-line Drugs

Isoniazid (INH or H)

Pharmacology: It has bactericidal action against *Mycobacterium tuberculosis* however, it does not inhibit most of the atypical mycobacteria. Though its mechanism of action is not clear but it probably inhibits synthesis of mycolic acid which is an essential component of mycobacterial cell wall. Combined with other antitubercular drugs, INH has good resistance preventing action unlike when used alone.

After oral administration, it gets distributed in all tissues and body cavities including tubercular cavities. It crosses placenta freely and its concentration in breast milk is same as in the plasma. Peak blood levels are reached in 1–2 hours. Onset of action occurs in 24–48 hours and duration of action lasts for up to 24 hours.

It is metabolized by acetylation to metabolite N-acetyl hydrazine in liver and is excreted in urine. The rate of acetylation is genetically determined and is responsible for hepatotoxic effects. The half-life may be prolonged in liver disease. The half-life in fast acetylators (seen in 30–40% of Indians) is 1 hour while it is 3 hours in slow acetylators (seen in 60–70% of Indians). Rate of acetylation has not been shown to

Table 10.1: Second line antitubercular drugs

Class	*Drug(s)*	
Broad spectrum	Cycloserine	
	Fluoroquinolones	Ofloxacin Levofloxacin Moxifloxacin Gatifloxacin
	Rifamycins	Rifabutin Rifapentine
	Macrolides	Clarithromycin Azithromycin
Narrow spectrum	Thiacetazone Para-aminosalicylic acid Ethionamide Clofazimine Kanamycin Amikacin Capreomycin	
Other drugs	Diaryquinolone, pyrrole Diamine Interferon-alpha Interleukin-12	

Table 10.2: Alternative classification of antitubercular drugs[2]

Group 1	First-line oral agents	Isoniazid, rifampicin, ethambutol, pyrazinamide
Group 2	Injectable agents	Streptomycin, kanamycin, amikacin capreomycin, viomycin
Group 3	Fluoroquinolones	Ofloxacin, levofloxacin, moxifloxacin, gatifloxacin, pefloxacin, sparfloxacin, moxifloxacin, prulifloxacin, gemifloxacin
Group 4	Second-line oral antitubercular drugs	Ethionamide, prothionamide, cycloserine, terizidone para-aminosalicylic, thiacetazone
Group 5	Agents with unclear efficacy*	Clofazimine Linezolid, amoxicillin/clavulanate Thioacetazone, imipenem/cilastatin Bedaquiline Clarithromycin

*Not recommended by WHO for routine use in MDR-TB

significantly alter the effectiveness of INH when taken daily. However, weekly regimes are less effective in fast acetylators and slow acetylation may to lead to toxicity with prolong use.

Fast acetylator is one whose 6 hours serum level of active INH following 4 mg/kg test dose is 0.2 mg/mL or less. The slow acetylator is one whose 6 hours serum level of active INH is 0.8 mg/mL or more after an equivalent dose.

Indication: It is used as first-line drug for tuberculosis.

Contraindications: Known hypersensitivity including drug, induced hepatitis and active hepatic disease. Hypersensitivity reaction is usually seen within 3–7 weeks of therapy. If seen drug should be discontinued and reinstituted gradually after the reaction subsides.

Dosage: 5 mg per/Kg body weight or 300 mg orally daily.

Adverse effects: It is a well-tolerated and is a safe drug.

Common: Asymptomatic elevation of serum hepatic enzymes.

Uncommon: Hepatitis is dose-related and is commonly seen in elderly. Pregnant women and postpartum women may be particularly at higher risk for hepatitis. Being a structural analog of pyridoxine, it promotes excretion of pyridoxine. Thus it causes peripheral neuritis. It is more frequent in undernourished, chronic alcoholics and diabetics. Pyridoxine administration in dose 10–50 mg/day has been recommended to prevent neurotoxicity in mother and fetus. Skin rash and vasculitis may occur.

Rare: Mental symptoms, fever, giddiness, convulsions, optic neuritis, hemolytic anemia, aplastic anemia, arthralgia, gynecomastia and lupoid reactions.

Interaction

- *Rifampicin*: Risk of hepatotoxicity is higher when both used together as compared to when used alone, more so in slow acetylators, with pre-existing liver disease and those receiving high dose.
- *Aluminum hydroxide gel*: Decreases absorption of INH, hence should be taken at least 1 hour before.
- *Antiepileptic*: INH inhibits hepatic clearance and increases toxicity of antiepileptics. Concurrent use requires serum monitoring of antiepileptic drug.
- *Oral anticoagulants*: There is increased effect of oral anticoagulants when used along with INH.
- *Alcohol*: Those who are alcoholic, have higher incidence of INH-related hepatitis.
- *Benzodiazepines*: Their activity is increased.
- *Ketoconazole*: Serum concentration of ketoconazole is decreased.
- *Disulfiram*: Concurrent use is avoided as it may lead to acute behavioral and co-ordination changes.
- *Enflurane*: It can lead to renal failure.
- *Halothane*: It can cause hepatotoxicity and hepatic encephalopathy.

Monitoring: Baseline LFT is performed. LFT is repeated if baseline is abnormal; patient is at high risk for adverse reactions or has symptoms. If SGPT is increased to more than 3 times the normal upper limit, the drug should be stopped. Ophthalmic examination should be performed in case of visual symptoms.

Safety during pregnancy and lactation: It is class C drug. Even though it crosses placenta, no significant teratogenic effects have been noted.

Rifampicin (R or RMP)

Pharmacology: It is a potent bactericidal drug. Both extra and intracellular organisms are affected. It has good sterilizing and resistance preventing actions. Its action is to inhibit DNA dependent RNA synthesis. Resistance to drug develops rapidly due to mutation in the gene which reduces its affinity for the drug. It is also effective against gram-positive and gram-negative bacteria.

After oral administration, it gets distributed in body tissues and also penetrates meninges, caseous masses and placental barrier. Its peak level reaches in 2–3 hours. Food interferes with its absorption. After metabolism in liver, it is converted into active deacetylated metabolite which is excreted in bile. It induces the microsomal enzymes of liver. High concentration is seen in bile and saliva.

It is largely excreted in feces. Small amount is excreted in urine unchanged. Hence dose adjustment is not needed in renal damage. Patient should be informed about the orange discoloration of the urine, feces, saliva, sputum, tears, sweat and even contact lenses.

Indication: Used as first line drug for tuberculosis.

Contraindication: Liver disease and jaundice.

Dosage: 10 mg/Kg body weight or 450 mg orally daily. Dose is 600 mg if body weight is more than 50 Kg.

Adverse Effects

Common: Pruritus.

Uncommon: Hepatitis, cutaneous hypersensitivity (flushing, pruritus, redness and watering of eyes), GI intolerance, thrombocytopenia, febrile reaction, Flu syndrome (chills, fever, headache, malaise and bone pain).

Rare: Respiratory syndrome (breathlessness which may be associated with shock and collapse). Hemolytic anemia, acute renal failure, thrombotic thrombocytopenic purpura.

Interaction

- *INH*: Risk of hepatotoxicity higher when both used together as compared to when used alone, more so in slow acetylators, with pre-existing liver disease.
  Rifampicin may reduce the efficacy of the following drugs by inducing the hepatic microsomal enzymes—acetoaminophen, barbitutares, benzodiazepines, beta blockers, corticosteroids, digitoxine, estrogens, oral anticoagulants, oral contraceptives, phenytoin, quinidine, sulphonylureas, etc.
- *Halothane*: Hepatoxicity and hepatic encephalopathy.
- *Ketoconazole*: Treatment failure of either ketoconazole or rifampicin.

Monitoring: CBC, platelets, and hepatic enzymes are tested. These are repeat if abnormal or when there are symptoms of adverse reaction.

Safety during pregnancy and lactation: It is class C drug. Although increase in limb defect have been observed in fetus of mother taking rifampicin, but the incidence is not high.

Ethambutol (EMB or E)

Pharmacology: It is a bacteriostatic and well-tolerated drug. It acts by inhibiting the enzyme arabinosyl transferase. It is active against fast multiplying bacilli and many atypical mycobacteria. In combination with other antitubercular drugs, it hastens the sputum conversion and prevents drug resistance. Oral absorption is good. It penetrates into erythrocytes which serve as the depot from where the drug is released into the circulation. Resistance to the drug develops slowly. It is excreted in urine. Caution is required in patient with renal disease.

Indication: It is used as first-line drug for tuberculosis.

Contraindications: Hypersensitivity, epilepsy, pre-existing optic neuritis from any cause.

Dosage: 15–25 mg/Kg body weight or 1200 mg orally daily.

Adverse effect: Acceptability is good and side effects are low.

Common: Optic neuritis, visual disturbance, color blindness is the most important dose-related adverse effects which are reversible after stopping the drug.

Uncommon: Cutaneous reactions and arthralgia.

Rare: Hyperuricemia, peripheral neuropathy.

Interaction: Aluminum salt reduces absorption of ethambutol.

Monitoring: Visual acuity and color vision should be checked at the beginning and then monthly.

Safety during pregnancy and lactation: It is class C Drug.

Pyrazinamide (PZA or Z)

Pharmacology: It is bactericidal drug, effective only against intracellular bacilli. It has good meningeal penetration. Mechanism of action is not exactly known. It is a prodrug and is converted into the active compound pyrazinoic acid which inhibits the synthesis of mycolic acid. Resistance develops fast if given alone, hence to be given with other antitubercular drugs. Rapidly absorbed after oral intake, has good penetration in CSF and is metabolized extensively in liver. Peak plasma levels are reached within 3–4 hours. The degradation products and the free drug are excreted in urine.

Indication: As first-line drug for tuberculosis.

Contraindications: Liver disease, hypersensitivity, acute gout.

Dosage: 25–35 per Kg body weight or 1500 mg orally daily.

Adverse Effects

Common: Anorexia, nausea, flushing, photosensitization and hyperuricemia.

Uncommon: Hepatitis, vomiting, arthralgia, cutaneous reactions.

Rare: Sideroblastic anemia and gout.

Interactions

- *Uricosurics*: Antagonistic effect on probenecid and sulfinpyrazone.
- *Antidiabetic agents*: It interferes with control of diabetes.

Monitoring: Baseline measurements of uric acid and hepatic enzymes.

Safety during pregnancy and lactation: No toxic effect of this drug in pregnancy has ever been found.

Streptomycin (SM or S)

Pharmacology: It is the first antitubercular drug. It is bactericidal and exerts its action by combining with bacterial ribosome and induces misreading of mRNA codons. It is not absorbed orally hence given by IM injection. It is excreted unchanged in urine. Half-life is prolonged in patients of renal failure.

Indication: As first line drug in TB.

Contraindications: Diseases of ear, kidney and hypersensitivity.

Dosage: 15 mg per/kg of body weight or 750 mg given by IM injection daily. Dose is 500 mg if age is more than 50 years.

Adverse Effects

Common: Cutaneous hypersensitivity, giddiness, numbness, tinnitus, pain at injection site.

Uncommon: Vertigo, ataxia, deafness.

Rare: Renal failure, aplastic anemia.

Interactions

Penicillin, cephalosporins, carbenicillin, ticaracillin: Causes antibiotic synergism.

Anesthetics, neuromuscular blocking agents: Risk of neuromuscular blockade and respiratory paralysis.

Furosemide, aminoglycosides, vancomycin, amphotericin B, bacitracin, cisplatin, cephalothin, methoxyflurane, bumetanide and mannitol—all these increased ototoxic, neurotoxic or nephrotoxic effects of streptomycin.

Monitoring: Hearing tests and kidney function tests.

Safety during pregnancy and lactation: Contraindicated during pregnancy, causes ototoxicity in the newborn.

Second-line Drugs

Ofloxacin (Ofl)

Pharmacology: It is bactericidal and inhibits the A subunit of DNA gyrase (topoisomerase) which is essential in the reproduction of bacterial DNA. Though it has no cross-resistance with other antitubercular drugs, but complete cross-resistance is seen between ofloxacin and ciprofloxacin. Oral absorption is 90–98%. It is widely distributed in body fluids. It crosses the placenta and is distributed in the breast milk. Eliminated mainly by the kidneys;

65–80% is excreted unchanged in the urine therefore it needs dose reduction in patients with severe renal impairment.

Indication of use: Multidrug resistant (MDR) TB.

Contraindications: Pregnancy, intolerance to ofloxacin.

Dosage: 600 mg orally daily, 800 mg daily if body weight is more than 45 Kg.

Adverse reactions: It is generally well tolerated.

Occasional: GI intolerance; CNS-headache, malaise, insomnia, restlessness, and dizziness.

Rare: Allergic reactions; diarrhea; photosensitivity; increased LFTs and peripheral neuropathy.

Drug interactions: Ofloxacin is known to inhibit hepatic metabolism and hence clearance of drugs, such as theophylline and caffeine.

Cations such as aluminum, magnesium, or iron reduce the absorption of ofloxacin and related drugs when given concomitantly.

The urinary excretion of ofloxacin and other fluoroquinolones is reduced by probenecid; plasma concentrations are not necessarily increased.

Monitoring: KFT.

Safety during pregnancy and lactation: Contraindicated in pregnancy.

Levofloxacin (Lfx)

Pharmacology: It is bactericidal and mechanism of action is same as ofloxacin; and is twice as active as ofloxacin. It is rapidly and completely absorbed orally, however it should not be administered within 4 hours of intake of drugs containing divalent cations. No interaction occurs with milk or calcium. It gets distributed well in lung tissues, kidneys, gallbladder, gynecological tissues, liver, lung, prostatic tissues, phagocytic cells, urine, sputum and bile. Hepatic metabolism is minimal; 87% of dose is excreted unchanged in the urine. Doses should be reduced in patients with severe renal impairment.

Indication: Multidrug resistant TB.

Contraindications: Hypersensitivity to levofloxacin.

Dosage: 500 mg orally daily, 750 mg daily if body weight is more than 45 Kg.

Adverse reactions: Generally well tolerated.

Occasional: GI intolerance; CNS-headache, malaise, insomnia, restlessness, dizziness, allergic reactions, diarrhea, photosensitivity.

Rare: Peripheral neuropathy.

Drug interactions:
- *Vitamins and minerals*: Containing divalent and trivalent cations such as zinc and iron decreases absorption of levofloxacin.
- *Antacids (magnesium, aluminum)*: Binds to levofloxacin resulting in decreased absorption and efficacy.
- *Sucralfate*: Decreases absorption by the chelation by aluminum ions contained in the sucralfate.
- *Probenecid*: Probenecid interferes with renal tubular secretion which may result in 50% increase in serum level of levofloxacin.

Monitoring: KFT

Safety during pregnancy and lactation: Class C drug. There are no adequate and well-controlled studies in pregnant women. Animal data demonstrated arthropathy in immature animals, with erosions in joint cartilage. Because of the potential for serious adverse effects from levofloxacin in nursing infants, decision should be made whether to discontinue nursing or to discontinue the drug, taking into account the importance of the drug to the mother.

Para-aminosalicylic Acid (PAS)

Pharmacology: It is a bacteriostatic and least active drug. However, inhibits the onset of resistance to streptomycin and INH. Oral absorption is 60–65% only, may requires increased dosage. It is well distributed in peritoneal fluid, pleural fluid, and synovial fluid except CSF (10–15%). Excreted by kidney after it gets acetylated in the liver.

Indication: Multidrug resistant TB.

Contraindications: Allergy to aspirin, severe renal disease and hypersensitivity.

Dosage: 10 g orally daily, 12 g daily if body weight is more than 45 Kg.

Adverse effects:

Common: GI intolerance because of which acceptability is poor; hypothyroidism.

Uncommon: Hepatitis (0.3-0.5%); allergic reactions; thyroid enlargement; malabsorption syndrome; increased PT. To be used carefully in patients with glucose-6-phosphate dehydrogenase (G6PD) deficiency.

Drug Interactions

- *Isoniazid*: Increased INH level is seen due to decreased acetylation, the dose may need to be decreased.
- *Digoxin*: Absorption is decreased.
- *Ethionamide*: Concurrent use increases risk of hypothyroidism; liver toxicity, monitor liver enzymes.

Monitoring: Liver and kidney function tests.

Safety during pregnancy and lactation: Safety class C drug. Congenital defects have been reported.

Ethionamide (Eto)

Pharmacology: It is a bacteriostatic drug and is effective against atypical *Mycobacterium*. Mechanism of action is not exactly known. Resistance develops rapidly if used alone and there is complete cross-resistance between ethionamide and prothionamide (partial cross-resistance with thiacetazone). It well absorbed orally and is widely distributed throughout body tissues and CSF. It crosses the placenta. It is extensively metabolized, probably in the liver, to the active sulfoxide and other inactive metabolites.

Indication: Multidrug resistant TB.

Contraindication: Hepatic impairment and hypersensitivity.

Dosage: 500 orally daily, 750 mg daily if body weight is more than 45 kg.

Adverse effects:

Common: Nausea, vomiting, anorexia, diarrhea, abdominal pain, excessive salivation, metallic taste; these effects may be minimized by decreasing dosage, by changing the time of drug administration, or by the concurrent administration of an antiemetic agent.

Uncommon: Hepatitis, drowsiness, cutaneous hypersensitivity, peripheral neuritis. Rare: Convulsion, depression, diplopia, alopecia and hypothyroidism especially when combined with PAS.

Interactions: It may increase the neurotoxic effects of other antitubercular drugs if administered concomitantly.

Monitoring: Liver and kidney function tests.

Safety during pregnancy and lactation: Class C drug. Newborns should be monitored for adverse effects.

Cycloserine (Cs)

Pharmacology: It is bacteriostatic and acts by competitively blocking action of an enzyme which incorporates alanine into an alanyl-alanine dipeptide which is an essential component of the mycobacterial cell wall. Oral absorption is good but decreased by food and thus it is best to take it empty stomach. It is widely distributed into body tissue and fluids including CSF. Mainly excreted unchanged in the urine hence doses should be reduced in patients with severe renal impairment.

Indication: Multidrug resistant TB.

Contraindications: Hypersensitivity, epilepsy, depression, severe anxiety, or psychosis. It should not be used in severe renal insufficiency and in alcoholics.

Dosage: 500 mg orally daily, 750 mg daily if body weight is more than 45 Kg.

Adverse reactions:

Common: Neurological and psychiatric disturbances, including headaches, tremors, confusion, dizziness irritability, aggression, and depression, restlessness, anxiety and sleep disturbances.

Uncommon: Visual changes, skin rash, numbness, tingling or burning in hands and feet and jaundice.

Rare: Seizures and suicidal thoughts.

Drug interactions: Isoniazid and ethionamide both have additive nervous system side effect. Vitamin B_6 in the dose of 150 mg/day may reduce neurotoxicity.

It may increase phenytoin level. There is increased risk of seizures if combined with alcohol.

Monitoring: Liver and kidney function tests.

Safety during pregnancy and lactation: Class C drug. If mother is breastfeeding then both mother and baby should be supplemented with vitamin B_6.

Kanamycin (Km)

Pharmacology: It is a bactericidal aminoglycoside. It irreversibly binds to 30S ribosomal subunit and inhibits protein synthesis. Oral absorption insignificant hence given by IM injections. It is distributed in extracellular fluid, abscesses, ascitic fluid, pericardial fluid, pleural fluid, synovial fluid, lymphatic fluid and peritoneal fluid. Not well distributed in sputum and CSF. It is excreted unchanged in the urine, hence to be used with caution in renal disease.

Indication: MDR TB.

Contraindications: Hypersensitivity to aminoglycosides and pregnancy as it causes congenital deafness.

Dosage: 500 mg orally daily, 750 mg daily if body weight is more than 45 kg.

Adverse reactions:

Common: Pain at injection site, renal failure, which is usually reversible.

Uncommon: Vestibular and auditory damage, though uncommon it is usually irreversible. Peripheral neuropathy and rash may occur.

Drug interactions: It Loop diuretics (like furosemide, torsemide)—It may have an additive auditory ototoxicity which is dose-dependent and may be increased with renal dysfunction. Avoid concomitant use.

Nondepolarizing muscle relaxants (like atracurium, pancuronium): Concomitant use to be avoided because of possible respiratory depression. Hence, if used, the dose of nondepolarizing muscle relaxant should be adjusted and neuromuscular function should be closely monitored.

Nephrotoxic agents (Amphotericin B, foscarnet, cidofovir): Additive nephrotoxicity hence coadministration should be avoided and if used together renal function should be monitored closely.

Monitoring: KFT, audiometry and vision check if indicated.

Safety during pregnancy and lactation: Contraindicated.

Clofazimine

Clofazimine a fat-soluble riminophenazine dye, although developed in the 1950s as an anti-TB drug, became established as a key drug for the treatment of leprosy. Clofazimine is presently being considered for the treatment of multidrug resistant (MDR) TB. It has been used with success in the treatment of MDR-TB.

New Drugs

Newer Fluoroquinolones

The newer fluoroquilones like moxifloxacin, gatifloxacin and sparfloxacin has same mechanism of action and pharmacokinetics like other fluoroquilones. These drugs are also active against nonreplicating, persistent mycobacteria; they are considered to be potentially useful and believed to be important for shortening the duration of TB drug. Sparfloxacin is more active against mycobacteria *in vitro*, but has been used clinically to a lesser extent.

Rifabutin

It is similar to rifampicin in mechanism of action; but less active against *M. tuberculosis* and more active against MAC. Adverse effects are GI intolerance, rashes, granulocytopenia, myalgia, and uveitis.

Macrolides

Newer macrolides, azithromycin and clarithromycin also have action against acid fast bacilli and are more active against MAC. They are used to treat MAC infection. Dose of azithromycin is 500 mg once a day and that of clarithromycin is 500 mg BD. Though both are equally efficacious, azithromycin has higher tissue and intracellular penetration.

Bedaquiline

It is a diarylquinoline that targets the proton pump of adenosine triphosphate (ATP) synthase, leading to inadequate synthesis of ATP. It is the first new treatment in 40 years and is US Food and Drug Administration (FDA) approved (2012). It is used to treat MDR-TB. It is to be used in a combination therapy for patients who have failed standard treatment and have no other options.

PA-824

The nitroimidazole-oxazine PA-824 is a derivative of metronidazole. It is hypothesized that PA-824 acts by inhibiting the synthesis of ketomycolates that are essential components of the mycobacterial cell wall; and by donating nitric oxide during enzymatic nitro reduction within *Mycobacterium tuberculosis*, thereby poisoning the respiratory apparatus. This drug is experimental compounds that are not commercially available.

Oxazolidinones

The oxazolidinones act via competitive inhibition of the enzyme that binds the incoming transfer ribonucleic acid (RNA) with the complementary codon on the messenger RNA and inhibiting translation. Cycloserine (4-amino-1,2-oxazolidin-3-one) was the first oxazolidinone that was used as an anti-TB drug. Another oxazolidinedione, linezolid, has been used off-label in the treatment of MDR-TB.

TREATMENT OF TUBERCULOSIS

Treatment of Active TB in Pregnancy

Principles of treatment: It should be promptly treated irrespective of period of gestation. Duration of treatment need not be modified because of pregnancy. Placenta should be examined for possible infection by *Mycobacterium tuberculosis*. Neonates should be closely examined and observed for development of TB.

Treatment of New Cases (former Categories I and III)

(New sputum smear-positive; New sputum smear-negative; New extrapulmonary tuberculosis and others).

Standard regime recommended by WHO are 4 drugs HRZE (for 2 months) in the initial phase and 2 drugs HR (for 4 months) in the continuation phase. Intermittent short course regimens that are administered thrice weekly have equivalent efficacy as daily regimens. In addition they have lower cost, greater feasibility for directly observed administration under ambulatory settings, and possibly also lower drug toxicity. Duration of treatment can be prolonged to 12 months for extrapulmonary TB. If sputum is positive after 2 months, IP is extended by 1 month due to risk of failure and relapse.

Previously Treated Cases (Former Category II)

(Sputum smear-positive relapse; sputum smear-positive failure; sputum smear-positive treatment after default; others that include patients who are sputum smear-negative or who have extrapulmonary disease who can have recurrence or resonance).

Relapse: Patients are said to have relapse if they have been cured earlier and come back as sputum positive pulmonary TB.

Treatment failure: Failed to respond to treatment (cough and sputum production persisting even after completing more than 5 months of treatment).

Default: Treatment was interrupted for one month for any reason.

Standard treatment regimen is 3 months Intensive phase + 5 months continuation phase-5 drugs at thrice-weekly schedule for initial 2 months followed by 4 drugs for next 1 month. Continuation phase-3 drugs at thrice-weekly schedule for remaining 5 months.

Treatment of Latent TB in Pregnancy

No treatment is given for latent TB in India. Under Revised National Tuberculosis Control Program (RNTCP) INH prophylaxis is given to children < 6 years who are in contact of sputum positive patient in household and HIV patients. WHO recommends INH 300 mg per day plus pyridoxine 10–25 mg per for 6 months.

Treatment of Drug-resistant Tuberculosis during Pregnancy

Multidrug resistant tuberculosis (MDR-TB) is defined as TB that is resistant at least to INH and RMP. Isolates that are multiresistant to any other combination of anti-TB drugs but not to INH and RMP are not classed as MDR-TB.

MDR-TB suspect can be any of the following: Any TB patient who fails an RNTCP Category I or II treatment; retreatment sputum positive case; contact of known MDR-TB cases; sputum negative retreatment cases; HIV TB case.

Treatment of MDR-TB must be done on the basis of drug sensitivity testing. The culture and drug sensitivity testing (DST) result should be from an RNTCP accredited laboratory. Various DST methods are:

- Conventional DST methods like Absolute Concentration Method, The Resistance Ratio and Proportion Method.
- Rapid molecular-based tests like GEN-X6 This test eliminate long wait for results of DST by other methods (weeks for liquid media methods or months for solid media methods). Results are available within 1–2 days.

Lok Nayak Hospital, TB Department has RNTCP accredited laboratory facility to carry out all these tests.

"MDR-TB" is treated with the RNTCP Category IV regimen containing second-line anti-TB drugs. It comprises of 6 drugs—kanamycin, ofloxacin (levofloxacin), ethionamide, pyrazinamide, ethambutol and cycloserine during 6–9 months of the intensive phase and 4 drugs—ofloxacin (levofloxacin), ethionamide, ethambutol and cycloserine during the 18 months of the continuation phase. Para-aminosalicylic acid (PAS) is included in the regimen as a substitute drug if any bactericidal drug (K, Ofl, Z and Eto) or 2 bacteriostatic (E and Cs) drugs are not tolerated.

Second-line drugs are associated with teratogenicity. If the duration of pregnancy is less than 20 weeks, the patient should be advised to opt for MTP in view of the potential severe risk to both the mother and fetus. However, good outcomes have been reported in children whose mothers were treated with aminoglycosides.[3-5] In the first trimester kanamycin and ethionamide are omitted from the category IV regimen and PAS is added. In case of completed the first trimester, kanamycin is replaced with PAS. Postpartum, PAS may be replaced with kanamycin and continued until the end of the intensive phase. Pregnant MDR-TB patients need to be monitored carefully both in relation to the category IV treatment and the progress of the pregnancy. This approach leads to good results, since the patient should be smear-negative at the time of parturition, and mother and infant do not need to be separated. Breastfeeding should be encouraged as long as the patient is sputum negative.

Treatment of Genital TB

Duration of treatment for genital TB in women remains controversial, as there are insufficient data regarding risk of relapse and failure in this population. In India, recommended treatment under RNTCP is category I regimen (2HREZ/4HR) for six months. After 6 months endometrial curettage is examined histologically and bacteriologically. In the setting of known infertility and genital TB, some experts advocate aggressive treatment for up to 1 year before advising patients to attempt spontaneous pregnancy or assisted reproductive technologies.

ANTITUBERCULOSIS TREATMENT AND CONTRACEPTION

Rifampicin induces the P-450 mixed function oxidase system that metabolizes oral contraceptives (OCP) and other drugs; therefore reliability of OCPs is diminished. Alternative contraceptive measures should be considered by postpartum women who require ATT.

DOTS AND DOTS-PLUS[6,7]

DOTS stands for "Directly Observed Treatment, Short-course" and is a major backbone in the WHO Global Plan to Stop TB. The DOTS strategy focuses on five main points of action-government commitment to control TB, diagnosis based on sputum-smear microscopy tests, direct observation short-course chemotherapy treatments, a definite supply of drugs, and standardized reporting and recording of cases and treatment outcomes. The WHO recommend all TB patients should have at least the first two months of their therapy observed (and preferably the whole of it observed). DOTS is used with intermittent dosing (thrice weekly or 2HREZ/4HR3).

The WHO extended the DOTS programme in 1998 to include the treatment of MDR-TB (called "DOTS-Plus"). Implementation of DOTS-Plus requires the capacity to perform drug-susceptibility testing (not routinely available even in developed countries) and the availability of second-line agents, in addition to all the requirements for DOTS. Monthly surveillance until cultures convert to negative is recommended for DOTS-Plus, but not for DOTS.

REFERENCES

1. Blumberg HM, Burman W, Chaisson RE, Etkind SC, et al. American Thoracic Society, Centres for Disease Control and Prevention and the Infectious Disease Society of America: Treatment of Tuberculosis. Am J Respir Crit care Med. 2003;167:603-62.
2. World Health Organisation. Guidelines for the programmatic management of drugs-resistant tuberculosis. WHO/HTM/TB/2006.361. Geneva: World Health Organisation; 2006.
3. Drobac PC, et al. "Treatment of Multidrug-Resistant Tuberculosis during Pregnancy: Long-Term Follow-up of 6 Children with Intrauterine Exposure to Second-Line Agents" Clin Infect Dis. 2005;40(11):1689-92.
4. Palacios E, Dallman R, Muñoz M, et al. "Drug-resistant tuberculosis and pregnancy: Treatment outcomes of 38 cases in Lima, Peru". Clin Infect Dis. 2009;48(10):1413-19.
5. Sharma SK, Mohan Allahabadi. Text book on Tuberculosis, second edition; 2009.
6. Treatment of Tuberculosis. WHO Guidelines; 2010.
7. Revised National Tuberculosis Control Programme DOTS-Plus Guidelines January; 2010.

CHAPTER 11

Urinary Tract Infection

Nalini Bala, Tanvi Raj, Krishna Agarwal

INTRODUCTION

Women are at increased risk of urinary tract infection (UTI) during pregnancy. UTI may present as asymptomatic bacteriuria, acute cystitis or pyelonephritis. Asymptomatic bacteriuria occurs in 2–10% of all pregnancies. If this is not treated, this can progress to cystitis in 30% cases and the infection may further ascend and cause pyelonephritis in 50% of these women.[1-3]

The American College of Obstetrics and Gynecology recommends that a urine culture be obtained at the first prenatal visit. A repeat urine culture should be obtained during the third trimester. Quantitative midstream urine culture is the gold standard for any type of suspected UTI and even in asymptomatic women. A colony count of 10^5 per mL is considered to be significant.

The causative pathogens for UTI are described in **Table 11.1**.

Antibiotic Treatment in Urinary Tract Infection

Antibiotic treatment of asymptomatic bacteriuria is effective in reducing the risk of pyelonephritis in pregnancy.[3] There is no clear consensus on the antibiotic choice or duration of treatment for urinary tract infection. Usually antibiotic is started empirically in all cases of UTIs and nitrofurantoin is the drug of choice except for pyelonephritis **(Table 11.2)**.

Penicillins, such as amoxicillin are commonly prescribed for the treatment of UTIs but resistance to these is very prevalent.

Fluoroquinolones like norfloxacin and ciprofloxacin are commonly used. These antibiotics have been associated with causation of arthropathy in animals; however it is rare in humans. Due to the risk of development of antibiotic resistance with the frequent use, these are not employed as first line agents and used according to the sensitivity pattern.[4,5]

Nitrofurantoin

Pharmacology: It acts by damaging bacterial DNA. It is given orally and is rapidly metabolized

Table 11.1: Causative organisms in UTI during pregnancy

Organism	*Frequency*
E. coli	70%
Gram positive organisms including streptococci	10%
Klebsiella and enterobacter	3%
Proteus	2%
Extended beta lactamase producing organisms	

Table 11.2: Empirical antibiotic treatment in UTI during pregnancy[3]

Type of infection	*First line*	*Second line*
Asymptomatic bacteriuria, recurrent bacteriuria* and cystitis	*Nitrofurantoin*: 100 mg 8–12 hourly daily for 5–7 days	*Amoxicillin*: 500 mg orally 8 hourly for 3–7 days or cephalexin 500 mg orally 6 hourly for 3–7 days
Persistent bacteriuria: If follow up urine culture shows growth of same bacteria	Nitrofurantoin 50–100 mg at bed time for the whole pregnancy if organism is susceptible to it	
Pyelonephritis		
Mild to moderate	*Ceftriaxone*: 1 g IV every 12–24 hours	*Aztreonam*: 1 g 8 hourly IV (If allergic to beta lactam) or Ampicillin 1–2 g IV 6 hourly plus 1.5 mg/kg IV gentamicin (Only given if intolerant to other drugs)
Severe	*Ticarcillin–Clavulanate*: 3.1 g IV every 4 hourly	*Piperacillin–Tazobactam*: 3.375 g IV every 6 hours or *Meropenem*: 500 mg IV every 8 hours

* *Recurrent bacteriuria*: If follow up urine culture is positive with different stain or one follow up culture becomes sterile after treatment and the next culture comes positive.

in liver leading to very low blood concentration. But urinary excretion is 40%, thus achieving bactericidal concentration in urine.

Indications of use: Refer to **Table 11.2**.

Contraindications: Patients with G6PD deficiency, severe renal impairment. It should be avoided after 36 weeks of gestation as it can rarely induce hemolytic anemia in the fetus or newborn, particularly in those with G6PD deficiency.

Dosage: Refer to **Table 11.2**.

Adverse effects: Most common side effects are nausea headache and flatulence. Less common are dyspepsia, diarrhea, dizziness, pruritus, hair loss, fever and chills. Rare adverse effects are amblyopia, acute pulmonary hypersensitivity reaction, interstitial pneumonitis, pulmonary fibrosis, hepatitis, cholestatic jaundice, hepatic necrosis, neuropathy with numbness and tingling (generally after 6 months of use), etc.

Drug interaction: Nitrofurantoin and quinolones are mutually antagonistic and the combination should be avoided. Similarly urinary alkalizers are safe in pregnancy; however they should not be used in combination with nitrofurantoin as it can reduce efficacy of nitrofurantoin.

Monitoring: Watch for any sign of pulmonary reaction or numbness and tingling in extremities. LFT KFT and CBC should be done in case of prolonged use.

Preparations

- *Martifur, urifast, uribid, nitfur*: 100 mg tablets.
- *Furadantin*: 50, 100 mg tablets.

Safety during pregnancy and lactation: It is category B drug in pregnancy. It should be avoided in first trimester and at this time use should only be limited to cases where no alternative antibiotic is available. It should also be avoided after 36 weeks of gestation.

During lactation, trace amount of drug gets secreted in breast milk and may cause diarrhea in the infants.

REFERENCES

1. McCormick T, Ashe RG, Kearney PM. Urinary tract infection in pregnancy. The Obstetrician and Gynaecologist. 2008;10:156-62.
2. Delzell JE, Lefevre ML. Urinary tract infections during pregnancy. American Family Physician. 2000;61:713-21.
3. Smaill F, Vazquez JC. Antibiotics for asymptomatic bacteriuria in pregnancy. Cochrane Database of Systematic Reviews 2007, Issue 2.
4. Loebstein R, Addis A, Ho E, Andreou R, Sage S, Donnenfeld AE, et al. Pregnancy outcome following gestational exposure to fluoroquinolones: a multicenter prospective controlled study. Antimicrob Agents Chemother. 1998;42(6):1336-9.
5. Wilton LV, Pearce GL, Mann RD. A comparison of ciprofloxacin, norfloxacin, ofloxacin, azithromycin and cefixime examined by observational cohort studies. Br J Clin Pharmacol. 1996;41(4):277-84.

Section IV

DRUGS USED DURING LABOR, DELIVERY AND PUERPERIUM

CHAPTERS

CHAPTER 12

Labor Analgesia

Sangeeta Bhasin, Reena Rani, Anju Bhalotra

"Delivery of the infant into the arms of a conscious and pain-free mother is one of the most exciting and rewarding moments in medicine."

Moir Br J Anaesth 1979

Labor is the most painful experience which most women go through in their lifetime. The experience varies for each woman and her request for labor pain relief is sufficient indication for its provision. Therefore, it is the responsibility of the obstetrician to formulate a plan for pain relief in consultation with the anesthesiologist. The different methods used to relieve pain depend upon the personal choice of the individual and the techniques available. These could be pharmacological or nonpharmacological. **Table 12.1** enlists the pharmacological methods of labor analgesia.

Table 12.1: Pharmacological methods of labor analgesia

Type	*Mode of administration*	*Drugs used*
Nonregional techniques	Inhalational analgesics	Nitrous oxide Sevoflurane Isoflurane
	Systemic analgesics-parenteral opioids	Pethidine Morphine Tramadol Fentanyl Remifentanil
	Patient-controlled analgesia (PCA)	Fentanyl
Regional techniques	Spinal analgesia	Bupivacaine Ropivacaine
	Lumbar epidural analgesia	
	Combined spinal-epidural (CSE) analgesia	
	Paracervical block	
	Pudendal block	

An ideal labor analgesic agent should have the following attributes:

- Relieves maternal anxiety and fatigue
- Does not cross the placental barrier and has minimal effects on fetus or neonate
- Easy to administer with minimal monitoring
- Provides adequate analgesia throughout the first and second stage with a minimum dose of drug
- Easily reversible if necessary
- Facilitates surgical anesthesia
- Has no motor effect and allows ambulation and maternal expulsive efforts
- Maintains uterine blood flow and preserves uterine contractility.

Inhalational Analgesics

Nitrous Oxide (N_2O)

Pharmacology: Nitrous oxide is a low potency anesthetic agent and causes minimal muscle relaxation. It is not metabolized in the body and is quickly removed from the body by lungs. It is a colorless, odorless and noninflammable gas supplied in steel cylinders.[1]

Entonox is a mixture of 50% nitrous oxide in oxygen. When administered it provides analgesia within 20–30 seconds of inhalation and maximum effect comes after about 45 seconds. Entonox does not eliminate the pain of contraction completely but diminishes its intensity. The analgesic efficacy is comparable to meperidine.

Indication of use: It is used for labor analgesia in low resource settings, where other options are not available.

Contraindication: Raised intracranial pressure, pneumothorax.

Dosage: It is generally administered via a mouth piece attached to a demand valve or through a face mask. Approximately 10 breaths of entonox inhalation during contractions are required by the parturient for adequate analgesic effect.

Adverse effects: Drowsiness, disorientation, nausea, vomiting, dryness of tongue may occur. There may be brief episodes of loss of consciousness and raised intracranial pressure. Prolonged use can cause peripheral neuropathy and bone marrow depression.

Drug interaction: No known drug interaction.

Monitoring: Patient herself can administer it. There is only minimal accumulation with intermittent use.

Preparation: For labor analgesia, nitrous oxide is typically administered as a mix of 50% N_2O and 50% O_2 using a portable unit with a gas mixer that is fed by small tanks of N_2O and O_2 or with a valve fed by a single tank containing a mixture of both N_2O and O_2.

Safety during pregnancy: It is safe for mother and fetus. Its use does not alter uterine contractility and does not have any impact on the Apgar score of the newborn.

FDA category: It is not FDA approved, however, the machine which delivers the nitrous oxide plus oxygen mixture is FDA approved.

Sevoflurane

Pharmacology: It is a polyfluorinated anesthetic agent. Absence of pungency makes it pleasant and administrable via mask. About 3% of absorbed sevoflurane is metabolized. It has a short onset of action and quick recovery from anesthesia.

Recent studies suggest that sevoflurane is an effective labor analgesic that can be used for patient controlled analgesia and provides better pain relief than Entonox.[2] However, it is costly and needs specialized equipment.

Indications of use: It can be used for labor analgesia and is being used for induction and maintenance of general anesthesia in patients undergoing surgery.

Contraindications: It should not be used in patients who have sensitivity to sevoflurane or to other halogenated agents, in patients with suspected malignant hyperthermia, confirmed hepatitis or a history of unexplained moderate to severe hepatic dysfunction.

Dosage: Used as 0.8% with O_2.

Adverse effect: Hypotension, respiratory depression, more intense sedation.

Drug interaction: It reacts with soda lime, so should not be used in a fully closed circuit.

Monitoring: Monitoring of the ECG, blood pressure, oxygen saturation is essential while using sevoflurane.

Preparation: Ultane.

Safety during pregnancy: Caution should be exercised in obstetric anesthesia due to the relaxant effect of sevoflurane on the uterus resulting in an increase in uterine hemorrhage and risk of respiratory depression in newborn.

It is FDA Category B.

Systemic Analgesics

Parenteral opioids are the most commonly used class of drugs for labor analgesia as they produce good analgesia and sedation. They can be given in intermittent doses or via patient controlled analgesia. They are inexpensive, easily available and easy to administer.

Their common side effects are nausea, vomiting, dysphoria and respiratory depression. Because of their ability to cross placenta, they cause fetal bradycardia, decreased beat-to-beat variability and neonatal respiratory depression. For reversal of neonatal effects naloxone is recommended.

Commonly used parenteral opioids are meperidine, morphine, tramadol, fentanyl, remifentanil, nalbuphine and butorphanol.

Meperidine (Pethidine)

Pharmacology: It is a synthetic compound and is well absorbed orally and parenterally. Onset of analgesia occurs in 45 minutes. It crosses placenta and after 2–3 hours of IM administration, highest fetal plasma concentration is reached. Effect on fetus gets aggravated by production of normeperidine leading to further sedation and respiratory depression. After birth these babies are sleepier, less attentive and have poor suckling but the Apgar score is normal. It is completely metabolized in the liver.[3]

Indications of use: Labor analgesia and for pain relief before gynecological minor surgical procedures.

Contraindications: Hypersensitivity to pethidine, raised intracranial pressure and head injury (opioid analgesics interfere with pupillary responses which are vital for neurological assessment), acute respiratory depression and obstructive airways disease. It may prolong the latent phase of labor and does not benefit labor in women with dystocia. The active metabolite normeperidine can cause convulsions and is contraindicated in those with severe pregnancy-induced hypertension.

Dosage: It is administered in dose of 100 mg (max 150 mg) IM injection initially and usually combined with IM injection promethazine 25 mg. A further dose of 50–100 mg of pethidine can be administered after 3–4 hours. If woman still demands pain relief, then another drug should be given. The last dose should be administered at least 3–4 hours prior to delivery in order to prevent neonatal depression.

Adverse drug reaction: The common adverse effects are delay in gastric emptying with increased gastric volume, sedation, confusion, drowsiness, dose-dependent respiratory depression, difficulty in passing urine and dryness of mouth in mother. In the newborn it can cause respiratory depression, impaired suckling and drowsiness. The active metabolite normeperidine on accumulation can lead to convulsions.

Drug interaction: Pethidine administered in patients taking selective serotonin reuptake inhibitor (SSRI, e.g. paroxetine and fluoxetine) may produce "serotonin syndrome" by enhancing serotonin release. This consists of a clinical syndrome of shivering, sweating, agitation, hallucinations, increased heart rate, dilated pupils, myoclonus (intermittent jerking or twitching), over responsive reflexes, and sometimes coma.

They should not to be taken with mono amine oxidase inhibitors, e.g. selegiline, phenelzine as they inhibit hydrolysis of pethidine leading to excess production of norpethidine.

Monitoring: Pulse, blood pressure, oxygen saturation, respiratory rate must be monitored regularly. Facilities for intermittent positive pressure ventilation must be immediately available.

Opioid antagonist naloxone is the drug of choice for reversing maternal and neonatal respiratory depression.

For maternal respiratory depression, it is given in the dose of 0.4 mg intravenously. However, it will also reverse the analgesic action. The half-life of naloxone is short and repeat administrations at intervals of 2–3 minutes to a maximum of 2 mg may be required.

For reversing the neonatal effects of maternal opioid administration, naloxone is best administered directly to the new born. The dose is 0.1 mL/kg intravenously after primary steps of resuscitation including intubation have been taken. Endotracheal administration of naloxone is not recommended.

Preparation: Demerol—It is available as 100 mg of pethidine HCL per 2 mL injection, for IM and IV use.

Safety during pregnancy: Pethidine should be used during pregnancy only when the need outweighs any possible risk to the fetus. (Category C).

FDA approval: FDA has approved pethidine for use in labor analgesia with warning regarding its side effects in mother and baby.

Morphine

Pharmacology: It is a strong opioid analgesic and it acts on μ opioid receptors. These receptors are specific for morphine and mediate analgesia, miosis, sedation, respiratory depression, bradycardia and decrease gastrointestinal transit. The effect increases with the increase in dose. Oral absorption is unreliable because of high and variable first pass metabolism. Oral bioavailability is 1/6 to 1/4 of the parenterally administered drug. Effect of parenterally administered drug lasts for 4 hours. The half-life of drug in the mother is one hour and in neonate is six hours. It has no active metabolites. Intramuscular (IM) injection acts in 15–20 minutes and the peak occurs in 40–60 minutes.[4]

Indications of use: Labor analgesia especially when benefits outweigh risks, e.g. in congestive heart failure and in heart disease patients.

Contraindications: It causes respiratory depression; therefore, should be avoided in conditions which cause poor respiratory reserve for example in bronchial asthma, emphysema, pulmonary fibrosis, head injury (which may cause carbon dioxide retention) and hypovolemia.

Dosage

- 5–20 mg IM every 4 hours. IM morphine is more effective in early labor.
- 3–5 mg IV slowly over 5 minutes repeated every 4 hours.
- 10–20 mg orally every 4 hours as needed.

Adverse drug reaction: It can cause respiratory depression, hypotension, delayed gastric emptying, vomiting, urinary retention, etc.

Drug interaction: Hypnotics and sedatives, tricyclic antidepressants, and phenothiazine enhance depressant effects of morphine. Buprenorphine, butorphanol, nalbuphine, or pentazocine may precipitate withdrawal symptoms in patients who have recently used morphine due to their antagonistic action.

Monitoring: Monitoring of vitals like respiratory rate, pulse rate, blood pressure and oxygen saturation is important.

Naloxone should be readily available for administration to the mother or neonate.

Preparation

- Neomorph 1 mL injection contains 15 mg/mL
- Rumorf 1 mL injection contains 10 mg/mL
- Duramor 10 mg tab.

Safety during pregnancy: Morphine rapidly crosses the placenta and can have more effect on fetus than the mother itself. Babies born 3 hours after an intramuscular dose of morphine have negligible amounts of the drug in cord blood.

It is category C drug and not recommended routinely and used only when the potential benefits outweigh the potential risks to the developing fetus.

Tramadol

Pharmacology: It is a centrally acting analgesic which not only acts on μ receptors but inhibits reuptake of 5 HT leading to activation of monoaminergic spinal inhibition of pain. Hence, action is only partially inhibited by naloxone. Onset of action occurs within 10 minutes and its effect lasts for 4–6 hours.

The placental permeability of tramadol is very high, however, it gets neutralized by the capacity of the neonatal liver to fully metabolize it.[5]

Indication of use: Useful for pain relief in first stage of labor, however, it has poor effectiveness in second stage. It is one-tenth as potent as morphine.

Contraindications: It should not be used in patients with previously demonstrated hypersensitivity to tramadol. It is not given in acute intoxication with alcohol, hypnotics, narcotics, centrally acting analgesics, opioids or psychotropic drugs. In these conditions, tramadol hydrochloride or any other opioid analgesic may worsen central nervous system and respiratory depression.

Drug dosage: It can be given as oral, IM, IV.

It is given in dose of 50–100 mg orally every 4 hourly.

50–100 mg IM every 4 hourly.

0.5–1 mg/kg IV every 4 hourly.

Adverse drug reactions: Nausea and vomiting are common side effects.

Drug interaction: Tramadol when injected in patient taking SSRI may produce "serotonin syndrome" autonomic instability (e.g. tachycardia, labile blood pressure, hyperthermia), neuromuscular aberrations (hyperreflexia and incoordination) and gastrointestinal symptoms (e.g. nausea, vomiting, diarrhea).

Monitoring: It requires monitoring of respiratory rate and oxygen saturation.

Preparations

- Tramazac 50 mg capule, 100 mg SR tablet
- Tramadol—50 mg/mL injection in 1 and 2 mL ampoules
- Maxitram 100 mg SR tablet.

Safety during pregnancy: Its use in pregnancy is generally avoided as it may cause some reversible withdrawal effects in the newborn. Its use as an analgesic during labor is generally avoided in second stage due to its long-onset of action (one hour). It is a category C drug.

FDA approval: Approved for labor analgesia.

Fentanyl

Pharmacology: It is highly potent, has a rapid onset of action and no active metabolite. It has high lipid solubility and enters the brain rapidly. Its peak effect appears within 3–5 minutes and analgesic effect remains for 30–60 minutes. It is 80–100 times more potent in producing analgesia as compared to meperidine.

It has a longer half-life than both meperidine and morphine, therefore, repeated dosing should not be done as it may result in drug accumulation in both the fetus and the mother.[6]

Indications of use: Because of its short duration of action it is generally used for patient-controlled analgesia (PCA) in labor.

Contraindications: Allergy to fentanyl, morbid obesity, uncontrolled hypotension, liver disease.

Dosage: It can be used as IV bolus or as patient controlled analgesia. Usual dose is 25–50 μg IV.

For patient controlled analgesia dose is 20 μg bolus with a 5 minute lockout.

Adverse drug reaction: Respiratory depression and transient decrease in fetal heart rate (FHR) variability are the common side effects.

Drug interaction: No significant drug interactions.

Monitoring: Close monitoring of respiratory rate and continuous oxygen saturation monitoring is essential. Neither initial nor subsequent doses should be administered to women with respiratory rate of less than 8 breaths per minute or an oxygen saturation of less than 94%. Naloxone should be kept ready while using fentanyl. Newborn must be monitored for at least 2 hours.

Preparation: Durogesic injection.

Safety during pregnancy: It is used during pregnancy only if the need outweighs any potential risk to the fetus.

It is FDA approved category C drug.

Remifentanil

Pharmacology: It is an ultrashort acting opioid with a half-life of 3–4 minutes. Blood and tissue esterases rapidly hydrolyze it and, therefore, it does not accumulate even after prolonged infusions. Fetal exposure is minimal. Its metabolism is not affected by hepatic or renal function.[7]

Indications of use: It is used for patient controlled analgesia. It is specially preferred when neuraxial block is contraindicated.

Contraindications: Allergy to opioid, baseline maternal oxygen saturation less than 95%.

Dosage: For patient-controlled analgesia (PCA), the dose is 0.25–0.5 μg/kg body weight and the lockout time (The time interval before the pump can provide the next dose) is 2–3 minutes.

As infusion the dose is 25 μg IV bolus followed by IV infusion of 0.05 μg/kg/minute and the lockout time is 5 minutes.

Adverse drug reaction: Nausea, vomiting, delayed gastric emptying and dose dependent maternal sedation are the common side effects.

Drug interaction: Alcohol, amiodarone, benzodiazepines (for example alprazolam), cimetidine, or sodium oxybate may increase the side effects of remifentanil.

Monitoring: Maternal oxygen saturation must be monitored continuously. Heart rate, BP, respiratory rate, sedation score, pain score and PCA pump parameters are monitored intermittently. Monitor the respiratory rate by actually counting breaths as the figure on the monitor may be inaccurate.

Preparation: Ultiva injection.

Safety during pregnancy: It is used during pregnancy only when the need outweighs any potential risk to the fetus.

It is FDA Category C.

Patient-controlled Analgesia

Patient-controlled analgesia (PCA) is an effective way of pain control. It uses an electronically controlled infusion pump which delivers a controlled dose of analgesic at set intervals of time when the patient presses a button. PCA is typically the term used for intravenous analgesia. If analgesia is established by means of epidural block, a special intravenous infusion catheter is connected to the epidural catheter and this is referred to as patient-controlled epidural analgesia (PCEA) and the patient can then self-administer further boluses as required. Fentanyl and more recently remifentanil are the drugs which are used for PCA.[8]

Dosage: The PCEA pump is programed at settings to deliver continuous infusion of 10 mL per hour and 5 mL bolus with 10 minute lockout interval. The solution for infusion is prepared by combining 0.08% bupivacaine and 2 μg of fentanyl per mL.

PCEA reduces the total amount of local anesthetic used and consequently it lessens unwanted effects such as motor block and hypotension. It also reduces the demands on staff on the labor floor, and it gives many of the parturients a feeling of satisfaction and empowerment. The woman should be instructed about the correct use of device.

Regional Analgesia

Central Regional Analgesic Techniques

Regional techniques like epidural and spinal are considered the gold standard for labor analgesia since they provide good pain relief with minimum maternal and neonatal side effects. The analgesic drugs are administered into a specific anatomical region (the lower neuraxis of central nervous system) so as to interrupt pain pathways, thereby producing pain relief. These modalities are therefore, also known as neuraxial techniques.

Because the drug is administered locally, small dose is required and the systemic drug concentration is low. The onset, duration and quality of analgesia can be enhanced by using small incremental doses and carefully monitoring early warning signs of toxicity.

Successful neuraxial block results in blockade of the sympathetic and sensory nerve supply of the birth canal and perineum. Onset of pain relief is accompanied by a decrease in endogenous catecholamines as well as peripheral vasodilatation.

Drugs used for epidural and spinal techniques: Various classes of analgesics are used for epidural and spinal block and these include following:

- *Local anesthetics*: They inhibit neural conduction by reversibly blocking axonal sodium channels. Bupivacaine and ropivacaine are commonly used.
- *Opioids*: They reversibly bind to opioid receptors in the dorsal horn of the spinal cord. Morphine, pethidine and fentanyl are commonly used.
- *Alpha-2 adrenergic agents*: They interact with alpha-2 adrenergic receptors in the spinal cord and within several brainstem nuclei. Clonidine hydrochloride is commonly used.
- *Cholinergic agonists*: They produce analgesia by increasing the concentration of acetylcholine proximate to muscarinic and nicotinic receptors in the superficial layers of the dorsal horn of the spinal cord. For example, neostigmine.

Peripheral Regional Analgesic Techniques

These include paracervical block and pudendal block. They involve blockade of cervical nerve plexus and pudendal nerve respectively by local anesthetic injection.

These techniques are uncommon because of complications like accidental injection into uterine artery, fetal bradycardia seen in 70% fetuses within 10 minutes of injection, accidental injection into fetal scalp or even fetal death. Sometimes, may cause uterine artery hematoma or cervical abscess.

Drugs used for paracervical and pudendal block are lignocaine, bupivacaine and ropivacaine.

Bupivacaine

Pharmacology: Bupivacaine is an local anesthetic with rapid onset of action (8–10 min), approximately 20 minutes are required to achieve peak effect. Duration of analgesia is approximately 90 minutes. Most of it (95%) is bound to plasma proteins, hence, has a low fetal/maternal ratio (0.2–0.4). It is metabolized in the liver and then excreted in the urine.

In low doses it produces sensory block (analgesia) with less pronounced motor block but at higher doses leads to anesthesia.[9]

Indications of use: Epidural, spinal and combined spinal epidural, paracervical and pudendal blocks.

Contraindications: It should be used with caution in patients with partial or complete heart block, patients on antiarrhythmic drugs and advanced liver disease.

Dosage

Spinal: 2.5–5 mg of 0.5% solution.

Epidural: Initial dose—10–15 mL of a 0.25%–0.125% solution; maintenance by continuous infusion—0.0625%–0.125% solution at rate of 8–15 mL/hour.

Paracervical block: 5–10 mL of 1% solution injected into cervix at 3 and 9 o' clock position.

Pudendal block: 3–10 mL of 1% lidocaine solution.

Adverse drug reaction: Common side effects are dizziness, paresthesia, nausea, vomiting, bradycardia, ventricular arrhythmia, urinary retention. Rarely, may lead to neuropathy, diplopia, respiratory depression, convulsions, and loss of consciousness. Levobupivacaine is less cardiotoxic than bupivacaine.

Acute systemic toxicity may occur with accidental intravenous injection, overdose or exceptionally rapid absorption of drug from highly vascular areas. This manifests as central nervous and cardiovascular systems effects. Central nervous system (CNS) effects occur first like light headedness, circumoral paresthesia, numbness of tongue, hyperacusis, tinnitus, dysarthria, muscle twitching and ultimately generalized convulsions, followed by loss of consciousness. Cardiovascular toxicity manifests later and is characterized by stimulation followed by depression; so there is hypertension and tachycardia followed by hypotension, bradycardia, ventricular arrhythmia, ventricular fibrillation, sudden cardiovascular collapse and cardiac arrest.

Drug interaction: Use of vasopressors or methylergometrine or administration of local anesthetic solutions containing epinephrine or norepinephrine may cause hypertension or cerebrovascular accidents.

Monitoring: Oxygen saturation, heart rate, BP, respiratory rate monitoring is essential.

Preparation: Sensorcaine, heavy marcaine.

Safety during pregnancy: It is a pregnancy category C drug. It crosses placenta and is excreted in breast milk. However, it is approved by FDA for use at term in obstetrical anesthesia.

Ropivacaine

Pharmacology: Ropivacaine is newer local anesthetic agent belonging to same class as bupivacaine. It is 40% less potent as compared to bupivacaine. However, latency and duration of action are similar to bupivacaine. Ropivacaine is less lipophilic than bupivacaine and is less likely to penetrate large myelinated motor fibers, resulting in a relatively reduced motor blockade. Therefore, the unique feature of ropivacaine is that it has a greater degree of motor sensory differentiation which is useful for labor analgesia because in these patients motor blockade is undesirable. This less lipophilicity is also responsible for lesser central nervous system toxicity and cardiotoxicity.[10]

Indications of use: Labor analgesia.

Contraindications: Hypersensitivity to ropivacaine.

Dosage

For labor analgesia: 10–20 mL epidural bolus of 0.2% ropivacaine followed by 20–30 mg top up injections or a continuous epidural infusion of 0.2% ropivacaine at rate of 6–10 mL/hour is given.

The addition of narcotics like fentanyl 2 µg/mL–0.1% solution of ropivacaine administered at rate of 10 mL/hour, significantly reduces local anesthetic concentration and the quality of analgesia is similar to ropivacaine 0.2% only solution or 0.2% ropivacaine plus fentanyl 2 µg/mL infused at a slower rate of 8 mL/hour. Addition of adjuvants like clonidine also significantly increases the duration of action of ropivacaine.

Adverse drug reaction: These are rare when it is administered correctly.

CNS effects are due to CNS excitation and may manifest as nervousness, dizziness, tingling around the mouth, tinnitus, blurred vision, tremor and seizures. These may be followed by CNS depression manifesting as drowsiness, loss of consciousness, respiratory depression and apnea. Cardiovascular effects may be hypotension, bradycardia, arrhythmias and may even lead to cardiac arrest.

Drug interaction: No significant drug interactions.

Monitoring: Oxygen saturation, heart rate, BP, respiratory rate monitoring is essential.

Preparation: Naropin.

Safety during pregnancy: Category B drug.

FDA approval: Not approved for intravenous use.

Newer Adjuvant Drugs

Clonidine and neostigmine are the two agents which have potential for use as labor analgesics:[11,12]

- Low dose clonidine along with 0.125% bupivacaine given as epidural dose produces a longer duration of analgesia as compared to bupivacaine and fentanyl.
- Addition of low dose clonidine to sufentanil and levobupivacaine leads to a better quality of anesthesia and reduces the dose of sufentanil with resultant decrease in side effects like pruritus.
- Addition of low doses of clonidine and *neostigmine* to intrathecal bupivacaine fentanyl mixture prolongs the duration of analgesia.

However, safety issues need to be addressed before routine use of multiple drugs for intrathecal administration is advocated. Although clearly effective for labor analgesia, FDA warns and states that it is not recommended for obstetrical, postpartum or perioperative pain management as the risk of hemodynamic instability may be unacceptable.

REFERENCES

1. Klomp T, van Poppel M, Jones L, Lazet J, Di Nisio M, Lagro-Janssen AL. Inhaled analgesia for pain management in labour. Cochrane Database Syst Rev. 2012;9:CD009351.
2. Yeo ST, Holdcroft A, Yentis SM, Stewart A, Bassett P. Analgesia with sevoflurane during labour: ii. Sevoflurane compared with Entonox for labour analgesia. Br J Anaesth. 2007;98(1):110-5.
3. Pereira RR, Kanhai H, Rosendaal F, van Dommelen P, Swaab D, Rodrigues Pereira E, van de Wetering B. Parenteral Pethidine for labour pain relief: 20-year follow-up cohort study in offspring. BMJ Open. 2012;2(3). pii: e000719.
4. Ullman R, Smith LA, Burns E, Mori R, Dowswell T. Parenteral opioids for maternal pain relief in labour. Cochrane Database Syst Rev. 2010;(9):CD007396. doi: 10.1002/14651858.CD007396.pub2.
5. Lee CR, McTavish D, Sorkin EM. Tramadol: A preliminary review of its pharmacodynamic and pharmacokinetic properties, and therapeutic potential in acute and chronic pain states. Drugs. 1993;46:313-40.
6. Anderson D. A review of systemic opioids commonly used for labor pain relief. J Midwifery Womens Health. 2011;56(3):222-39.
7. Remifentanil for labour analgesia: a meta-analysis of randomised controlled trials. Eur J Anaesthesiol. 2012;29(4):177-85.
8. Campbell DC. Labour analgesia: what's new and PCEA too. Can Janesth. 2003;50:R1-R7.
9. Belfrage P, Berlin A, Raabe N, Thalme B. Lumbar epidural analgesia with bupivacaine in labor. Drug concentration in maternal and neonatal blood at birth and during the first day of life. Am J Obstet Gynecol. 1975;123:839-44.
10. NganKee WD, Ng FF, Khaw KS, Lee A, Gin T. Determination and comparison of graded dose-response curves for epidural bupivacaine and ropivacaine for analgesia in laboring nulliparous women. Anesthesiology. 2010;113:445-53.
11. Kizilarslan S1, Kuvaki B, Onat U, Sağiroğlu E. Epidural fentanyl-bupivacaine compared with clonidine-bupivacaine for analgesia in labour. Eur J Anaesthesiol. 2000;17(11):692-7.
12. Owen MD1, Ozsaraç O, Sahin S, Uçkunkaya N, Kaplan N, Magunaci I. Low-dose clonidine and neostigmine prolong the duration of intrathecal bupivacaine-fentanyl for labor analgesia. Anesthesiology. 2000;92(2):361-6.

CHAPTER 13

Cervical Ripening Agents

Krishna Agarwal, Swati Priya

INTRODUCTION

Preinduction cervical ripening is the most important predictor of successful labor induction.[1] Labor induction is an exhausting process, unripe cervix is associated with higher chances of chorioamnionitis, prolonged labor and cesarean delivery.[2] The most commonly used index to assess cervical favorability is Bishop's score. The success of induction depends on five components, consistency, position, effacement and dilatation of cervix and the station of presenting part. Each parameter is scored out of 2 or 3 and total score is given out of 13. Poor Bishop's score (<6) is indicator of unfavorable cervix and thus the need for cervical ripening agents. Thus, cervical ripening facilitates more successful outcome during induction of labor.[3] **Table 13.1** enlists the drugs used for preinduction cervical ripening.

Table 13.1 Agents used for preinduction cervical ripening

Drug(s)		*Use in clinical practice*
Prostaglandins	Dinoprostone (PGE2)	Effective and commonly used
	Misoprostol (PGE1)	Effective but not recommended, should be used only in research setting
Relaxin		Used only in research setting
NO (nitric oxide) donors		

Prostaglandins

Prostaglandin analogs are most commonly used for the purpose of cervical ripening. Prostaglandins facilitate cervical ripening by mainly altering the extracellular ground substance of the cervix and increasing the activity of collagenase in the cervix. Risks associated with the use of prostaglandins include uterine hyperstimulation and maternal side effects such as nausea, vomiting, diarrhea and fever.

Dinoprostone (PGE2)

Pharmacology: Dinoprostone is a derivative of prostanoic acid. PGE2 has an important role in the events leading to the initiation of labor. The half-life of dinoprostone is 2.5–5 minutes. The rate limiting step for inactivation is regulated by the enzyme 15-hydroxyprostaglandin dehydrogenase. Any PGE2 that escapes local inactivation is rapidly cleared to the extent of 95% on the first pass through the pulmonary circulation.

PGE2 is endogenously secreted in the body by the fetal membranes and placenta and play an important role in spontaneous initiation of labor.

It acts as a local hormone and enables ripening of the cervix by a number of different mechanisms. It softens the cervix by altering the extracellular ground substance of cervix by increasing the activity of collagenase in the cervix, thus causes an increase in elastase, glycosaminoglycan, dermatan sulfate, and hyaluronic acid levels. The relaxation of cervical smooth muscle facilitates dilation. It also causes an increase in intracellular calcium levels, leads to gap junction formation, necessary for the coordinated uterine contractions during labor.[4-10]

Indications of use

- Most common use is for preinduction cervical ripening at term pregnancy
- Used for cervical ripening in following conditions
  - Termination of pregnancy from 12 to 20 gestational weeks
  - Missed abortion or intrauterine fetal death
  - Nonmetastatic gestational trophoblastic disease.

Contraindications

These are some of the relative contraindications:

- Asthma.
- Increased intraocular pressure, e.g. glaucoma.
- Compromised CVS, renal or hepatic function.

Adverse effects: It is generally a safe drug and has few adverse effects:

- Nausea, vomiting and fever
- Placental abruption and scar dehiscence due to uterine hyperstimulation may sometimes occur if drug is inappropriately introduced high up beyond internal Os of cervix.

Drug interactions: Dinoprostone may increase activity of oxytocin, therefore both should not be used concomitantly. After intracervical gel instillation, oxytocin infusion should only be started after atleast 6–8 hours.

Dosage and preparations: Dinoprostone is available in many preparations. It is available as gel for both intracervical and intravaginal use, vaginal tablets (pessary, suppositories) and vaginal inserts.

Intracervical gel: This 0.5 mg dinoprostone is available in 2.5 mL base in prefilled syringe. The dose may be repeated every 6 hours to a maximum of 3 doses in 24 hours.[6]

Method of instillation: It should be confirmed that the patient is not febrile, there is no active vaginal bleeding and FHR pattern is reassuring. The fetal heart rate and uterine activity should be closely monitored 15–30 min before and 30–120 min after instillation of dinoprostone. Gel should be inserted below the internal Os, in the cervical canal, either blindly or under visualization with speculum. Patient should remain recumbent for 30 minutes after PGE2 gel instillation.

Preparations: Cerviprime gel, dinoripe gel—all contain 0.5 mg dinoprostone.

Intravaginal gel: In cases of unfavorable cervix in primigravida, one application of 2 mg dinoprostone gel is inserted into the vagina. A repeat dose of 2 mg can be used after 6 hours. Maximum of only 2 doses are recommended.

Preparation: Prostin E2 contains 2 mg dinoprostone.

Intravaginal tablet: Vaginal tablet containing 3 mg dinoprostone is inserted followed by another tablet after 6–8 hours if necessary. Maximum dose of 6 mg can be given.

Preparation: Prostin E2 vaginal tablet contains 3 mg dinoprostone.

Intravaginal insert: It is a controlled-release prostaglandin E2 vaginal insert. It contains 10 mg dinoprostone which is released slowly at rate of 0.3 mg per hour for 24 hours. Vaginal insert is a thin polymeric wafer held within a polyester sac, with a long tail to allow easy removal. The patient is kept recumbent for 2 hours after insertion under strict FHR and uterine activity monitoring. It is removed after 12 hours or with labor onset. It is used as a single dose and a single application **(Fig. 13.1)**.

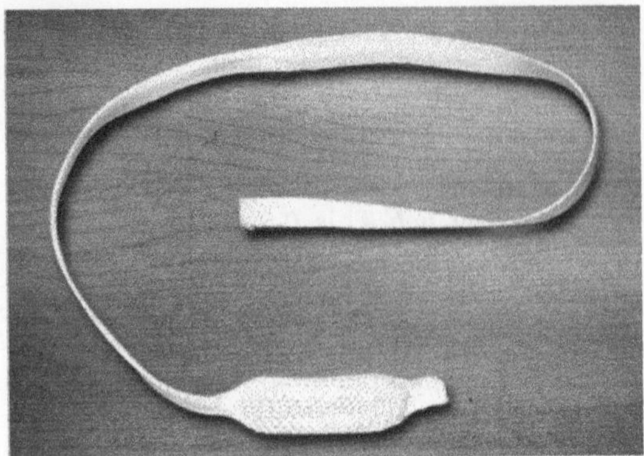

Fig. 13.1 Intravaginal insert

It is approved and available for use in USA, Canada and Europe.

Preparation: Cervidil contains 10 mg dinoprostone.

Stempel et al. conducted a randomized trial for comparing efficacy and safety of intracervical versus intravaginal gel for preinduction cervical ripening and found intravaginal gel to be more favorable as compared to intracervical gel **(Table 13.2).**[11]

Storage/Stability: Dinoprostone gel is stored in refrigerator at 36°–46°F. Suppository is stored in freezer below –4°F and inserts between –4° and –14°F. Inserts are stable for a period of 3 years when stored in a freezer.

Monitoring: The fetal heart rate and uterine activity should be closely monitored 15–30 minutes before and 30–120 minutes after instillation of dinoprostone.

Safety during pregnancy: It a FDA category C drug. It is used only when termination of pregnancy is indicated. It is not used during lactation.

Misoprostol

Misoprostol is a synthetic PGE1 analog that has been found to be effective and inexpensive agent for cervical ripening as well as labor induction.

Although it has been used as an effective agent for that purpose in viable pregnancies, it is not approved by the US Food and Drug Administration for cervical ripening and labor induction.[12,13]

The Royal College of Obstetricians and Gynaecologists recommends that until the best dose regime is determined, misoprostol use should be confined to clinical trials.[13]

Pharmacology: The initial effect of both vaginal and oral misoprostol is increase in uterine tonus. The onset of action of oral misoprostol is more rapid and initial increase is more pronounced. Oral misoprostol has a rapid onset of action and peak and shorter duration of action than misoprostol administered by vaginal route. The half-life of oral misoprostol is 30 minutes and time to peak plasma concentration is 30 minutes as compared to 80 minutes of vaginal misoprostol. Thus, vaginal misoprostol has a more sustained action.[14]

Indications of Use

- Used for cervical ripening and labor induction.
- Used for medical association.

Table 13.2 Comparison of efficacy of intracervical and intravaginal dinoprostone for preinduction cervical ripening

Parameter	*Intravaginal dinoprostone*	*Intracervical dinoprostone*
Achievement of vaginal birth within 24 hours	More efficacious	Increased risk of vaginal birth not achieved
Risk of uterine hyperstimulation and tachysystole	More frequent (5%)	Less frequent (1%)
Recommendation	Low doses (1–2.5 mg) of vaginal dinoprostone is preferred over intracervical gel for preinduction cervical ripening	

Contraindication: Misoprostol is contraindicated for induction of labor in women with previous cesarean section.[14]

The use of misoprostol in prior uterine surgery or cesarean delivery is avoided in third trimester.

Dosage: The 25–100 μg doses have been tried and compared in various trials, with different dosing intervals Usually 25 μg every 4–6 hours interval to a maximum of 6 doses is given.[9]

Routes of administration: Misoprostol may be administered orally or vaginally. Although it can be used by buccal or sublingual routes, these routes are not recommended.

Adverse effects: Uterine hyperstimulation (3–8%).

Use of misoprostol may lead to adverse fetal heart changes, twice as compared to dinoprostone. The incidence is closely related to the dose and frequency of misoprostol.[15]

When used for cervical ripening and labor induction, it significantly reduces cesarean rates and need for oxytocin induction. In addition, it results in shorter intervals to vaginal delivery thus increasing the number of vaginal births within 12–24 hours.[11,15] However, use of oral misoprostol in trials have shown lower risk of Apgar score <7 at 5 minutes of life.

Since the best dose and route of misoprostol for labor induction with a live fetus are not known and there are concerns regarding hyperstimulation, misoprostol use for induction of labor should be within clinical trials.

Relaxin and Nitric Oxide

The hormone relaxin facilitates cervical ripening. Further studies are required to support its use as cervical ripening agent.[15]

NICE 2008 does not recommend the use of relaxin, NO donors as cervical ripening agents.[2]

REFERENCES

1. Xenakis EM, Piper JM, Conway DL, Langer O. Induction of labor in the nineties: Conquering the unfavorable cervix. Obstet Gynecol. 1997;90:235-9.
2. Induction of labor. Evidence-based Clinical Guideline Number 9. Royal College of Obstetricians and Gynecologists. 2001.
3. Brindley BA, Sokol RJ. Induction and augmentation of labor: basis and methods for current practice. Obstet Gynecol Surv. 1988;43:730-43.
4. Witter FR. Prostaglandin E2 preparations for preinduction cervical ripening. Clin Obstet Gynecol. 2000;43:469-74
5. Induction of labor. ACOG Practice Bulletin no. 107. Obstet Gynecol . 2009;114:386-97.
6. Arias F. Pharmacology of oxytocin and prostaglandins. Clin Obstet Gynecol. 2000;43:455-68.
7. Rayburn WF. Prostaglandin E2 gels for cervical ripening and induction of labor: a critical analysis. Am J Obstet Gynaecol. 1989;160:529-34.
8. Induction of labor. WHO 2011.
9. Induction of labor. ACOG 2000.
10. Induction of labor. Clinical Guideline No. 16 Royal College of Obstetricians and Gynecologists. 1998.
11. Stempel JE, Prins RP, Dean S. Preinduction cervical ripening: a randomized prospective comparison of the efficacy and safety of intravaginal and intracervical prostaglandin E2 gel. Am J Obstet Gynecol. 1997;176(6):1305-9.
12. Khan RU, El-Refaey H, Sharma S, et al. Oral, rectal, and vaginal pharmacokinetics of misoprostol. Obstet Gynecol. 2004;103:866-70.
13. Sanchez-Ramos L, Kaunitz AM. Misoprostol for cervical ripening and labor induction: a systematic review of the literature. Clin Obstet Gynecol. 2000;43:475-88.
14. Sanchez-Ramos L, Gaudier FL, Kaunitz AM. Cervical ripening and labor induction after previous cesarean delivery. Clin Obstet Gynecol. 2000;43:513-23.
15. Kelly AJ, Kavanagh J, Thomas J. Relaxin for cervical ripening and induction of labor. Cochrane Database Syst Rev. 2002;2:CD003103.

CHAPTER 14

Oxytocics

Poonam Sachdeva, Binni Makkar

INTRODUCTION

Oxytocics are the drugs of varying chemical nature that have the power to excite contraction of the uterine muscles.

Different types of oxytocics which are used in clinical practice are given in **Table 14.1**.

Oxytocics Used in Obstetrics

Oxytocin

Oxytocin is on WHO list of essential medicines, a list of most important medications required for basic health system.[1] It is a hormone produced endogenously in the body in the supraoptic and paraventricular nuclei of hypothalamus. It is stored in posterior pituitary gland from where it is released in the blood circulation. Synthetic oxytocin can be administered from outside to enhance the action of endogenous oxytocin.

Table 14.1: Oxytocics used in obstetrics

Oxytocin	
Ergot derivatives	Methergine, ergometrine
Prostaglandins	PGE2 analog-Misoprostol PGF2 alpha-Carbopost

Pharmacology: Endogenous or administered oxytocin predominantly affects the uterine smooth muscles. Its interaction with the myometrial cell membrane receptor promotes the influx of calcium ions from extracellular fluid and from sarcoplasmic reticulum into the cell, this increase in cytoplasmic calcium stimulates the uterine contractions. Oxytocin is the prime mediator of myometrial contractility during labor. Near term, there is 100–200 fold increase in the expression of oxytocin receptors in uterine smooth muscle cells. These cells become increasingly sensitive to stimulant action of oxytocin. Also there is stimulation of prostaglandin synthesis. Oxytocin causes increase in both force and frequency of contractions mainly at the fundal region which, in turn, is associated with cervical relaxation

In small doses oxytocin produces vasodilation by direct relaxation of vascular smooth muscle. Transient hypotension and flushing followed by tachycardia are observed.

In high concentrations, due to activation of vasopressin receptor, oxytocin has a weak antidiuretic and pressor activity.

In lactating mothers, it acts at the mammary glands causing the milk to be "let down" into the subareolar tissue from where it can be excreted via nipple.

Oxytocin is not bound to plasma proteins and is eliminated by kidney and liver. Its half-life is 5 minutes in pregnant women due to presence of the enzyme oxytocinase in placenta, uterus and plasma. Circulating half-life is 10–15 minutes in nonpregnant women.

Indications

Early pregnancy
- To accelerate abortion
- For induction of abortion
- In molar pregnancy at the time of evacuation

Late pregnancy
- To induce labor
- For cervical ripening

Labor
- Augmentation of labor
- Uterine inertia
- Active management of 3rd stage

Puerperium
- Control of postpartum hemorrhage (PPH).

Contraindications

It should not be given in:
- Malpresentations
- Contracted pelvis
- Cephalopelvic disproportion
- Previous hysterotomy
- Obstructed labor
- Incoordinate uterine contractions
- Fetal distress when delivery is not imminent and in
- Hypertonic uterine contractions.

Dosage

Augmentation of labor

Controlled intravenous infusion: It is safer to use oxytocin by infusion pump as it causes minimum fluid overload and the dose is also more regulated. It is always started at a lower dose rate of (1–2 mIU/min) and should be increased gradually.

It is prepared by diluting 1 mL vial containing 5U oxytocin in 4 mL saline resulting in 1 U/mL preparation. Two milliliter of this has to be diluted in 500 mL of 5% dextrose or 500 mL of ringer lactate and started at a drip rate of 15 drops/min which is equivalent to 2 mIU/min **(Table 14.2)**.

Table 14.2: Dose of oxytocin in mIU and its correlation with drop rate per minute

Unit of oxytocin per 500 mL of saline	Infusion of drops per minute 15	30	60
	Oxytocin dose in mIU/minute		
1	2	4	8
2	4	8	16
4	8	16	32

1 unit = 1000 mIU, and 15 drops = 1 mL

Induction of labor: It should be started at the rate of 1-2 mIU/min and be escalated at an interval of 20–30 minutes till optimum contractions numbering 3 in 10 minutes lasting for 40 seconds is achieved. The same rate should continue till delivery and at least 30-60 minutes beyond that.

Regulation of the drip can also be done manually by counting the drops manually which is commonly practiced where infusion pumps are not available. The drip rate can be started at a low dose of 1-2 mIU/minute and escalated by 1–2 mIU/minute every 20 minutes up to 8 mIU/minute. In majority of cases 16 mIU/minute (2 units in 500 mL Ringer Lactate with drop rate of 60 per minute) is enough to achieve optimum contractions. The maximum dose is 32 mIU/minute.

Active management of third stage of labor: The 10 IU of oxytocin is given intramuscular (IM) after the delivery of the anterior shoulder of the baby.[1]

Control of postpartum hemorrhage: The 40 IU of oxytocin in 1000 mL of normal saline or ringer lactate to be started at 60 drops per minute.[1]

Adverse effects : Serious toxicity of oxytocin is rare, if used in controlled manner.

Its injudicious use may cause complications like uterine rupture (as seen in grand multipara, previous cesarean and patients with contracted pelvis), placental abruption and fetal bradycardia subsequent to excessive uterine stimulation.

Hypotension may occur due to transient vasodilatation. To avoid this, it should be administered IV as dilute solutions at controlled rate.

Inadvertent activation of vasopressin receptors may occur, when it is given in high doses (40-50 mIu/minute) resulting in excessive fluid retention. This may lead to seizures and coma. Sometimes it may cause nausea and vomiting.

Monitoring: During augmentation of labor, it requires close monitoring:

- Before starting one should ensure correct fetal position and size and rule out all contraindications to the drug.
- Fetal heart rate (FHR) auscultation should ideally be continuous and if not feasible then every 15-30 minutes for 60 seconds, during first stage is essential.
- In second stage every postcontraction FHS should be monitored.
- Maintain partogram including monitoring of maternal pulse, BP and uterine contractions.
- Infusion should be stopped if contractions last more than 60 seconds or are less than 2 minutes apart.
- Maintain intake output chart as its anti-diuretic effect may cause fluid overload, seizures and coma.

During treatment of postpartum hemorrhage, patient should be monitored for hypotension and signs of water intoxication.

Preparation

- Pitocin—5 IU per mL in 1 mL vial, 5 mL per 0.5 mL in 1 mL vial.
- Syntocinon—5 IU per mL in 1 mL vial.
- Gynotocin—5 IU per mL in 1 mL vial.
- Oxytocin—5 IU per mL in 1 mL vial.

Safety during pregnancy and lactation: Oxytocin belongs to FDA category X. It is only used during pregnancy when termination of pregnancy is decided.

Ergometrine and Methylergometrine

Ergometrine is an ergot derivative which is detoxified in the liver and excreted in the urine. Methylergometrine is a synthetic analog of ergometrine. Both have same effects.

Pharmacology: While it acts at alpha adrenergic, dopaminergic and serotonin receptors, it exerts on the uterus a powerful stimulant effect not clearly associated with a specific receptor type. Uterine contraction with methylergometrine is so frequent that uterus is in a state of spasm without relaxation in between contractions.

Indications

- Given as a routine prophylaxis to prevent PPH after delivery of the placenta.[1,2]
- In management of atonic postpartum hemorrhage and bleeding following abortion or H mole evacuation.

Contraindications

- History of allergy and hypersensitivity
- Chronic and gestational hypertension[1,2]
- In heart disease patients. It may cause congestive heart failure in patients with heart disease.[1,2] Because it increases preload by sudden uterine contraction which squeezes blood into systemic circulation and afterload by causing vasoconstriction.
- During pregnancy because it stimulates strong uterine contractions.
- Rh negative mothers because there is more risk of Feto maternal transfusion
- In multiple pregnancies, it is contraindicated after delivery of first baby because it may cause fetal compromise in the second twin due to tetanic uterine contraction.

Dosage: For prophylaxis of postpartum hemorrhage, it is given as 0.25 mg IM or IV injection immediately after delivery of placenta.

In management of postpartum hemorrhage—0.25 mg IV injection is given, repeated every 15 minutes if bleeding is not controlled, maximum 5 doses can be given.

Adverse effects: It can cause headache, dizziness and tinnitus. Patient may complain dyspnea, palpitation, chest pain and may have transient rise in blood pressure due to its vasoconstrictor action. Patient may have nausea, vomiting diarrhea and hematuria. There may be thrombophlebitis at the injection site. High doses can lead to severe peripheral vasoconstriction and gangrene of toes.

Monitoring: Pulse and blood pressure monitoring should be done every 15 minutes for one hour.

Preparations

- Methylergometrine maleate—1 mL injections contain 0.2 mg per mL
- Emergen—1 mL injections contain 0.2 mg per mL
- Utergin—0.125 mg tablets
- Methergine—0.125 mg tablets.

Safety during pregnancy and lactation: It is FDA category C drug.

Prostaglandins

Misoprostol: It is a synthetic PGE1 analog used for variety of indications in the practice of obstetrics and gynecology. Chief advantages include ease of administration, cost-effectiveness and easy storage.

Pharmacology: It binds to myometrium cells causing strong uterine contractions leading to expulsion of contents. The agent also causes cervical ripening, softening and dilatation of cervix.

It may be given orally, rectally or vaginally. It is extensively absorbed and gets de-esterified to its free acid, which is the active moiety. Elimination half-life is 20–40 minutes

Indications: It is used "off label" for variety of indications which include:

- *Medical abortion*: Misoprostol is usually used in combination with mifepristone. There is evidence of excellent efficacy up to 63 days of gestation. The method is cheaper, simpler and less invasive as compared to surgical evacuation. This method of medical abortion is approved by government of India.[3]
- It is used for induction of abortion in cases of miscarriage and for completion of abortion in incomplete abortions up to 12 weeks of gestation. Various regimens which are used include single dose of 600 µg orally, 800 µg vaginally or 400 µg sublingually.[3,4]
- It is also an effective cervical ripening agent prior to 1st trimester surgical abortion.
- It is a used for induction in second trimester for termination of pregnancy and for induction of labor in case of intrauterine fetal death. The most frequently used regimen is 400 µg vaginally every 4 hours up to a maximum of six doses. However this is an off label use and should be tried only when the conventional methods have failed.[4]
- It is used for cervical ripening and induction of labor for a viable fetus, 25 micrograms of vaginal misoprostol every 4-6 hours up to a maximum of six doses can be given. However this is an off label use, there is risk of fetal distress and uterine rupture and the patient should be properly counseled before its use.[4]
- It may also be used for prevention of PPH in dose of 800 µg per rectally and for treatment of PPH, 1000 micrograms rectally.[1,5]

Contraindication: It should not be used in patients with allergy to misoprostol, during pregnancy and lactation.

Side effects: It cause nausea, vomiting and diarrhea. Patient may have fever with chills and may have uterine cramps.

Monitoring: Patient on misoprostol should be carefully monitored for any side effects like diarrhea and fever which may require medication. Risk of rupture is always more as compared to oxytocin since it causes very strong uterine contraction. There should always be high index of suspicion and the patient should be under close watch for this complication.

Preparations

- Misoprost—25, 100, 200 and 600 mcg tablet
- Zitotec—200 mcg tablet

- Prestakind—200 mcg tablet
- Cytolog—25, 100, 200 mcg tablet

Safety during pregnancy and lactation: It is contradicted for use during pregnancy and it is FDA category X drug.

The DCGI has not approved misoprostol for use beyond 63 days of pregnancy and any use for termination of pregnancy beyond this limit is off-label use.

Carboprost Tromethamine

It is a synthetic analog of PGF2 alpha.

Pharmacology: It acts directly on the myometrium and directly stimulates uterine contractions but this has not been completely established. Because of its effect on smooth muscles of lungs, vasculature and gastrointestinal tract it may cause bronchospasm, rise in blood pressure and diarrhea.

Indications

- It is used in treatment of postpartum hemorrhage caused by uterine atony and not controlled by other medical methods.[1,5]
- Also used in termination of pregnancy during 2nd trimester.

Contraindications

- Severe cardiovascular, renal and hepatic disease.
- Hypersensitivity to prostaglandins.
- Exert caution in asthmatic patients.

Dose: Injection carboprost in a dose 250 mcg IM, can be repeated every 15 minutes and maximum dose of up to 8 doses can be given.

It can be given intramyometrial during cesarean section.

It is never given intravenously.

Adverse effects: These are nausea vomiting, diarrhea, hypotension, arrhythmia, dyspnea, chest pain, headache, paresthesia, syncope, weakness, dizziness.

Monitoring: Patient on carboprost also should be carefully monitored for any side effects such as diarrhea and fever which may require medication. Risk of rupture is always more as compared to oxytocin since it is also very effective in causing uterine contraction. There should always be high risk of suspicion and patient should be under close watch for this complication.

Preparations

- Prostadon—injection 125 mcg per mL in 0.5 mL vial, 250 mcg per mL in 1 mL vial
- Deviprost—250 mcg per injection
- Evacarb—125, 250 mcg per injection.

Safety during pregnancy and lactation: It belongs to FDA category C.

REFERENCES

1. WHO recommendations for the prevention of postpartum hemorrhage. Geneva: World Health Organization; 2007.
2. Liabsuetrakul T, Choobun T, Peeyananjarassri K. Prophylactic use of ergot alkaloids in the third stage of labour. Cochrane Database Syst Rev. 2007;18(2)CD005456.
3. Tang J, Kapp N, Dragoman M, de Souza JP. WHO recommendations for misoprostol use for obstetric and gynecologic indications. Int J Gynaecol Obstet. 2013;121(2):186-9.
4. Goldberg AB, Greenberg MB, Darney PD. Misoprostol and pregnancy. N Engl J Med. 2001; 344(1):38-47.
5. Gülmezoglu AM, Forna F, Villar J, Hofmeyr GJ. Prostaglandins for preventing postpartum haemorrhage. Cochrane Database of Systematic Reviews 2007;Issue 4.

CHAPTER 15

Galactagogues and Lactation Suppressants

Nalini Bala, Tanvi Raj

INTRODUCTION

Drugs which safely and effectively promote or suppress lactation are few and enumerated in **Table 15.1**.

Galactagogues

Galactagogue is a medication that helps in promoting lactation or increasing breast milk production if it is inadequate. Prior to prescribing galactagogues one should try to find out the cause of lactation failure as various conditions may not require any medical treatment.

- There could be adequate milk production but poor milk extraction, which can be improved by educating mother about proper latching technique and correcting anatomical abnormalities like retracted nipples.
- Stop medications that suppress milk production for example, Combined oral contraceptive pills, ergot derivatives, etc.

Table 15.1: Drugs which modify lactation

Galactagogue	Metoclopramide Domperidone
Lactation suppressants	Cabergolin Pyridoxine (vitamin B_{12})

- Exclusive breast feeding on demand, at least 10–12 times a day.
- Proper emptying of breast with each feed. Mother advised to feed on one breast till it is empty and only then switch over to other side.
- Improving general condition and nutrition of mother.

Metoclopramide and domperidone are being used as galactagogues, but these medications are not approved for this use and such use is considered as "off-label use".[1]

Metoclopramide

Pharmacology: Prolactin, the most important galactopoietic hormone is regulated by the presence of prolactin-inhibiting factor (dopamine). Metoclopramide is a dopamine receptor antagonist and works by blocking D2 receptors in anterior pituitary, resulting in an increase in prolactin levels. Studies have shown it can increase milk production by an average of 60%.[2]

Metoclopramide is rapidly and well absorbed when given orally. It is metabolized in liver and eliminated in the urine.

Indications of use: It is commonly used to treat nausea, vomiting and gastroesophageal reflux disease. Increasing breast milk secretion is an additional benefit of the drug.

Contraindications: It is contraindicated in patients with pheochromocytoma, suspected bowel obstruction, epilepsy, bowel surgery in past 3–4 day or history of intestinal perforation or obstruction.

It is to be used with caution in patients with Parkinson's disease and patients with clinical depression as it may worsen their condition.

Dosage

For promoting lactation: 10 mg orally, three times a day for up to 3 weeks (off label use).

For nausea and vomiting: 10 mg orally up to three times a day depending upon severity of symptoms. For acute and severe symptoms parenteral dose (IM or IV) 10–20 mg given slowly over 1–2 minutes, can be repeated up to 3 times a day.

For GI reflux disease: 10–15 mg orally up to 4 times a day, 30 minutes before meals, and maximum duration of therapy is 12 weeks.

Adverse drug reaction: Common side effects include tiredness, diarrhea and restlessness (akathisia). Due to its ability to penetrate the blood-brain barrier, metoclopramide can cause central nervous system side-effects such as depression, involuntary body movements (tardive dyskinesia), neuroleptic malignant syndrome, extrapyramidal side effects like oculogyric crisis. Infrequently it can cause hypertension, hypotension, headache, agranulocytosis, supraventricular tachycardia, and hyperaldosteronism.

These side effects are seen only with prolonged usage. It is thus rarely recommended to take the medication for longer than twelve weeks. Side effects have been observed more frequently in women and more so during pregnancy and lactation so prolonged use for more than three weeks should be avoided. Extrapyramidal side effects are more common when high doses are given intravenously for treating chemotherapy induced vomiting. If acute dystonia occurs then 50 mg diphenhydramine can be given.

Drug interaction: Additive sedative effects can occur when used with alcohol, sedatives, hypnotics or narcotics. It releases catecholamines and should be used cautiously in patients receiving MAO inhibitors as it can cause hypertensive crisis. Absorption of some drugs from the stomach may be diminished (e.g. digoxin) by metoclopramide, whereas the rate and/or extent of absorption of drugs from the small bowel may be increased (e.g. acetaminophen, levodopa, ethanol, cyclosporine). As it influences the delivery of food to the intestines and thus the rate of absorption, insulin dosage or timing of dosage may require adjustment.

Monitoring: No specific monitoring is required for short term use. Patient taking long term therapy should be monitored for side effects.

Preparations

Perinorm: Tablet 10 mg, injection 5 mg per mL available in 2 mL vial.

Reglan: Tablets 5 mg, 5 mg per mL available as 2 mL vial.

Safety during pregnancy and lactation: It is FDA Category B drug.

DCGI approval: It is not approved for use as a galactagogue.

Domperidone

Pharmacology: Domperidone is another dopamine receptor antagonist which can be used as an alternative to metoclopramide for enhancing lactation. It has similar mechanism of action but unlike metoclopramide, domperidone does not cross the blood-brain barrier and does not tend to cause drowsiness, depression and other neurological side effect.

Indication of use: In the United States, domperidone is not approved for use as galactagogue.[3,4] By contrast, Australian guidelines consider domperidone to be the preferred galactagogue when nonpharmacological approaches have been proved to be insufficient.[5] The American Academy of Pediatrics has rated domperidone as "usually compatible with breastfeeding."

A study called the EMPOWER trial has been designed to assess the effectiveness and safety of domperidone in assisting mothers of preterm babies to supply breast milk for their infants.

Contraindications: It should be avoided if the mother or infant has a cardiac disorder as it can prolong QT interval. It is also contraindicated in patients with intestinal obstruction or those with prolactin secreting tumors.

Dosage

As galactagogue: 10–20 mg orally, 3–4 times a day (maximum up to 80 mg/day) for up to 3 weeks.

Nausea and vomiting: 10–20 mg, orally 3–4 times a day for a maximum of 80 mg daily.

Gastrointestinal motility disorder: 10 mg oral, 3–4 times a day, 30 minutes prior to meals.

Adverse drug reaction: It can cause dry mouth, skin rash, itching, headache, abdominal cramps, drowsiness, prolongation of QT interval or arrhythmias.

Drug interaction: It interacts with drugs known to affect the QT interval, e.g. ketoconazole or erythromycin.

Monitoring: No monitoring is required for short term use. Renal functions and ECG to be monitored in patients on prolonged treatment or those predisposed to QT prolongation.

Preparation

- *Domstal*: 5, 10 mg tablets
- *Motilium*: 10 mg tablet
- *Avomit*: 5, 10 mg tablets
- *Dolium*: 5, 10 mg tablets

Safety during pregnancy and lactation: There are no reports of any adverse effects in the breastfed infants and it is a FDA category C.[6]

DCGI/FDA approval: It is not approved for use as a galactagogue by FDA.

Other Drugs which May Increase Lactation

Some antipsychotics such as risperidone, chlorpromazine and sulpiride.[7,8]

Hormones such as oxytocin, growth hormone, thyrotropin releasing hormone and medroxyprogesterone acetate.[7,8]

Various herbal remedies, including milk thistle and fenugreek, have been suggested to improve poor milk supply. However, there is insufficient evidence of safety or efficacy to recommend such use.

Various granules and powders to enhance lactation are available in market for example, lactare granules, lactonic granules, etc. which contain *Asparagus* and cumin as the main ingredient apart from several other herbal components. The efficacy and side effects of these supplements are not well studied.

None of these drugs are recommended for use for lactation promotion.

Lactation Suppressant

Many pharmacological and nonpharmacological methods have been attempted to suppress lactation, but there is no evidence-based guidance on the most effective approach although pharmacological and nonpharmacological measures appear to be better than no treatment at all.[9] Most of them act by reducing prolactin. For this reason they only work in the early stages of lactation when prolactin levels are high. They are much less effective if used after weeks or months of breastfeeding.

Cabergolin and pyridoxine are two commonly used and safe drugs for lactation suppression.

Cabergoline

Pharmacology: Cabergoline is a dopamine ergoline derivative, with potent and long-lasting prolactin-lowering activity which inhibits breast milk production.[10]

Indications of use: Lactation suppression is desired in mothers who have had still birth or neonatal death. Certain other conditions may sometimes require lactation suppression like if mother has acute febrile conditions or is critically ill, in HIV positive woman if she desires not to breastfeed the baby, in cases of breast abscess, open cases of tuberculosis and if woman is on antithyroid or anticancer drugs.

Some conditions of baby desire stopping of breastfeeding and lactation suppression. For example, in cases of breast milk jaundice, cleft lip or palate and metabolic disorders like galactosemia, etc.

Contraindications: It should not be given if there is hypersensitivity to the drug or any other ergot alkaloids, pre-eclampsia or postpartum hypertension. It is also contraindicated in patients with history of pulmonary or pericardial fibrotic disorder, severe hepatic insufficiency, history of postpartum psychosis and Raynaud syndrome.

Dosage

Prevention of onset of lactation: 1 mg as a single dose given on the first day postpartum, preferably within the first 12 hours of birth.

Established lactation suppression: 0.25 mg every 12 hours for 2 days for a total of 1 mg.

Adverse effects: Headache, dizziness, fatigue, orthostatic hypotension, nose bleed and hypertension.

Drug interactions: It interacts with antiemetics commonly used in the postpartum period. Other dopamine antagonists such as metoclopramide, the phenothiazines, butyrophenones and thioxanthines when used with it may reduce its prolactin lowering effects. There may be aggravation of symptoms of psychosis when used with antipsychotic medications.

Monitoring: Patient is monitored for development of any side effects.

Preparation
- *Caberlin*: 0.25, 0.5, 1 mg tablets
- *Cabgolin*: 0.5 mg tablets
- *Parcar*: 1 mg tablets

Safety during pregnancy and lactation: It is FDA category B, however contraindicated during lactation.

DCGI/FDA approval: It is not approved for use as lactation suppressant.

Pyridoxine (Vitamin B_6)

Pharmacology: The exact mechanism is not known but pyridoxal phosphate promotes conversion of preformed DOPA to Dopamine by acting as a co-enzyme. High doses of pyridoxine may help suppress lactation but studies are inconclusive.[11]

Indications of use
- Lactation suppression
- Pyridoxine deficiency.

Contraindications: Allergy to Pyridoxine.

Dosage: No specific dose regimen is documented for this indication but the usual regimen includes 200 mg orally thrice daily for 4 days followed by 100 mg thrice daily for 3 days.

Adverse drug reaction: It can cause allergic reactions, drowsiness, numbness and tingling of feet and around mouth, decreased sensation of touch, temperature and vibration.

Drug interaction: Pyridoxine decreases the effectiveness phenytoin.

Monitoring: Patient should be closely for monitored for side effects.

Preparation: B long—100 mg pyridoxine sustained release tablets.

Safety during pregnancy and lactation: FDA category C.

Various other Drugs Used in Past for Lactation Suppression

Estrogen alone or in combination with androgen and/or progestogens.

Dopaminergic drugs (bromocriptine lisuride).

Antiserotonergic drugs (cyproheptadine, methysergide and metergoline).

Clomiphene, pyridoxine, prostaglandin E2, frusemide, 2-mercaptopropionylglycine.

Estrogens alone or in combination with androgens show variable effectiveness and are indirectly associated with high percentage for lactation rebound, thrombosis, or pulmonary embolism or both of the later during puerperium.

Bromocriptine was used in past but has been implicated in serious puerperal complications such as cerebral accident, myocardial infarction and thromboemblic complications. Bromocriptine is associated with lactation rebound in 18–40%. In 1989, the United States Food and Drug Administration recommended against the routine use of bromocriptine for suppression of postpartum lactation, noting that while there was no clear proof of adverse effects, there were also no proven health benefits.

REFERENCES

1. National health services, UK. Drug treatment for inadequate lactation. March 2012. *www.evidence.nhs.uk.*
2. Gabay M. Galactogogues: medicatons that induce lactation. J Hum Lact. 2002;18(3):274-9.
3. Da Silva OP, Knoppert DC. "Domperidone for lactating women". CMAJ. 2004;171(7):725-6.
4. FDA warns against women using unapproved drug, domperidone to increase milk production." US Food and Drug Administration 7 June 2004.
5. Amir LH, Pirotta MV, Raval M. "Breastfeeding—evidence based guidelines for the use of medicines". Aust Fam Physician. 2011;40(9): 684-90.
6. US National Library of Medicine Drugs and Lactation Database (Lactmed)—*http://toxnet.nlm.nih.gov.*
7. Donovan TJ, Buchanan K. Medications for increasing milk supply in mothers expressing breastmilk for their preterm hospitalised infants. Cochrane Database Syst Rev. 2012.pp.14-3.
8. Anderson PO, Valdes V. A critical review of pharmaceutical galactagogues. Breastfeed Med. 2007;2:229-42.
9. Oladapo OT, Fawole B. Treatments for suppression of lactation. Cochrane Database of Systematic Reviews. 2009, Issue 1 Art. No.: CD005937.
10. Bracco PL, Armentano G, Pellegrini A, Sugliano GC, Tornatore GP. Cabergoline in the inhibition of lactogenesis and suppression of lactopoiesis. Minerva Ginecol. 1997;49(10):469-73.
11. Scaglione D, Vecchione A. Pyridoxine for the suppression of lactation-a clinical trial on 1592 cases. Acta Vitaminol Enzymol. 1982;4(3): 207-14.

CHAPTER 16

Preterm Labor

Reva Tripathi, Meenoo S

INTRODUCTION

Preterm birth is a significant cause of perinatal morbidity and mortality. The annual incidence of preterm birth is approximately 10%. Preterm labor is responsible for 85% of perinatal morbidity and mortality.[1] Not too many drugs are used in preterm labor as the most common cause is idiopathic **(Table 16.1)**.

Table 16.1: Drugs used in preterm labor

Therapeutic	Maternal aspect	Progesterone
		Tocolytic therapy
	Fetal-corticosteroids aspect	
Prophylactic	Progesterone	

Maternal Aspect Drugs

Progesterone

Progesterone is used in prevention of preterm labor as it causes uterine muscle quiescence.

Pharmacology: Progesterone has been extensively studied and found to act at various levels detailed below:

Myometrium and cervix: Progesterone differentially regulates expression of 2 major isoforms viz progesterone receptor (PR)-A and PR-B. At term, there is alteration of PR-A/PR-B ratio that favors myometrial contractility and cervical effacement.2 It also alters the expression of PR coactivators and histone acetylation within myometrial cells, which are key regulators of myometrial contractility. Further it interferes with oxytocin binding and signalling in a nongenomic fashion by binding with transmembrane oxytocin receptor.3

Placenta: It interferes with cortisol-mediated regulation of placental gene expression. The most important result of this is increase in corticotropin releasing hormone (CRH)4 which thereby regulates the timing of labor.

Amniotic fluid: It increases endogenous inhibitor of phospholipase A2 thereby decreasing the availability of arachidonic acid5 which ultimately leads to decreased production of prostaglandins.

The half-life of vaginal progesterone is 13 hours. It has high bioavailability.

The half-life of injectable 17-HPC is 7 days.

Indications

- Women with previous history of preterm delivery.[6]
- Asymptomatic women with short cervical length of less than 16 mm in routine ultrasound done in 2nd trimester between 20 and 24 weeks.[6]

Contraindications

- Current or past history of thrombophlebitis, thromboembolic disorders or cerebral apoplexy.
- Liver dysfunction or disease.
- Known or suspected malignancy of breast or genital organs.

Dosage

- In cases of prior spontaneous preterm birth, injection 17-hydroxyprogesterone caproate 250 mg IM is given weekly from 16–20 weeks through 36 weeks.[7]
- In patients with short cervical length, progesterone suppository of 90–200 mg vaginally is advised since diagnosis through 36 weeks.[8]

Adverse Drug Reactions

Common side effects include fatigue, headache, malaise.

Preparations

- Micronized progesterone that can be used either orally or intravaginally (Preparations—Nidagen, Susten, Endogest, Wisrone)
- Injectable 17-hydroxyprogesterone caproate (HPC) (injection proluton depot, HPC depot, proguard, uniprogestin depot 250 or 500 mg).

Progesterone is not recommended in multiple gestation as it neither prolongs gestation nor improves perinatal outcome.[9]

Tocolytic Therapy

Medications to suppress premature uterine contractions. These drugs **(Flow chart 16.1)** are generally used for short-term for transfer of patients to centers where NICU facilities are available. Generally tocolytics are given for a period of about 48–72 hours to enable a steroid cover for the baby as it improves lung maturation and most of the tocolytics have their respective side effects if used more than 48 hours. The evidences if tocolytic drugs improve perinatal outcome or if whether they are associated with reduction in perinatal morbidity and mortality are not very clear. So tocolysis must be mainly advised in women who are in very preterm labor and those needing transfer to a hospital with NICU facilities or to complete steroid course.

Flow chart 16.1 Commonly used tocolytic drugs

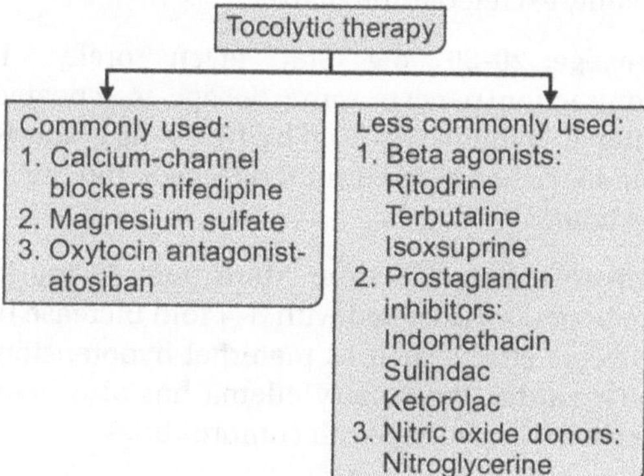

Contraindications

- Chorioamnionitis/sepsis.
- Significant antepartum hemorrhage.[10]
- Cervical dilatation > 4 cm.
- Placental insufficiency.
- Pre-eclampsia/eclampsia.
- Congenital malformation/Intrauterine fetal demise.

Calcium-channel Blockers

Of all the calcium-channel blockers (CCBs), nifedipine is most widely used as it is safe and effective and is better tolerated and has fewer side effects. It is the recommended first-line tocolytic agent.[11]

Pharmacology: Voltage-gated Ca^{++} channels (VGCCs) mediate the Ca^{++} influx in response to membrane depolarization and regulate intracellular processes. Ca^{++} binds to calmodulin and activates the enzyme myosin light chain kinase (MLCK) in the myometrial cells and therefore leads to the phosphorylation of serine 19 on myosin light chains which initiates subsequent cross-bridge cycling and subsequent myometrial contraction. Nifedipine blocks these voltage gated L type calcium channel.[12]

The half-life of nifedipine is 8 hours. It is mainly excreted through liver.

Dosage: 20–30 mg stat given orally. If contraction persists same dosage is repeated after 30 minutes followed by 10–20 mg 6 hourly for 48–72 hours. Maximum dosage is 160 mg in 24 hours.

Adverse drug reaction: More than 60 mg in 24 hours is associated with 3–4 fold increase in adverse effects such as maternal hypotension, tachycardia. Pulmonary edema has also been reported in patients with comorbidities.

Monitoring: Pulse rate should be checked before every dosage and if more than 120/min dosage should be withheld.

Contraindications: Cardiac disease, renal disease, tachycardia >120 bpm, BP <100/60, SpO_2 <95%.

Caution

Nifedipine should never be used with magnesium because it enhances neuromuscular blocking effects and interferes with pulmonary and cardiac function.[13]

Preparations: Depin, Nicardia retard, nifedine, depicor.

Magnesium Sulfate

Pharmacology: It suppresses intracellular calcium influx by inhibiting myosin light chain kinase activity. Magnesium competes for the binding site with calcium on the sarcoplasmic reticulum and thus reduces intracellular calcium. Magnesium also increases cGMP (cyclic guanosine monophosphate), and thus causes muscle relaxation.[14]

The onset of action is immediate in IV administration and lasts for 30 minutes. It is excreted only through kidneys.

Contraindications: Myasthenia gravis is an absolute contraindication,[15] while heart disease and renal disease are relative contraindications.

Dosage: 4 g bolus IV followed by 2 g/hr infusion for 24 hours.

Adverse drug reaction: Flushing, pulmonary edema, nausea, headache, blurring of vision, respiratory distress.

Toxicity: While giving magnesium sulfate, monitoring of serum levels is suggested but need not be necessarily done. The **Table 16.2** shows various serum levels of magnesium and its consequences.

Preparations

Injection solution 4% (elemental magnesium 0.325 mEq/L).

Injection solution concentrate 8% (elemental magnesium 0.65 mEq/L).

Injection solution concentrate 50% (elemental magnesium 4 mEq/mL).

Chloromag, Epsom salt, Sulfamag.

Some workers have claimed it is not effective in preterm birth and has no apparent advantages over other tocolytics.[16] On the other

Table 16.2: Serum levels of magnesium and its various effects

Effects	*Serum levels of magnesium*
Normal	0.8–1 mmol/L
Therapeutic levels	1.7–3.5 mmol/L
Prolonged PR interval and wide QRS	2.5–5 mmol/L
Loss of tendon reflexes	5–7.49 mmol/L
Respiratory paralysis	7.5–11.9 mmol/L
Cardiac arrest	≥12 mmol/L

hand, some authors believe that magnesium sulfate used as tocolytic in early preterm labor also seems to have an effect on neurocognitive development of the baby by reducing the risks of cerebral palsy.[17] The opinion of magnesium sulfate being ineffective in preterm birth might change in future.

Oxytocin Antagonist

As the name suggests, this is most physiological and logical drug that is available in western countries for prevention of preterm labor but is yet to be available in India.

Atosiban is a synthetic nonapeptide.

Pharmacology: It downregulates oxytocin receptors and inhibits uterotonic action in a competitive and dosage dependent manner by inhibiting the oxytocin-mediated release of inositol triphosphate from the myometrial cell membrane. As a result, there is reduced release of intracellular, stored calcium from the sarcoplasmic reticulum of myometrial cells, and reduced influx of Ca^{++} from the extracellular space through voltage-gated channels. In addition, It also suppresses oxytocin-mediated release of PGE and PGF from the decidua.[18] These actions lead to decreased myometrial contractility. The half-life of atosiban is 18 minutes.

Dosage: 6.75 mg IV stat over one minute followed by an infusion of 18 mg/hr for 3 hours and then 6 mg/hr for up to 45 hours. Total duration not more than 48 hours and total dosage not more than 330 mg.[19]

Effect: It decreases contractions by 75% in 3 hrs.

Adverse drug reaction: Common side effects include tachycardia, palpitations, hypotension, chest pain, dyspnea, vomiting, headache.

Contraindications: Hepatic and renal disorder.

Preparations: Tractocile, antocin.

Prostaglandin Inhibitors (Cox-2 Inhibitors)

It is well known that prostaglandins are used in induction of labor and termination of pregnancy by softening the cervix by stimulating gap-junctions and sensitizing the myometrium for oxytocin, thereby leading to a progressive cervical dilatation.[20]

Cyclooxygenase 2 (COX-2) is an enzyme which converts arachidonic acid to prostaglandin H_2. Indomethacin, Sulindac and Ketorolac **(Table 16.3)** are inhibitors of COX-2 and thereby cause decreased production of prostaglandins and hence cause decreased myometrial contractility.

Beta Agonists

These compounds act on beta 2 receptors in myometrial cell membrane and cause increase in cGMP and inhibit myosin light chain kinase **Table 16.4**.

Nitric Oxide Donors

Nitroglycerine

Pharmacology: Forms free radical (nitric oxide) which activates the enzyme guanylate cyclase resulting in increased GMP in smooth muscle and other tissues. This causes dephosphorylation of myosin light chain kinase, which is responsible for the contractility of smooth muscle and thus acts as smooth muscle relaxant of vessels, gut and uterus.

Route of administration: Sublingual, transdermal, intravenous.

The serum half-life of transdermal nitroglycerine is 3 minutes. It undergoes mainly hepatic metabolism.

Contraindications: Obstructive hypertrophic cardiomyopathy, pronounced hypovolemia, inferior myocardial infarction with right ventricular involvement, raised intracranial pressure, cardiac tamponade.

Table 16.3: Various prostaglandin inhibitors in preterm labor

Drugs	*Route*	*Dosage*	*Indication*	*Side effects*	*Contraindications*
Indomethacin (Preparations—Indmecin, Indocid SR, Inocin)	Oral, rectal	50 to 100 mg followed by 25–50 mg every 4–6 hours for maximum of 14 days. Max 200 mg/day	Mostly indicated in preterm labor associated with polyhydramnios. (it requires serial monitoring of AFI)	Premature closure of ductus arteriosus, oligo (as it causes reversible decrease in renal function), increased incidence of respiratory distress, bronchopulmonary dysplasia	1. Peptic ulcer 2. Drug-induced asthma 3. Coagulation disorders
Sulindac (Preparations—Lindac, Sulidac, Sulin)	Oral	200 mg OD or BD for 24–48 hrs.			
Ketorolac (Preparations—Cadolac, Kelac, Ketlac, Ketorol)	Intramuscular	60 mg IM followed by 30 mg IM every 6 hours for 24–48 hours.			

Table 16.4: Beta agonists in preterm labor

Drugs	*Route*	*Dosage*	*Side effects*	*Contraindications*
Ritodrine (Preparations—Ritolan, Ritodin, Ritopar UR, Tocopar, Utodin)	Intravenous/ Oral	50 µg/min and increase every 20 min to a maximum of 350 µg/min for 48–72 hours	Tachycardia, palpitations, headache, hyperglycemia, maternal hallucinations, pulmonary edema (causes retention of sodium and water)	Diabetes, cardiac disease, MI, hypertension
Terbutaline (Preparations—Asmaterb, Bricanyl, Brontline, Tetrasma)	Oral SC IV	2.5 mg–5 mg every 4–6 hrs for 48–72 hours 250 µg SC every 20–30 min 4–6 dosages for 48–72 hours 5–10 µg/min increased every 10–15 min to a max of 80 µg/min for 48 hours	Hyperglycemia, hyperinsulinemia, tremors, pulmonary edema, sudden maternal death. There is also an evidence of myocardial necrosis after long-term use. It also causes fetal tachycardia, fetal hyperglycemia, hyperinsulinemia	
Isoxsuprine[21] (Preparations—Duvadilan, Adilin, Bioprin, Dulovas)	Oral IV/IM	10–20 mg every 6 hours for 48 hours 200–500 mcg/min IV infusion till control is achieved then 10 mg IM injection every 8 hourly for one week	Same as other beta 2 agonists	

Dosage: 100 µg bolus IV followed by 1 µg/kg/min. In general, IV is not preferred as it is neither superior nor effective compared to other tocolytics and is associated with more side effects of which the most common is maternal hypotension. So the preferred route is 50 µg for 24 hours as transdermal patch. Transdermal nitroglycerin is found to be more effective than β2-adrenergic receptor agonists though there is no current evidence to support its routine use as a tocolytic agent for the treatment of preterm labor. Further trials are needed.[22]

It is unclear if a combination of multiple tocolytic agents with different modes of action are for more advantageous than single agent due to lack of large well-designed trials.[23]

Preparations: Nitrostat, Nitroquick, Tridil, Nitro-bid.

Fetal Aspect Drugs

Corticosteroids

Pharmacology: These drugs have no maternal role in preterm labor. They are used for the benefit that accrues to the fetal lung.

The lungs are among the last of the fetal organs to mature, a process that involves the formation of surface-active phospholipids (surfactants) in the alveolar spaces.[24] In the mature fetal lung, the surfactants reduce the surface tension within the alveolar spaces after delivery, which allows the alveoli to stay open for gas exchange. Before delivery, the surfactants are released into the amniotic fluid and are a biological marker of fetal lung maturity. Preterm delivery may result in respiratory distress syndrome due to decreased surfactant of the newborn which may have unfavorable long-term outcomes.

Mechanism of action: Corticosteroids stimulate the pulmonary beta receptors and help in synthesis and release of surfactants into the alveolar spaces.[24]

Indications

- Generally used in patients with period of gestation less than 34 weeks in active labor or with threatened preterm labor.
- PPROM with patients less than POG 34 weeks.[25]
- In patients with fetal growth restriction between 24 and 35 + 6 weeks.
- In all elective cesarean sections done before 38 + 6 weeks.

Contraindications: Chorioamnionitis, sepsis.

Dosage: Injection dexamethasone 6 mg IM per dosage, a total of 4 dosages given 12 hours apart is used.

Injection betamethasone 12 mg per dosage, a total of 2 dosages given 24 hours apart is used.

If the patient is in active labor, delivery should preferably be delayed as long as possible with tocolytics so as to give adequate time for effect of steroids on fetus.

There has been much debate whether fetal outcomes are better with dexamethasone or betamethasone. According to UN commission, both dexa and betamethasone are similar based on efficacy and safety. Betamethasone and Dexamethasone have no significant difference in reducing perinatal morbidity and mortality however dexamethasone shows less incidence of intraventricular hemorrhage and shorter NICU stay.[26,27]

The recommended formulation of betamethasone should be a mixture of long acting betamethasone acetate and fast acting betamethasone phosphate which is not available in India. The available salt in India is betamethasone phosphate which is only short acting and this salt of betamethasone has no added advantage over dexamethasone sodium phosphate. Further betamethasone is more costly and less stable at higher temperatures and dexamethasone sodium phosphate is easily available in India and is 20 times cheaper compared to betamethasone.[28,29] So the preferred corticosteroid is dexamethasone especially in Indian scenario.

Repeated courses: Refers to administration of repeated courses of glucocorticoid dosage when delivery becomes imminent or more than 7 days have elapsed since previous course. It is not recommended as there is increased risks of respiratory distress and evidence of small reduction in size at birth.[30]

Preparations: Decadron, Dexasone, Dexona, Dexicol.

REFERENCES

1. Norwitz ER, Caughey AB. Progesterone supplementation and prevention of preterm birth. Rev Obstet Gynecol. 2011;4(2):60-72.
2. Oh SY, Kim CJ, Park I, et al. Progesterone receptor isoform (A/B) ratio of human fetal membranes increases during term parturition. Am J Obstet Gynecol. 2005; 193: 1156-60.
3. Grazzini E, Guillon G, Mouillac B, Zingg HH. Inhibition of oxytocin receptor function by direct binding of progesterone. Nature. 1998;392:509-12.
4. Karalis K, Goodwin G, Majzoub JA. Cortisol blockade of progesterone: a possible molecular mechanism involved in the initiation of human labor. Nat Med. 1996;2:556-60.
5. Norwitz ER, Wilson T. Secretory component: a potential regulator of endometrial-decidual prostaglandin production in early human pregnancy. Am J Obstet Gynecol. 2000;183:108-17.
6. Dan Farine, Mundle WR, Jodie Dodd. The Use of Progesterone for prevention of preterm birth. SOGC technical update. No. 202, Jan 2008.
7. ACOG Committee Opinion number 419 October 2008 (replaces no. 291, November 2003). Use of progesterone to reduce preterm birth. Society for Maternal Fetal Medicine Publications Committee. Obstet Gynecol. 2008;112(4):963-5.
8. Hassan SS, Romero R, Vidyadhari D, et al. for the pregnant Trial. Vaginal progesterone reduces the rate of preterm birth in women with a sonographic short cervix: a multicenter, randomized, double-blind, placebo-controlled trial. Ultrasound Obstet Gynecol. 2011;38:18-31.
9. Meis PJ, Klebanoff M, Thom E, et al. National Institute of Child Health and Human Development Maternal-Fetal Medicine Units Network. Prevention of recurrent preterm delivery by 17 alpha-hydroxyprogesterone caproate. N Engl J Med. 2003;348:2379-85.
10. Clinical practice guideline for tocolytic treatment in pregnancy. Royal College of Physicians of Ireland.
11. Brown RG, MacIntyre DA. CCB are effective as first line tocolysis in management of preterm labor. Evid Based Med. 2014; 19:214.
12. Wray S, Jones K, Kupittayanant S, Li Y, Matthew A, Monir-Bishty E, Noble K, Pierce SJ, Quenby S, Shmygol AV. Calcium signaling and uterine contractility. J Soc Gynecol Investig. 2003;10:252–264. doi: 10.1016/S1071-5576(03)00089-3.
13. Jorgensen JS, Weile LK, Lamont RF. Preterm labor: Current tocolytic options for the treatment of preterm labor. Expert Opin Pharmacother. 2014;15(5):585-8.
14. Fawcett WJ, Haxby EJ, Male DA. Magnesium: Physiology and pharmacology. Br J Anaesth. 1999;83(2):302-20.
15. American College of Obstetricians and Gynecologists (ACOG). Management of preterm labor. Washington (DC): 2003 May. 9 p. (ACOG practice bulletin; no. 43).
16. Crowther CA, Brown J, Mckinley CJ, Middleton P. Magnesium sulfate for preventing preterm birth in threatened preterm labor. Cochrane Database Syst Rev. 2014;8:CD001060.
17. Magee l, Sawchuck D, Synnes A, Von Dadelszen P. SOGC Clinical Practice Guideline. Magnesium Sulfate for fetal neuroprotection. J Obstet Gynaecol Can. 2011;33(5):516-29.
18. Sanu O, Lamont RF. Critical appraisal and clinical utility of atosiban in the management of preterm labor. The Clin Risk Manag. 2010;6:191-9.
19. Tocolysis for women in preterm labor. Green top guideline No. 1b.
20. Husslein P. Causes of labor initiation in man and role of oxytocin and prostaglandins. Z Gebutshife Perinat. 1985:189(3):95-102.
21. Giorgino FL, Egan CG. Use of isoxsuprine hydrochloride as a tocolytic agent in the treatment of preterm labor: a systematic review of previous literature. Arzneimittelforschung 2010;60(7):415-20.doi:10.1055/s-0031-1296305.
22. Conde-Agudelo A, Romero R. Transdermal nitroglycerin for the treatment of preterm labor: a systematic review and metaanalysis. Am J Obstet Gynecol. 2013;209(6): 551.e1-551.e1.

23. Vogel JP, Nardin JM, Dowswell T, West HM, Oladapo OT. Combination of tocolytic agents for Preterm labor. Cochrane Database Syst Rev. 2014;11.7.CD006169.
24. American College of Obstetricians and Gynecologists. ACOG educational bulletin number 230, November 1996: assessment of fetal lung maturity. Int J Gynaecol Obstet 1997: 56:191-5.
25. Miracle X, Carlo G Di Renzo, Stark A, Fanaroff A, X. Carbonell-Estrancy, et al. Guideline for the use of antenatal corticosteroids for fetal maturation. J Perinat Med. 2008;36:191-6.
26. Brownfoot FC, Gagliardo D, Bain E, Middleton P, Crowther CA. Different Corticosteroids and regimens for accelerating fetal lung maturation for women at risk of preterm birth. Cochrane Database Syst Rev. 2013;8: CD006764.
27. Elimian A, Garry D, Fiqueroa R, Spitzer A, Wiencek V, Quirk JG. Antenatal betamethasone compared with dexamethasone (betacode trial): a randomized controlled trial. Obstet Gynecol. 2007; 110(1):26-30.
28. Dexamethasone versus Betamethasone as an antenatal corticosteroid (ACS). UN Commission/ Born too soon care Antanatal Corticosteroids Working group. August 20,2013.
29. Use of antenatal corticosteroids in preterm labour (under specific conditions by ANM). Operational guidelines, june 2014. Child health division, Ministry of health and family welfare, Government of India.
30. Crowther CA, Mckinlay CJ, Middleton P, Harding J. Repeated DOSAGEs of prenatal corticosteroids for women at risk of preterm birth for improving neonatal health outcomes. Cochrane Database Syst Rev 2011; 6: CD003935.
31. RCOG. Green top guidelines No.44; 2006. Preterm Premature rupture membranes.

Section V

DRUGS USED IN MEDICAL DISORDERS OF PREGNANCY

CHAPTERS

CHAPTER 17

Anemia

Renu Tanwar, Ankita Pal

INTRODUCTION

Anemia during pregnancy is a major problem in the low income countries. It is one of the major causes of maternal morbidity and mortality.[1-4] **Table 17.1** summarizes the drugs which are commonly used for treatment and prophylaxis of anemia during pregnancy.

Iron Therapy

Iron deficiency anemia is the most common cause of anemia during pregnancy and most common cause for iron deficiency is poor nutrition. Iron can be given orally or parentally.

Table 17.1: Drugs used in treatment of anemia during pregnancy

Type of anemia	*Drug(s)*
Iron deficiency anemia	Iron
	Folic acid
	Vitamin C
	Anthelmintics
Megaloblastic anemia	Vitamin B_{12}
	Folic acid
Anemia of chronic renal disease	Erythropoietin
Sideroblastic anemia	Pyridoxine

Oral Iron Therapy

Oral iron is treatment of choice because it is cheap, easily available and easy to administer.

Pharmacology: Ferrous sulfate form of iron is better absorbed than ferric sulfate form. Iron absorption occurs in distal duodenum and jejunum.

The absorption is facilitated by acid in stomach and situations leading to acidic medium like vitamin C ingestion. Before absorption iron gets converted to ferrous form from ferric form. Acidic medium facilitates this conversion and hence absorption.

At brush border of intestinal cells ferric gets reduced to ferrous form, which then gets transported via divalent metal transporter-1 to the cell, where it reconverts to ferric form, which binds to apotransferrin leading to formation of transferrin (transport form of iron). This complex goes to clathrin coated pits on hepatocytes and gets bound and used in heme formation. The excess iron binds to apoferritin to form ferritin (storage form of iron) and gets stored mainly in liver and bone marrow.[5]

Indications of use: It is used for prophylaxis and treatment of iron deficiency anemia during pregnancy. Patients of chronic kidney disease who are on dialysis and erythropoietin therapy also need iron supplementation.

Contraindications: Hypersensitivity, hemosiderosis, hemochromatosis, etc.

Dosage

Prophylaxis: A daily dose of 100 mg of elemental iron during pregnancy is recommended by World Health Organization (WHO) for prevention of anemia.[6]

National Iron Plus Initiative of Ministry of Health and Family Welfare, Government of India 2013, recommends 100 mg of elemental iron and 500 mcg of folic acid for 100 days during pregnancy after the first trimester (14–16 weeks) and for 100 days in postpartum period.[7]

Treatment

For treatment of anemia, 2–3 mg/kg/day or 200 mg of elemental iron is given in three divided doses. An oral tablet of 325 mg of ferrous sulfate taken thrice a day provides 195 mg iron. National Anemia Control Program (1987) recommends a dose of 100 mg of elemental iron with 500 mcg of folic acid should be taken twice a day till hemoglobin becomes normal and should be continued for another 12 weeks for iron stores to be replenished.[8]

Iron absorption is better if taken empty stomach because chemicals in food hinder its absorption and reduce its bioavailability. It should be given in divided doses and preferably before meals (2 hour before and one hour after). However, if patient does not tolerate iron, then it can be given after meals.

Delayed and extended release tablets are irrational as iron is absorbed in proximal intestine. Hence these should be avoided. Salts which have been promoted to have reduced side effects usually have lesser amount of elemental or bioavailable iron.

Adverse effects: They are usually mild. They are related to iron content of the preparation and include staining of teeth, metallic test, nausea, vomiting, heart burn, mild gastrointestinal disturbance, and constipation (astringent action), diarrhea (irritant action), discoloration of stool, etc.

At times, side effects are troublesome enough to cause intolerance and require switching over to a different salt or to a parenteral preparation.

Iron toxicity could be seen in children who have taken iron syrup in high quantity or those who have hemochromatosis, etc.

Drug interaction: Iron reduces absorption of following drugs if taken simultaneously and thus decreases their efficacy:
- Fluoroquinolones
- Penicillamine
- Tetracycline
- Methyl dopamine, levodopa
- Levothyroxine
- Bisphosphonates.

It should not be given within 2 hours of antacid administration.

Monitoring: Clinically, the effectiveness of iron therapy is best evaluated by tracking the reticulocyte response and the rise in the hemoglobin or the hematocrit. An increase in the reticulocyte count is not observed for at least 4–7 days after beginning of therapy. An increase in the hemoglobin level takes even longer. Decision regarding the effectiveness of treatment should not be made until 3–4 weeks after the start of treatment, when an increase in the hemoglobin concentration up to 2 g% is considered a positive response. There is no justification for continuing oral iron therapy beyond 3–4 weeks if a favorable response has not occurred.

The average response to oral iron is not proportional to the dose administered. **Table 17.2** shows the relation of total dose of iron and the rate of absorption and increase in hemoglobin concentration. Therefore 200–300 mg of elemental iron in two divided doses is sufficient for oral treatment of iron deficiency anemia and further increment in oral intake is not cost effective.

Poor response to oral iron therapy occurs in following conditions:
- Inappropriate choice and administration of iron preparation
- Noncompliance

- Insufficient duration of therapy
- Concurrent oral administration of inhibitors of iron absorption like antacids, H2 receptor blockers, calcium salts and phytates in food
- Co-existing vitamin B_{12} and folic acid deficiency
- Chronic inflammatory conditions
- Ongoing blood loss.

Preparation: In a review on use of iron salts, it was observed that ferrous ascorbate is better suited for Indian diet which is normally rich in inhibitors of iron absorption.[9] Various oral iron preparations available are given in **Table 17.3.**

Safety in pregnancy: Iron is safe in pregnancy. FDA category N (not classified).

Table 17.2: Average response to oral iron therapy

Total dose of iron (mg/day)	*Estimated absorption mg/day (% of oral intake)*	*Increase in hemoglobin (gm/L) per week*
35	14 (40%)	0.7
105	25 (24%)	1.4
195	35 (18%)	1.9
390	45 (12%)	2.2

Parenteral Iron

Principles of parenteral iron therapy:[10,11]

- All parenteral iron preparations are iron salts with carbohydrates.
- Reaction to one kind of iron salt increases risk of sensitivity to others, however reactions are not necessary across salts.
- Parenteral iron in plasma gets picked up by reticuloendothelial cells, where iron is separated from carbohydrate moiety and gets transported by transferring to liver, spleen and bone marrow and to erythrocyte precursor cells. Absorption, storage and rate of metabolism depend upon iron status, reserves and stores in body.
- The administration of any of available preparations can be associated with acute chestpain, bonepains without accompanying

Table 17.3: Commonly used oral iron compounds and preparations

Iron compound (mg/tab)		*Elemental iron mg/tab (% of iron compound)*	*Iron preparations*	*Specific features*
Ferrous sulfate hydrous	300	60 (20%)	Fersolate, Fesofor Z, Irosoft SR	Drug of choice
Ferrous sulfate (dried)	200	65 (32.5%)	LG Fol, Ferrito SR	
Ferrous succinate	100	35 (35%)	Ferfol	
Ferrous gluconate	300	36 (12%)	Livogen	Better tolerated
Ferrous fumarate	200	66 (33%)	Autrin, livogen	Metallic taste
Carbonyl iron	100	98 (98%)	Karion, ironifol, iron C	Elemental form
Na-feredetate	231	33 (14%)	Ewioc	
Iron hydroxide polymaltose		100	Globac PM, mumfer, hemglo	
Elemental iron		100	Ferium, ferium XT, ferobest, globac, nicofer, orofer XT	
Ferrous ascorbate		100 (13.5%)	Figo XT, lyron XT, ferri XT, livogen XT	Better absorption[9]

hypotension, wheezing, stridor or periorbital edema. With iron dextran, this usually is seen after the test dose.

Parenteral iron is administered either intramuscularly or intravenously.

Intramuscular preparations are:
- Iron sorbitrate citrate complex
- Iron dextran.

Intravenous preparations are:
- Iron sucrose
- Iron dextran
- Sodium ferric gluconate complex in sucrose.

Calculation of the Dose

Any one of the three formulae can be used:
1. 4.4 × body weight in kg × hemoglobin deficit (g/dL)
2. Body weight in kg × (desired hemoglobin *Patient's hemoglobin) × 2.21 + 1000 mg *Usually the dose is calculated by taking desired hemoglobin of 14 gm/dL
3. 250 mg of elemental iron for each gm of hemoglobin deficit and add another 50% for iron store replenishment.

For patients who are treated chronically with parenteral iron, it is important to monitor iron storage levels to avoid the serious toxicity associated with iron overload.

Iron Sorbitol Citric Acid

Pharmacology: Iron sorbitol citrate is a low molecular weight complex, hence the absorption is easy.

Difference between iron sorbitol citrate and iron dextran is given in **Table 17.4**.

Table 17.4: Differences between iron dextran and iron sorbitol citrate complex

Iron dextran (50 mg/mL)	*Iron sorbitol citrate complex (50 mg/mL)*
High molecular weight	Low molecular weight
Can be given IM or IV	Only for IM use
Absorbed through lymphatics	Directly absorbed in circulation
10-30% gets locally bound when given IM	No local binding
Does not bind to transferrin	Binds to transferrin
Taken up by macrophages and slowly distributed	Directly available for RBC formation
Does not get excreted	30% gets excreted in urine
FDA Category C	FDA Category B

Indications of use: Parenteral iron therapy is used in following conditions:
- Oral iron therapy fails or is not tolerated
- Patient is noncompliant
- After 32 weeks of gestation: ensures compliance
- Failure to absorb oral iron in malabsorption, inflammatory bowel disease, chronic inflammatory illness
- Along with erythropoietin.

Contraindications: It should be cautiously used in patients of asthma, heart disease, hemoglobinopathies, history of allergy, underweight people, etc.

Dosage: Its recommended dose is 1.5 mg/kg/day after test dose. Single daily injection of more than 2 mL is not recommended. Multiple injections are required to meet iron deficiency.

Z technique is used for intramuscular injection in the gluteus maximus. In Z technique, the skin and tissue at the injection site, is pulled and held firmly and then a long needle is inserted deep in the muscle. After injecting the drug, skin and tissues are loosened so they come back to their original position. Now when the needle is withdrawn, a track forms which is a zig-zag track. It prevents spillage of drug and discoloration of skin.

Adverse drug reaction: Because it is given intramuscularly, the patient may have pain, local irritation, flushing, swelling, staining of skin, transient metallic taste, headache, dizziness, diarrhea and abscess formation at injection site. Severe systemic side effects and anaphylactic reactions are rare but noted.

Drug interaction: Oral iron needs to be discontinued with parenteral iron as it overwhelms the iron receptor.

Monitoring: For test dose, 0.5 mL of drug is injected at site of injection using 2–3 inch long 22 G needle 1 minute before the injection.

Preparation (See Table 17.5): Jectocos—available as 1.5 mL vials, contains 50 mg/mL, stored at room temperature in shade.

Jectocos Plusavailable as 1.5 mL vial, contains iron-sorbitol-citric acid complex 75 mg, folic acid 750 mcg, vitamin B_{12} 75 mcg.

Safety during pregnancy: FDA category B drug.

Iron Dextran

Pharmacology: It is a preparation of colloidal ferric oxyhydroxide which is complexed with polymerized dextran. Iron dextran is available in two forms: high and low molecular weight iron dextran.

High molecular weight dextran was the first parenteral iron form and was used. However, it was associated with significant sensitivity reaction, which led to development of low molecular weight dextran.

All parenteral iron are metabolized in reticuloendothelial system. If intravenous dose is less than 500 mg it gets cleared within 6 hours however if dose exceeds 1 g IV as a total dose, it undergoes reticuloendothelial cell clearance at constant rate of 10–20 mg/hour. This slow clearance results in brownish discoloration of plasma for 1–2 weeks.

Indications of use: It is same as mentioned in iron sorbitol citric acid.

Contraindications: In patients suffering from chronic inflammations like history of allergies, strict vigilance is required for signs of delayed hypersensitivity. Use with extreme caution in patients with rheumatoid arthritis or other connective tissue disorder. If any signs of hypersensitivity is observed, drug should be abandoned.

Dosage: Total dose of iron requirement is calculated and 100 mg injection is given as follows:

- 100 mg elemental iron daily by deep IM injection till total dose is given
- 100 mg elemental iron daily as slow IV injection daily till total dose is given
- 100 mg elemental iron dissolved in 100 mL of NS and transfused slowly over 2–3 hours daily till total dose is given
- Total dose infusion by dissolving total iron requirement in 500 mL of normal saline and given slowly over 5–6 hours. If total dose exceeds 1500 mg, it is given in two sittings.

Adverse drug reaction: Acute anaphylactic reaction which manifests as respiratory distress, hypotension, tachycardia, chest pain, urticaria, arthralgia, lymphadenopathy, etc.[12]

Patient may have injection site pain, cellulitis, phlebitis, sterile abscess, brown skin pigmentation.

Systemic side effects include dyspnea, urticaria, itching, arthralgia, myalgia and diaphoresis. Hypersensitivity is reported to occur in 2.47%, however anaphylaxis is usually seen in less than 1% of patients. Patients may have paresthesia, headache, weakness, syncope, dyspnea, broncospasm, leucocytosis, lymphadenopathy, pancytopenia, thrombocytopenia, nausea, vomiting, diarrhea or metallic taste.

Delayed reactions may occur 1–2 days after administration of iron dextran, manifested by arthralgia, backache, myalgia, fever, chills, dizziness, headache, nausea and/or vomiting. The etiology of these reactions is unknown. Delayed reactions tended to subside within 2–7 days. More common after total dose infusion, although still may occur after intramuscular injection. The severity or frequency of delayed reactions may be reduced by lowering the dose or increasing the dosing interval.

Drug interaction: It is same as mentioned in iron sorbitol citric acid.

Monitoring

Test dose: It is given in form of 0.5 mL of undiluted iron dextran or equivalent to 25 mg of elemental iron diluted in saline. Observe the patient till one hour for immediate and any signs of hypersensitivity.

It is usually not given as intramuscular preparation due to its erratic absorption by this route. It is preferably given by intravenous route. Iron dextran is associated with more systemic complications than iron sorbitol. Absorption of iron dextran occurs over a period of 3-4 weeks.

Preparation: Dexferrin, dexferrum, INFeD—available as 2 mL vial and contain 50 mg elemental iron/mL **(Table 17.6)**.

Iron Sucrose

Pharmacology

Indications of use: It is currently the most commonly used iron preparation. It has low molecular weight hence of better use in patients on hemodialysis.[13,14]

Contraindications: Hypersensitivity, hemosiderosis, hemochromatosis, etc.

Dosage: Single max dose is 200 mg and can be repeated up to 3 doses per week.

It can be given undiluted as IV bolus of 1 mL/min with maximum dose of 100 mg over 5 minutes. It can also be given in dilution with normal saline however the concentration should not be less than 1 mg/mL. This diluted form remains stable up to 7 days. The solution is infused over a period of 20 minutes with initial 20-25 mL as slow infusion to observe for reactions.

Adverse drug reaction

Common: Change in taste, nausea, vomiting diarrhea, muscle cramps, pain in arms and legs, burning sensation at injection site.

Less common: Body ache, abdominal pain. Patient may develop hypotension or hypertension.

Drug interaction: Oral iron should be discontinued before starting parenteral preparation.

Monitoring: No test dose is required, sensitivity reactions are less common, although serious hypersensitivity and anaphylactic reactions have been noticed.

Preparation: Venofer, xenofer, hemofer—available as 5 mL ampoule and contains 20 mg elemental iron/mL.

Safety during pregnancy: FDA category B. It should be avoided in first trimester and can be given later if absolutely indicated.

FDA Approval: Iron sucrose is FDA approved.

Administration guidelines for parental iron preparation is given in **Table 17.5.**

Sodium Ferric Gluconate Complex

Iron gluconate is preferred intravenous iron preparation in patients of chronic kidney disease who are on dialysis. It can be safely administered to patients who are sensitive to iron dextran.[15-17]

The recommended route of administration is by intravenous injection or infusion. The rate of administration should not exceed 12.5 mg per minute so a standard dose of 125 mg may be administered over 10 minutes. It is available as 5 mL ampoule and each ampoule contains 62.5 mg of iron. 10 mL of solution is diluted in 100 mL normal saline to make 12.5 mg/mL of infusion which is given over 60 minutes. It does not require a test dose.

The common intravenous iron preparations are summarized in **Table 17.6.**

Newer Injectable Iron Preparations[19]

Ferric Carboxymaltose

Ferric carboxymaltose is first of newer agents which is approved for rapid administration of large doses. It is approved for use in Europe and Asia.

It is given in infusion and not more than 1000 mg is given in single dose.

Multiple studies are going on and several have proven it to be safe in patients with chronic heart disease, on dialysis and with iron intolerance.

Table 17.5: Administration guidelines for commonly used parental iron preparations[18]			
	Iron dextran (low molecular weight)	*Iron sucrose*	*Iron gluconate*
Concentration	50 mg/mL (2 mL vial)	20 mg/mL (5 mL vial)	12.5 mg/mL (5 mL ampoule)
Maximum infusion rate	50 mg/min	20 mg/min	12.5 mg/min
Test dose	Required on first infusion	Not mandatory	Not mandatory
Mode of test dose	25 mg slow IV	25 mg slow IV	25 mg slow IV or 25 mg in 50 mL of NS IV over 60 min
Dosing	100 mg	100 mg	125 mg
IV injection	100 mg over 2–5 minutes	100 mg over 5 minutes	125 mg IV over 10 minutes
Infusion of dilute dose	100 mg in 100 mL normal saline and infused over 2–3 hours	100 mg in 100 mL NS, infuse IV over 15 minutes	125 mg in 100 mL of NS IV over 1 hour
Maintenance dose	Daily until calculated total amount required has been administered	1–3 times per week	1000 mg over 8 dialysis sessions
Minimum cumulative dose	Based on iron replacement calculations	1000 mg	1000 mg
Total dose infusion*	Yes	No	No

**Total dose infusion*: Total iron requirement is calculated and the total dose is administered by IV infusion in a single sitting

Table 17.6: Summary of common intravenous iron preparations						
Trade name	*Iron compound*	*Iron concentration per mL (mg/mL)*	*Available as vials*	*Test dose required*	*Maximum single dose (mg)*	*FDA category*
Dexferrum	High molecular weight iron dextran	50	1,2 mL	Yes	100	C
INFeD	Low molecular weight iron dextran	50	2 mL	Yes	100	C
Ferricit	Iron gluconate	12.5	5 mL	No	125	B
Venofer	Iron sucrose	20	5 mL	No	200	B
Feraheme	Iron polyglyconate	30	17 mL	No	510	C

FDA approval for the drug is pending investigation of unexplained hypophosphatemia following infusion in patients with chronic kidney disease and rise in number of adverse cardiac events.

Ferumoxytol

It is one of the newer agents which got FDA approval in 2009 for treatment of iron deficiency anemia in chronic kidney disease. Test dose is not required and 510 mg dose can be given in less than 20 sec.

Safety trials are in progress currently and results are yet to be published.

Iron Isomaltose

It is the latest addition in the list of parental iron preparations. It is approved in Europe for use in doses of up to 20 mg/kg.

It does not require test dose. Characteristic feature of this drug is that iron is strongly bound to carbohydrate moiety which ensures slow and controlled release of bioavailable iron and minimizes free iron release. Adverse effect profile is similar to other intravenous agents.

Vitamins in treatment of Anemia

Folic Acid

Pharmacology: Folate from diet is usually absorbed in duodenum and upper jejunum. Liver takes up most of folic acid from the diet and secretes, methyl tetrahydrofolic acid in bile, most of which gets reabsorbed from enterohepatic circulation. Total body stores range from 5 mg to 10 mg.

Indications of use

- Megaloblastic anemia
- *Prophylaxis for neural tube defects*: Periconceptional folic acid is known to reduce neural tube defects. In women with a history of a pregnancy complicated by a neural tube defect, a larger dose of 4 mg/day has been recommended.

Contraindications: Intolerance to drug.

Dosage

- Therapeutic dose is 2–5 mg/day orally
- Prophylactic dose is 0.5 mg/day orally.

Adverse drug reaction: It is nontoxic and there are no known side effects.

Drug interaction: Anticonvulsant action of phenytoin is antagonized and increase in dose of phenytoin may be required.

Monitoring: No special monitoring is required.

Preparation: Folvite, foliage, folcin, folat, folera—5 mg tab.

Safety during pregnancy: It is safe during pregnancy and lactation and is a category A drug.

National Nutritional Anemia Control Program (NNACP)

This folifer tablet which contains 100 mg elemental iron along with 500 mcg folic acid for at least 100 days. It needs to be continued till lactation.

National Iron Plus Initiative (NIPI)[7]

This program was initiated by Government of India in collaboration with state. Folifer tablet for 100 days during pregnancy from 2nd trimester and for 100 days in postpartum.

WHO Recommendations

Sixty mg elemental iron and 400 mcg folic acid is given for 6 months during pregnancy and to be continued for 3 months postpartum.

Vitamin C

This vitamin is responsible for general growth and development. It is also involved in the pathway of hemoglobin synthesis therefore in patients with nutritional anemia this vitamin is also given along with iron and folic acid.

Dosage: 500 mg, 2–3 times a day.

Preparations: Celin 500, ascorbic acid 500, redoxon 500 mg tablets.

Vitamin B_{12} (Cyanocobalamin)

Pharmacology: Vitamin B_{12} and folic acid are essential vitamins. Deficiency of both impair DNA synthesis in any cell in which chromosomal replication and division occurs, hence cells undergoing rapid turnover are very sensitive. Therefore most dramatic changes are observed in hematopoietic system.

Intracellular vitamin B_{12} is maintained in form of two active coenzymes: methylcobalamin and deoxy-adenosylcobalamin. Deficiency of vitamin B_{12} and folate decreases the synthesis of methionine and S-adenosyl methionine (SAM) thus interferes with protein biosynthesis, number of methylation reaction and hence leading to inadequate nuclear and cellular development, maturation and replication.

Deficiency of vitamin B_{12} leads to folate trapped as methyl tetrahydrofolate and hence functional deficit of folic acid leading to hematological abnormality.

Vitamin B_{12} in diet in presence of gastric acid and pancreatic protease gets released and combines with intrinsic factor in stomach and transports to terminal ileum. At site of terminal ileum in presence of bile, sodium bicarbonate and extrinsic factor releasing factor releases B_{12} in combination with transcobalamin 2. It transports vitamin B_{12} to liver where 1–10 mg is stored.

The 3 mcg of vitamin B_{12} is excreted in bile per day of which 50–60% is permanently lost and is not available for enterohepatic circulation.

Indications of use: Megaloblastic anemia and pernicious anemia.

Contraindications: Sensitivity to vitamin B_{12}

Dosage: Dosage in nutritional vitamin B_{12} deficiency and pernicious anemia is as follows:

- *Vitamin B_{12} nutritional deficiency*: It can be given orally as intranasal spray or intranasal gel or by IM injection.
  - Orally 1500 microgram of cynacobalamin is given once daily for three months.
  - For intramuscular injection 25–250 microgram daily in thigh.
  - For intranasal spray or gel 250 mcg in one nostril once a week.

  This treatment may be required for long period may be for lifelong if vitamin B_{12} deficiency persists.
- *Pernicious anemia*: 1000 mcg intramuscular once a day for 7 days, if clinical improvement is seen and reticulocyte count show a rise then 1000 mcg IM on alternate day for 7 days and then twice a week for 2–3 weeks. Once clinical improvement is established then 100–1000 mcg IM once a month lifelong to be given.
- Nasal spray 500 mcg in one nostril once a week can be given lifelong.

Iron and folic acid need to be supplemented with vitamin B_{12} administration as isolated vitamin B_{12} deficiency generally does not occur. Therefore vitamin B_{12} administrations alone will unmask deficiency of iron and folic acid.

Adverse drug reaction: It occurs in form of mild reactions like transient diarrhea, itching and exanthema. Significant side effects are rare but include peripheral venous thrombosis, polycythemia vera, pulmonary edema, congestive cardiac failure and anaphylactic shock.

Drug interaction: It interacts with chloramphenicol.

Monitoring: Initial response to therapy manifests as symptomatic relief closely followed by increase in reticulocyte count which starts by 5–7 day and gets established by 15 day. Increase in hemoglobin concentration and RBC indices are observed in 2–3 weeks, with normalization of hematological profile over next 6–8 weeks.

Preparation

Oral

- Nurokind—1500 microgram tablet
- Methycobal—1500 microgram tablet

Injectable

- Cobal 1000—available as vial 10 mL with 1000 mcg cynocobalamin per mL.
- Methycobal—500 mcg/mL methycobalamin

Nasal spray: Hydroxocobalamin is usually preferred due to better retention; however it has been shown to induce antibody formation, leading to reduction in metabolically available B_{12}. It is not used in US however being used in UK and India.

Safety during pregnancy: It crosses placenta and gets concentrated in the fetus. It is also secreted in breast milk. It is FDA category C drug.

Antihelminths

One of the common cause of iron deficiency anemia is worm infestation therefore in all cases diagnosed as iron deficiency anemia are prophylactically given de-worming drugs. The common drugs which are used during pregnancy are imidazole group which includes mebendazole and albendazole.

Albendazole

Pharmacology: It inhibits microtubule polymerization by binding to beta-tubulin. This group of drugs binds preferentially to parasitic protein than mammalian protein. Its active agent acts on both larval and adult stage.

Albendazole is variably absorbed after oral administration. A fatty meal increases absorption. It is not detectable immediately after consumption in blood and gets metabolized to its active sulfoxide metabolite. Both positive and negative enantiomers of its metabolite are active biologically. Almost 70% of albendazole is protein bound in circulation. Due to its metabolites and protein binding properties, half-life is variable (4–15 hours). It gets metabolized and is excreted in urine.

Indications of use: It acts on *Necator americanus* and *Ancylostoma duodenale.* It is the treatment of choice for endemic nematode intestinal infection in India. It acts on blood feeding adult hookworms in intestines.

Contraindications: Sensitivity to albendazole, abnormal liver function tests, severe anemia, neutropenia.

Dosage: Albendazole 400 mg single dose HS.

Adverse drug reaction: Mild gastrointestinal symptoms in less than 1% have been observed.

Drug interaction: It causes significant reaction with phenytoin and minor reaction with dexamethasone.

Monitoring: With single dose no specific monitoring is required.

Preparation: Abel, Aban, Abide.

Safety in pregnancy and lactation: It has been proven to be embryotoxic and teratogenic in rats. However, not proven in humans but its better avoided in first trimester.

FDA drug category: Category C.

Mebendazole

This drug has same properties as albendazole and can be used alternatively. It is given in dose of 100 mg twice a day for 3 days or 500 mg single dose.

Miscellaneous

Recombinant Human Erythropoietin (Epoietin Alpha)[20]

Pharmacology: Recombinant human erythropoietin is a 165-amino acid glycoprotein produced by a recombinant DNA method with the same biologic effects as endogenous erythropoietin. It is used to stimulate red blood cell production. Some studies suggest it may be cerebroprotective in cerebral malaria and schizophrenia.

Indications of use: It is used in following conditions:

- Anemia of chronic renal disease, patients of renal transplant or patients requiring dialysis.
- Patients of myelodysplastic syndrome or on chemotherapy. However, its use is under consideration as FDA has issued concerns regarding higher incidence of mortality in some cancers.

Contraindications: All patients should receive adequate iron supplementation. Iron supplementation should be started at the start of treatment with epoetin alfa and should continue throughout the duration of therapy. Dose should be reduced by 25% if hemoglobin increases greater than 1 g/dL in any 2 week period or hemoglobin reaches a level needed to avoid RBC transfusion.

Dosage: 50–150 IU/kg of body weight given subcutaneously twice or thrice weekly. Dosage varies according to the indication for which it is used.

Adverse drug reaction: Epoietin alfa is generally well tolerated. Common side effects include high blood pressure, headache, severe migraine (resistant to remedies), joint-pain and clotting at the injection site.

Rare cases of stinging at the injection site, skin rash and flu like symptoms (joint and muscle pain) may occur within few hours of administration. More serious side effects include allergic reactions, seizures and thrombotic events (e.g. heart attacks, strokes and pulmonary embolism).

Drug interaction: When EPO is used with cyclosporine there is greater risk of high blood pressure and EPO may lead to variability in blood levels of cyclosporine.

ACE inhibitors may interfere with hematopoiesis by decreasing the synthesis of endogenous erythropoietin or decreasing bone marrow production of red blood cell.

Monitoring: Patient should be monitored for development of any adverse reaction at the time of injection. Blood pressure is monitored during administration and for 1 hour after the administration.

Preparation

- Epofer—6000 IU per vial
- Celpoietin—10,000 IU per vial
- Eprex (0.4 mL)—4000 IU in 0.4 mL
- Epox (1 mL)—4000 IU/mL.

Safety during pregnancy and lactation: Recent investigations have demonstrated lack of placental passage of recombinant epoietin alfa across the human placenta. Of concern with epoetin alfa is the inability to differentiate between epoetin alfa associated hypertension and that of preeclampsia. Epoetin alfa is only recommended for use during pregnancy when there are no alternatives and benefit outweighs risk.

There are no data on the excretion of epoetin alfa into human milk, so should be cautiously used in nursing women.

FDA category C.

FDA approval: FDA notes significant risks associated with erythropoietin use. These agents should be used only in patients with cancer when treating anemia specifically caused by chemotherapy, and not for other causes of anemia.

Pyridoxine

Patients with sideroblastic anemia characteristically have impaired Hb synthesis and accumulate iron in the perinuclear mitochondria of erythroid precursors, so-called ringed sideroblasts. Oral therapy with pyridoxine is of proven benefit in correcting the sideroblastic anemias associated with the antituberculosis drugs isoniazid and pyrazinamide, which act as vitamin B_6 antagonists. A daily dose of 10–25 mg of pyridoxine completely corrects the defect without interfering with treatment, and routine pyridoxine supplementation is recommended.

REFERENCES

1. Stevens G, Finucane M, De-Regil L, Paciorek C, Flaxman S, Branca F, et al. Nutrition Impact Model Study Group (Anaemia). Global, regional, and national trends in haemoglobin concentration and prevalence of total and severe anaemia in children and pregnant and non-pregnant women for 1995–2011: a systematic analysis of population-representative data. Lancet Glob Health. 2013;1:e16-e25.
2. National Family Health Survey-III Available at *http://www.rchiips.org/nfhs/nutrition_report_for_website_18sep09.pdf.*

3. *http://www.who.int/vmnis/indicators haemoglobin.pdf.*
4. CDC pregnancy and paediatric nutritional surveillance system: *http://www.cdc.gov/pednss/what_is/pednss_he99999alth indicators.htm.*
5. The Goodman Gilman manual of pharmacology and therapeutics: 11th edition, p.698-700.
6. Picciano MF. Pregnancy and Lactation: Physiological Adjustments, Nutritional Requirements and the Role of Dietary Supplements. J Nutr. 2003;133:61997S-2002S.
7. National Iron-plus Initiative guidelines for control of iron deficiency anaemia in India, 2013 Available at- http://www.unicef.org/ india/10._National_Iron_Plus_Initiative_Guidelines_for_Control_of_IDA.pdf.
8. Kumar A1 National nutritional anaemia control programme in India. Indian J Public Health. 1999;43(1):3-5, 16.
9. Allahabadia, Shroff, Aggarwals. Review of Indian clinical experience with ferrous ascorbate. In Fogsi Times. 2006.p.15.
10. Sharma JB. Nutritional anaemia during pregnancy in non-industrialised countries. Studd J. Progress in Obstetrics and Gynaecology: Churchill Livinstone. 2003.pp.103-22.
11. Fahmy K Systemic reactions with total dose infusion of iron dextran complex in obstetric patients. Int J Gynaecol Obstet. 1978;16:170-2.
12. Hart GD, Soots M. An anaphylactic reaction complicating total dose infusion therapy of iron deficiency. Appl Ther. 1969;11:645-6.
13. Auerbach M, Ballard H. Clinical Use of Intravenous Iron: Administration, Efficacy, and Safety. Am J Hematol. 2010.pp.338-47.
14. NFK-DOQI clinical practice guidelines for the treatment of anemia of chronic renal failure. National Kidney Foundation-Dialysis Outcomes Quality Initiative. Am J Kidney Dis. 1997;30(4): S192–S240.
15. Bastani B, Rahman S, Gellens M. Lack of reaction to ferric gluconate in hemodialysis patients with a severe reaction to iron dextran. ASAIO J. 2002;48(4):404-6.
16. Fishbane S, Ungureanu V, Maesak JK, Kaupke CJ, Lim V, Wish J. The safety of intravenous iron dextran in hemodialysis patients. Am J Kidney Dis. 1996;28(4):529-34.
17. Folkert VW, Michael DO, Agarwal R, et al. Chronic use of sodium ferric gluconate complex in hemodialysis patients: safety of higher-dose (_250 mg) administration. Am J Kidney Dis. 2003;41(3):651-7.
18. Scott B. Silverstein and George M. Rodgers: Parenteral Iron Therapy Options. Am J Hematol. 2004;76:74-8.
19. The Goodman Gilman manual of pharmacology and therapeutics: 11th edition 938-45
20. Fibach E, Rachmilewitz EA. Does erythropoietin have a role in the treatment of β-hemoglobinopathies? Hematol Oncol Clin North Am. 2014;28(2):249-63. *www.cdc.gov/tb/publications/ltbi/treatment.htm.*

CHAPTER 18

Hypertensive Disorders of Pregnancy

Sangeeta Gupta

HYPERTENSIVE DISORDERS

Hypertensive disorders during pregnancy are one of the leading causes of maternal and fetal morbidity and lead to maternal mortality.

Treatment

Antihypertensive treatment is offered when BP is 150/100 mm Hg or more, that is, moderate and severe hypertension.[1] On antihypertensive treatment, target is to keep diastolic blood pressure between 80 mmHg and 100 mm Hg systolic blood pressure less than 150 mm Hg.[1]

Management of severe hypertension is important as it decreases cerebral arterial vasospasm and prevents eclampsia. Oral or parenteral antihypertensive drugs can be used for managing severe hypertension.[2]

Methyldopa

Methyldopa is the alfa-methyl analog of dopa, the precursor of dopamine and nor adrenaline. It has good safety profile during pregnancy and lactation.

Pharmacology

Pharmacokinetics: About one-third of orally administered drug is absorbed. Majority of the drug which is absorbed is excreted in the urine. The plasma half-life of methyldopa is about 100 minutes.

Mechanism of action: The primary site of action is central. The antihypertensive effect of methyldopa is due to its metabolism in the brain to an active form, which then lowers arterial pressure by stimulation of central inhibitory alpha-adrenergic receptors.

The maximum decrease in blood pressure occurs four to six hours after oral dosage. Once an effective dosage level is attained, a smooth blood pressure response occurs in most patients in 12–24 hours.[3] Blood pressure usually returns to pretreatment levels within 24–48 hours after stopping therapy.

Indications: It has been safely and successfully used to treat hypertension during pregnancy and is the treatment of nonemergent hypertension during pregnancy. It is started in doses of 250 mg tds and gradually escalated to maximum dose of 500 mg qid till BP is lowers to the desirable range. The target diastolic BP after treatment is between 80 mmHg and 100 mm Hg and systolic BP of less than 150 mm Hg.[1]

Contraindications

- Active hepatic disease, such as acute hepatitis and active cirrhosis
- Liver disorders previously associated with methyldopa therapy

- On therapy with monoamine oxidase (MAO) inhibitors.

Dosage

Oral administration: 250 mg tds, maximum dose: 2 grams per day in four divided doses.

Adverse effects[3]

- Sedation, lethargy and reduced mental capacity
- Dryness of mouth, nasal stuffiness and headache
- Fluid retention and weight gain
- Mild postural hypotension
- Positive Coomb's test and hemolytic anemia
- Fever, rash, hepatitis, 'flu' like illness, thrombocytopenia and rarely lupus syndrome.

Drug interaction: Monoamine oxidase (MAO) inhibitors.

Caution: If a woman has taken methyldopa to treat hypertension in antenatal period, stop within 2 days of birth as it may cause postpartum depression.[1]

Preparations: Tablet aldomet 250 mg.

FDA category: Category B when administered orally.[4]

Labetalol

Labetalol is an adrenergic receptor blocker. It works by blocking both alpha and beta receptors in the body, which lowers blood pressure. It is a selective alfa-1 and nonselective beta blocking agent.

Pharmacology

Pharmacokinetics: The peak plasma levels of labetalol are achieved after 1 to 2 hours of oral administration. It undergoes extensive first-pass metabolism in the liver and hence only 25% of drug is available in systemic circulation. The plasma half-life of labetalol following oral administration is about 6 to 8 hours. Duration of action after 100 mg doses is 8 hours and after 300 mg dosage is 12 hours. The maximum response of the drug on BP after oral, twice-a-day dosing schedule occurs within 24-72 hours.

When administered intravenously, onset of action is in 2.5 minutes and peak effect is achieved in 15 minutes. The half-life is 5.5 hours.

Labetalol is metabolized by conjugation to glucuronide metabolites. These metabolites are excreted in the urine and feces. In patients with hepatic and renal impairment, elimination of labetalol is not altered. However, in hepatic impairment the relative bioavailability of drug is increased due to decreased first pass metabolism in liver.

Labetalol has been shown to cross the placental barrier in humans.[1]

When administered intravenously, onset of action is in 2.5 minutes and peak effect is achieved in 15 minutes. The half-life is 5.5 hours.

Indications

- Oral preparation is used as first line treatment of nonemergent control of hypertension during pregnancy. It is usually effective when administered alone, but may be combined with other antihypertensive agents.
- Intravenous administration for lowering BP during hypertensive crisis.

Contraindications[5,6]

- Asthma
- Heart block
- Congestive heart failure.

Dosage

Chronic hypertension and preeclampsia: 100 mg orally 12 hours initially; increased by 100 mg 12 hours every 2–3 days, Maximum dose not to exceed 2400 mg per day.

Hypertensive emergency: 20 mg intravenously over 2 minutes initially, repeat 40 mg after 20 minutes, then 80 mg and 80 mg till BP controlled. BP should be monitored every 10 minutes and maximum permissible dose is 220 mg.[7]

Adverse drug reactions

Side effects

- Maternal
  - Fatigue and weakness
  - Difficulty in sleeping
  - Orthostatic hypotension
  - Lupus like rash
  - Rarely, respiratory distress

- Fetal:
  - Reduced frequency of fetal heart rate accelerations
  - Preterm birth and FGR[8]
  - Neonatal hypoglycemia.[9]

Drug Interactions: Calcium channel blockers (e.g., verapamil because they may increase the risk of labetalol's side effects.

Caution

Diabetes mellitus and hypoglycemia: Beta-adrenergic blockade may prevent the appearance of premonitory signs and symptoms (e.g., tachycardia) of acute hypoglycemia. This is especially important with labile diabetics. Beta-blockade also reduces the release of insulin in response to hyperglycemia; it may therefore be necessary to adjust the dose of antidiabetic drugs.[1]

FDA category: Category C.[4]

Hydralazine

Pharmacology

Pharmacokinetics: Hydralazine is absorbed via gastrointestinal tract. When administered orally, it undergoes acetylation during first pass metabolism. Thus, the drug requires dose adjustment, fast acetylators need higher doses than slow acetylators. However, the intravenous administration of drug is independent of acetylator phenotype and hence, half-life does not differ in slow or fast acetylators. The half-life of hydralazine is 1 hour, its duration of action is 12 hours and peak plasma concentration.[10]

Mechanism of action

- It relaxes the arterial smooth muscle directly leading to peripheral vasodilation. It interferes with the calcium movement in the vascular smooth muscle.
- It increases cardiac output and renal blood flow.

Indication: Hypertensive emergency in pregnancy.

Contraindications: Coronary artery disease,[5,6,11] mitral valve disease.[5,6]

Disadvantages: Delayed onset of action, variable peak effect and fetal distress.

Dosage: Initial dose of 5 intravenously over 2 minutes, repeat 5–10 mg dose at 15–20 minute interval until satisfactory response.[5] Maximum dose is 40 mg. Target response is decrease in DBP to 90–110 mm Hg.

Drug interaction: MAO inhibitors

Adverse drug reactions

Side effects

- Maternal:
  - Nausea and vomiting
  - Hypotension, headache and dizziness, flushing and nasal congestion.
  - Palpitation
  - Lupus like syndrome[5,6]
- *Fetal:* Late decelerations[12]
- *Fetal:* Thrombocytopenia.

FDA category: Category C.[4]

Nifedipine

Pharmacology: Nifedipine is a dihydropyridine.[4]

Pharmacokinetics: After oral absorption, bioavailability is 30–60%.[4] Half life of nifedipine is 2 hours.[13]

Mechanism of action: Calcium-channel blocking agent leading to arteriolar vasodilator.

Indications

- High efficacy for control of acute pregnancy-related hypertension.[14]
- Treatment of chronic HT and preeclampsia.

Contraindication: Myocardial infarction.[5,6,15]

Dosage

- 10 mg initial dose to be repeated in 30 minutes up to 3 doses if necessary. Once controlled doses are scheduled every 6 hourly.[10]
- Sublingual nifedipine no longer recommended.

Drug interactions: Simultaneous use of magnesium sulfate is hazardous due to synergistic effects.

Adverse drug reactions

Side effects: Hypotension, headache, ankle edema, tachycardia, coronary steal phenomenon and inhibition of labor.

FDA category: Category C.[4]

Magnesium Sulfate

Magnesium sulfate is not given to treat hypertension.[16] It is used in severe preeclampsia and eclampsia to prevent convulsions.

Pharmacology

Mechanism of Action

- It has an anticonvulsant action but the mechanism of action is controversial
  - *Peripheral action:* Blocks neuromuscular transmission by
    - Decreased acetylcholine release from nerve endings
    - Decreased motor end plate sensitivity to acetylcholine
    - Competitive inhibition of calcium channels, thereby reducing calcium influx
  - *Central action:* Causes vasodilatation of cerebral blood vessels, thereby avoiding vasospasm and tissue ischemia
- It also acts as a tocolytic by direct depressant action on uterine muscle.

Indications

- For prevention of seizures in severe preeclampsia and eclampsia-drug of choice
- As a tocolytic agent in preterm labor.

Contraindications

- Myasthenia gravis
- Impaired renal function.

Dosage: Intramuscular route is as effective as intravenous administration.

For prevention and treatment of seizures

- *Pritchard's regime:*[17]
  Loading dose: 4 g IV (20 mL of 20% solution) over 3–4 minutes followed by 10 g (20 mL of 50% solution) deep IM, 5 g in each buttock.
  Maintenance dose: 5 g (10 mL of 50% solution) deep IM on alternate buttock every 4 hours.
  Maintenance dose to be continued till 24 hours after delivery or last seizure; whichever is later.
- *Intravenous regimen*[18]
  Loading dose: Give 4 g (20 mL of 20% solution) in 100 mL normal saline over 15–20 minutes.
  Maintainance dose: Add 10 g of magnesium sulfate (two 10 mL amp of 50%) to 1000 mL of normal saline and give at the rate of 1 g per hour.

When magnesium sulfate is given to arrest eclamptic seizures, 10–15% women will have a subsequent convulsion. If so, additional 2 g dose (20% solution) is slowly given IV In a small woman, this additional 2 g dose may be used once, but it can be given twice if needed in a larger woman.

Therapeutic level of serum magnesium = 4–7 mEq/L.

Monitoring for Magnesium Toxicity

- Deep tendon reflexes should be present → disappearance of patellar reflex is the first sign of impending toxicity. Patellar reflexes disappear at 10 mEq/L.
- Respiratory rate >14/min. Breathing weakens at levels >10 mEq/L. Respiratory paralysis and arrest follows at ≥12 mEq/L.
- Urine output ≥30 mL/hr (as magnesium is eliminated by kidneys)
- Pulse oximetry >96%.

Management of Toxicity[16]

- Withold magnesium sulfate administration
- Injection calcium gluconate (10 mL of 10% solution IV over 3 minutes)
- For severe respiratory depression and arrest, prompt tracheal intubation and mechanical ventilation are lifesaving.
- Loading dose achieves the desired therapeutic level, and infusion maintains the steady-state level. In cases of diminished glomerular filtration rate as indicated by serum creatinine levels, only the maintenance infusion rate should be altered. When plasma creatinine is >1.0 mg/dL, serum magnesium levels are measured to guide the infusion rate.

Adverse drug reactions

Side effects

- Maternal
  - Flushing
  - Perspiration
  - Headache
  - Muscle weakness
  - Decreased vital capacity
  - Pulmonary edema
  - Cardiac arrhythmias
  - Increased blood loss during delivery
- Fetal
  - Small but significant effect on fetal heart rate pattern.1[9,20]
- Neonatal[21]
  - Lethargy
  - Hypotonia
  - Hyporeflexia
  - Respiratory depression.

Drug interaction: It acts synergistically with muscle relaxants used for general anesthesia, hence smaller doses to be used.

Antihypertensive Treatment for Acute Management of Severe Hypertension[11]

The drugs used for rapid lowering of BP are hydralazine, labetalol and nifedipine. Labetalol is the treatment of choice for control of acute hypertension (intravenous) and maintenance therapy with oral form. It is preferred as it is effective and has low incidence of side-effects. Hydralazine is less preferred because it causes abnormal FHR patterns. In the meta-analysis by Magee et al,[22] evidence did not support use of hydralazine as first line treatment of acute hypertension. However, the cochrane review 2013[23] found no major difference between the 3 medications and recommended each one be started based on patient individual characteristics and clinical scenario, adverse effects, and clinicians own experience.

Pregnant Women with Chronic Hypertension

American college of obstetricians and gynecologist (ACOG)[5] recommends that in pregnant women with 150–160/100–110 mm Hg should be treated with drugs and BP should be lower than 150/100 mm Hg. NICE guidelines[1] also recommend treatment with aim to keep lower than 150/100 mm Hg. However, DBP should not be below 80 mm Hg. In pregnant women with end organ damage secondary to chronic hypertension, treatment should be given to maintain BP below 140/90 mm Hg, thus reducing risk of further end organ damage.

Preeclampsia

Antihypertensive treatment is recommended in moderate preeclampsia to keep BP <150/80–100 mm Hg. NICE the first line treatment is labetalol. Alternative therapies are methyldopa and nifedipine, depending on choice of clinician.

Antihypertensives are indicated in mild preeclampsia if it is associated with heavy proteinuria, liver dysfunction or hematological dysfunction[18] or in co-morbid conditions like diabetes, chronic hypertension or renal disease.[24]

REFERENCES

1. National Institute for Health and Clinical Excellence (NICE). Hypertension in Pregnancy: The management of hypertensive disorders during pregnancy. NICE clinical guideline. 2010; 107:1-295.
2. Podymow T, August P. Update on the use of antihypertensive drugs in pregnancy. Hypertension. 2008;51:960-9.
3. Tripathi KD. Antihypertensive drugs. Tripathi KD. Essentials of Medical pharmacology. 7th edn. Jaypee Brothers Medical Publishers; 2013.
4. Benowitz NL. Antihypertensive agents. Katzung BG. Basic and clinical pharmacology. 12th edn. McGraw Hill; 2012.
5. American College of Obstetricians and Gynecologists Taskforce on Hypertension in Pregnancy. Hypertension in Pregnancy. Washington, DC: ACOG; 2013.
6. Marik PE, Rivera R. Hypertensive emergencies: an update. Curr Opin Crit Care. 2011;17:569-80.
7. Chobanian AV, Bakris GL, Black HR, et al. The seventh report of the Joint National Committee on Prevention, Detection, Evaluation, and Treatment of High Blood Pressure: the JNC 7 report. JAMA. 2003;289:2560-72.

8. Meidahl Petersen K, Jimenez-Solem E, Andersen JT, et al. β-Blocker treatment during pregnancy and adverse pregnancy outcomes: a nationwide population-based cohort study. BMJ Open. 2012; 2:1-7.
9. Davis RL, Eastman D, McPhillips H, Raebel MA, Andrade SE, Smith D, Yood MU, Dublin S,Platt R. Risks of congenital malformations and perinatal events among infants exposed to calcium channel and beta-blockers during pregnancy. Pharmacoepidemiol Drug Saf. 2011;20:138-45.
10. Vadhera RB, Simon M. Hypertensive emergencies in pregnancy. Clin Obstet Gynecol. 2014;57(4): 797-805.
11. Bansal V, damania KR. Hypertenive disorders in pregnancy. Bhide A, et al. High Risk Pregnancy & Delivery. 4th edn. Elsevier; 2015.
12. Alexander JM, Wilson KL. Hypertensive emergencies of pregnancy. Obstet Gynecol Clin North Am. 2013;40(1):89-101.
13. Holford NHG. Pharmacokinetics and pharmacodynamics: Rationale dosing and the time course of drug action. Katzung BG. Basic and clinical pharmacology. 12th edn. McGraw Hill; 2012.
14. Firoz T, Magee LA, MacDonell K, Payne BA, Gordon R, Vidler M, von Dadelszen P; Community Level Interventions for Pre-eclampsia (CLIP) Working Group. Oral antihypertensive therapy for severe hypertension in pregnancy and postpartum: a systematic review. BJOG. 2014;121(10):1210-8.
15. Katzung BG. Vasodilators and treatment of angina pectoris. Katzung BG. Basic and clinical pharmacology. 12th edn. McGraw Hill; 2012.
16. Cunningham HG, et al. Hypertensive disorders. Cunningham HG, et al. Williams Obstetrics. 24th edn. McGraw hill Education; 2014.
17. Walfisch A, Hallak M. Hypertension. James D. High Risk Pregnancy. 4th edn. Elsevier; 2011.
18. Royal College of Obstetricians and Gynaecologists: the management of severe pre-eclampsia. RCOG Guideline; 2006. p. 10.
19. Hallak M, Martinez-Poyer J, Kruger ML, Hassan S, Blackwell SC, Sorokin Y. The effect of magnesium sulfate on fetal heart rate parameters: A randomized, placebo-controlled trial. Am J Obstet Gynecol. 1999;181:1122-7.
20. Duffy CR, Odibo AO, Roehl KA, Macones GA, Cahill AG. Effect of magnesium sulfate on fetal heart rate patterns in the second stage of labor. Obstet Gynecol. 2012;119(6):1129-36.
21. Abbassi-Ghanavti M, Alexander JM, McIntire DD. Neonatal effects of magnesium sulfate given to the mothers. Am J perinatol. 2012; 29:795.
22. Magee L, Cham C, Waterman E, Ohlsson A, von Dadelszen P. Hydralazine for treatment of severe hypertension in pregnancy: meta-analysis. BMJ. 2003;327:955-60.
23. Duley L, Meher S, Jones L. Drugs for treatment of very high blood pressure during pregnancy. Cochrane Database Syst Rev. 2013.
24. SOGC Practice Guidline No.206, March 2008. Diagnosis, evaluation and management of the hypertensive disorders of pregnancy. J Obstet Gynecol. 2005;193:1591-8.

CHAPTER 19

Diabetes in Pregnancy

Asmita M Rathore, Shailja Singh

Pregnancy is a diabetogenic state, for maintaining an uninterrupted supply of glucose to growing fetus and for catering to metabolic needs of mother. The post-prandial values are affected to greater extent compared to fasting ones. Uncontrolled maternal diabetes is associated with maternal and fetal/neonatal adverse effects. Pedersen suggested that maternal hyperglycemia leads to transplacental transfer of glucose and results in increased secretion of insulin by beta cells in fetus and eventually causing macrosomia. The intrauterine environment during fetal life determines the health of the individual in adult life. So optimal maternal blood glucose control is required to reduce perinatal morbidity and mortality. Also blood glucose control helps in reduction of disease like heart disease, diabetes, etc. in adult life.

Control of blood sugar levels is the main stay of management of diabetes in pregnancy, but treatment of comorbid conditions and complications associated with diabetes in pregnancy is also important. In this chapter, we have discussed the drugs used for glycemic control during pregnancy and antenatal corticosteroids, which may be required in diabetic woman for treatment of complications (prematurity) and may affect glycemic control.

DRUGS USED FOR CONTROLLING BLOOD SUGAR LEVELS

The drugs used for glycemic control are:

- Insulin
- Oral hypoglycemic agents.

INSULIN

Insulin has remained the sole hypoglycemic agent used during pregnancy for long-time and is still preferred for glycemic control during pregnancy. The classification and pharmacokinetics of insulin are given in **Table 19.1.**

Rapid-acting insulin: Insulin lispro is produced by reversing proline and lysine at the carboxy terminus B28 and B29 positions and in Insulin aspart proline at B28 is replaced by aspartic acid. These changes decrease the ability to form hexamers and leading to rapid absorption. Advantage with these rapid-acting insulin analogs is that they can be given immediately before meal. Moreover, they have greater stability and consistency of action.

Short-acting insulin: Regular insulin need to be taken at least 30 minutes before taking meal. It is stabilized by small amount of zinc. At the concentration of injectible solution, the

Table 19.1: Classification and pharmacokinetics of insulin

Type	*Onset (hour)*	*Peak (hour)*	*Duration (hour)*
	Rapid Acting		
Insulin Lispro	0.2–0.4	1–2	3–5
Insulin Aspart	0.2–0.4	1–1.5	3–5
	Short Acting		
Regular (soluble) Insulin	0.5–1	2–4	6–8
	Intermediate Acting		
Insulin Zinc Suspension or Lente	1–2	8–10	20–24
Neutral Protamine Hagedorn (NPH)	1–2	8–10	20–24
	Long Acting		
Protamine Zinc Insulin (PZI)	4–6	14–20	24–36
Insulin Glargine	2–4	5–12	24

insulin molecules form hexamers around zinc ions. When subcutaneous injections are given, monomers are released slowly.

Intermediate-acting insulin: NPH insulin has slow onset and long duration of action; hence it is suitable for providing basal requirement of insulin.

Long acting insulin: It includes the analogs Insulin glargine and detemir. In insulin glargine, at position A21, asparagine is replaced by glycine and two arginines are added at the C-terminus of the B-chain (B31 and B32). As a result of these changes, insulin glargine is more soluble in acidic PH compared to neutral environment. When it is injected as subcutaneous injection, they form stable hexamers which have slow dissolution and absorption in neutral environment at the injection site. In Insulin detemir, there is addition of a C14 fatty acid side chain at position B29. These long-acting Insulin analogs have peak less action for 24 hours.

Current Evidence

In a meta-analysis (2011), 8 cohort studies done on 702 women were reviewed to study the safety of insulin glargine in pregnancy. It was shown that insulin glargine does not cause increase in adverse fetal outcome.[1] In a randomized controlled trial (2014), insulin detemir was found to be well tolerated and safe for use in pregnant women with type1 diabetes.[2]

Table 19.2: Insulin requirement according to gestational age

Weeks gestation	*Total daily insulin (μ/kg/d)*
First trimester	0.7–0.8
Second trimester	0.8–1
Third trimester	0.9–1.2

Dosage

Insulin is given as injection because it is a protein and if given orally it will be digested in stomach before absorption. Initial starting dose of insulin is calculated taking maternal weight and gestational age **(Table 19.2)** into account and later dose adjustments are made according to blood sugar controls.[3] Also insulin requirement increases in times of stress, sepsis, steroids administration, etc.

In commonly used regimen for insulin administration, total insulin requirement is calculated using above table and out of the total dose calculated, 2/3 dose given in morning (2/3 NPH and 1/3 regular insulin) and 1/3 dose in evening (½ as NPH and ½ as regular insulin).

NPH is given before breakfast and at bed-time (to avoid nocturnal hypoglycemia, if given pre dinner). Insulin requirement in type 2 DM is higher during each trimester as compared to type 1 DM patients.[4] In early pregnancy, insulin requirement is almost same for both type 1 and type 2 DM. However, the required dose of insulin increases by 10% in type 1 DM and 33% in type 2 DM, during the second trimester and in last trimester insulin requirement increases up to 40% in type 2 DM.

Others regimens include basal-bolus regimen and continuous subcutaneous infusion.

In basal-bolus regimen regular insulin is given prior to 3 major meals for catering to postprandial hyperglycemia and NPH is given at bed time to provide basal control of blood sugar. This is considered more appropriate for gestational diabetes which is characterized by postprandial hyperglycemia and is more physiological. The major problem with this basal-bolus regimen is that multiple injections have to be given per day.

Continuous subcutaneous infusion requires lesser dose of insulin and provides effective control of blood sugar and is recommended in pregnancy if adequate glycemic control is not achieved by MOI of insulin without causing hypoglycemia.[5]

Regardless of the regimen used, blood glucose monitoring is important for proper titration of dose and to avoid hypoglycemia. According to ACOG (2015) target capillary blood glucose levels are tasting (<95 mg/dL), preprandial (≤100 mg/dL), 1-hr postprandial (≤140 mg/dL) 2-hr postprandial (≤120 mg/dL) and 2 am–6 am (≥60 mg/dL).[6]

Routes of Administration

Subcutaneous, intravenous.

Contraindications

There are no contraindications as such for use of insulin in pregnancy but care should be taken so as to avoid hypoglycemia. Insulin should be avoided in case of allergy to insulin.

Adverse Drug Reaction

Hypoglycemia is most commonly seen and serious problem associated with insulin therapy. The response to hypoglycemia occurs by two mechanisms-sympathetic stimulation and neuroglucopenic effect. These responses may be less pronounced in conditions such as long standing diabetes, concomitant use of drugs, e.g. beta-blockers, etc.

Insulin causes movement of potassium into the cells, leading to hypokalemia that if not treated promptly may lead to respiratory paralysis, ventricular arrhythmia, and death.

Local reactions: Redness, pain and swelling in injection site.

Allergic Reaction

Lipodystrophy: Lipodystrophy is not a problem with newer preparations.

Drug Interactions

Beta-blockers: Beta-blockers (especially nonselective blockers) mask the response to hypoglycemia.

Certain drugs may increase insulin requirement: Progesterones thiazides, glucocorticoids, thyroid hormones and sympathomimetics.

Certain drugs may decrease the requirement of insulin: Oral hypoglycemic agents (OHA), theophylline, lithium, salicylates, alcohol and nonselective beta-blockers.

Safety During Pregnancy

Insulin lispro, Regular, NPH and detemir are FDA pregnancy category B drugs while insulin aspart and insulin glargine are FDA pregnancy category C drug.

Preparation

Insulin Regular, NPH and Mixtard 30/70 come in 40U and 100U strength and are available as vials or cartridges.

ORAL HYPOGLYCEMIC AGENTS

Insulin although safe in pregnancy, has certain disadvantages associated with its use. Apart from the fact that multiple daily injections are required, insulin has a risk of hypoglycemia. To overcome these problems over past two decades, many oral hypoglycemic drugs have been studied to achieve glycemic control during pregnancy. **Table 19.3** shows classification of oral hypoglycemic agents. Out of these drugs, only two oral hypoglycemic agents have been recommended for use at present in pregnancy—glyburide and metformin. Further studies are required to recommend the use of other oral hypoglycemic agents (thiazolidinediones, meglitinide and alpha-glucosidase inhibitors).

GLYBURIDE

First generation sulfonylureas are not used in pregnant population as there has been concern about risk of neonatal hypoglycemia and increase in congenital malformations. Glyburide has been widely studied for use in diabetes in pregnancy.

Pharmacology

Mechanism of Action

Glyburide has following effects on carbohydrate metabolism.

- Glyburide has an inhibitory effect on ATP-sensitive potassium channel located on the pancreatic islet cell membrane, as a result of which voltage, gated calcium channels are opened and there is intracellular influx of calcium. Finally, β-cells of the pancreas are stimulated to release insulin
- It Increases peripheral glucose utilization and decreases hepatic gluconeogenesis.
- It causes increase in the number and sensitivity of insulin receptor.

Pharmcokinetics

It is metabolized in the liver. Its metabolites exert a small clinically insignificant hypoglycemic effect. Glyburide metabolites are excreted in urine and feces. Glyburide is well absorbed orally and significant absorption of glyburide occurs within one hour, peak drug levels at about four hours, and low but detectable levels at 24 hours. The decrease glyburide level in the serum of normal healthy individuals is biphasic; initial distribution half-life of roughly 30 min and a terminal elimination half-life of approximately 10 hours. Thus, the overall elimination half-life of glyburide is approximately 4 hours. Glyburide has a small volume of distribution (0.2 L/kg). In pregnancy, clearance of glyburide is increased significantly (two fold).

Current Evidence

In a randomized controlled trial performed on 404 singleton pregnancies between 11 weeks to 33 weeks by Langer O and coworkers

Table 19.3: Classification of oral hypoglycemics
Sulfonylureas *First Generation*: Tolbutamide, Chlorpropamide *Second Generation*: Glibenclamide (Glyburide), Glipizide, Gliclazide, Glimepiride
Biguanides: Metformin
Meglitinide: Repaglinide, Nateglinide
Thiazolidinediones: Rosiglitazone, Pioglitazone
Alpha-Glucosidase Inhibitors: Acarbose, Miglitol
Dipeptidyl peptidase (DPP-4) inhibitors: Sitagliptin
Glucagon-like peptide (GLP-1) analog: Exenatide

a comparison was done between glyburide and insulin and no significant difference in fetal or neonatal outcome was seen, although 8 (4%) of the patient on glyburide required insulin.[7] According to two recent meta-analyses (2014, 2015) done to compare the outcomes associated with use of glyburide with metformin and insulin, it was found that as compared to insulin, in glyburide group the birth weight of babies was higher. Also macrosomia and neonatal hypoglycemia (an effect that may be due to maternal to fetal transfer of glyburide) were more commonly associated with use of glyburide. Maternal hypoglycemia was comparatively more common in insulin group. When compared to metformin, maternal weight gain was more common in women taking glyburide. Moreover babies born to these mothers (glyburide group) had higher birth weight, and were more prone for having macrosomia.[8,9] Treatment failure was slightly higher in metformin group. It has been found that out of all patients receiving glyburide 20% will have treatment failure. Glyburide is found to be safe during lactation.

Contraindications

- Allergy to glyburide.
- Type 1 diabetes mellitus.
- Diabetic coma and diabetic ketoacidosis.
- Liver disease or renal impairment.
- Glyburide should be given with caution in conditions like adrenal insufficiency, G6PD deficiency, and autonomic neuropathy.

Dosage

2.5 mg to 5 mg, taken daily with meals, dose can be increased by 2.5 mg per week. Maximum dosage is 20 mg per day.

Adverse Drug Reactions

Side Effects of Glyburide

- Hypoglycemia
- Allergic reactions such as itching, redness, hives and bruising.
- Anemia, decrease in platelets and white blood cells.
- Drowsiness, dizziness, blurred vision and joint/muscle pain.

Drug Interactions

Certain drugs may potentiate the action of glyburide by displacing it from protein binding (phenylbutazone, salicylates), by inhibiting its metabolism or excretion (warfarin, alcohol intake) and by synergistic role (salicylates, propanolol, lithium and theophylline).

Certain drugs may decrease the action of glyburide by inducing metabolism (phenobarbitone, phenytoin, rifampicin and by antagonizing its action (thiazide, furosemide, corticosteroids, oral contraceptives).

Preparations

Glyburide is available in tablet form in 1.25 mg, 2.5 mg, 5 mg strength.

Safety During Pregnancy

Glyburide is a FDA pregnancy Category B Drug.

METFORMIN

Metformin is a second generation biguanide. Apart from being an insulin sensitizer, metformin has antiatherosclerotic, anticancer and hypotensive effect also. Metformin crosses placenta but no teratogenic effect has been noted. Minimal amount of drug is transferred in breast milk and there is no harmful effect on baby.[10]

Pharmacology

Mechanism of Action

It causes activation of AMP-activated protein kinase (AMPK) leading to following effects:

- Decreased intestinal absorption of glucose
- Increased uptake of glucose into the cells
- Decrease in plasma fatty acid concentration
- It also inhibits gluconeogenesis

- Metformin has a favorable effect on plasma lipid profile, reduces oxidative stress, and increases plasma fibrinolytic activity.

Pharmacokinetics

Absorption of metformin takes place throughout the gastrointestinal tract. Metformin has a good oral bioavailability of metformin (50–60%) and it has large volume of distribution. Metformin does not significantly bind to plasma proteins and steady state plasma concentration is reached in 24–48 hours and it is <1 mcg/mL. Plasma half-life of metformin is around 6.2 hours while blood elimination half life is 17.6 hours. Metformin does not undergo hepatic metabolism and over 90% of the drug is excreted unchanged in the urine (mainly tubular secretion). Pregnancy may associated with increased tubular secretion of the drug but further studies are required to evaluate the effect of pregnancy on pharmacokinetics of metformin.

Current Evidence

MiGTrial (2008), a RCT on 751 patients with gestational diabetes mellitus has concluded that metformin does not cause any increase in perinatal complications moreover metformin was preferred by these women over insulin but supplemental insulin was required in 46% cases.[11] The same set of workers reviewed babies of these women at age of 2 years (MiG the offspring follow-up) and compared body composition of babies in these two group. It was seen that babies in metformin group had more subcutaneous fat but total body fat remained same in both the groups. So there was less visceral fat in babies in metformin group, thus higher insulin sensitivity is expected.[12]

In a meta-analysis (2013) that included 5 RCTs involving 1270 participants' metformin was compared with insulin for treatment of diabetes in pregnancy, and metformin was found to provide glycemic control that is comparable to insulin.[13] Moreover, it has the advantages of not causing any hypoglycemia, favorable effect on maternal weight gain and a protective effect on the development of pre-eclampsia. Metformin was found to be better for treatment of mild GDM. In another meta-analysis, it was found that the current evidence do not support the fact that metformin causes reduction in incidence of diabetes in polycystic ovarian syndrome patients.[14] The neonatal effect of metformin was similar to insulin although babies born to mothers on metformin weighed less at birth compared to insulin group. Metformin has also been found safe for use in breastfeeding mothers.

Contraindications

Metformin is contraindicated in patient kidney disease, cardiogenic shock, ischemic with heart disease, and septicemia. Metformin should not be given in patients who have history of metformin hypersensitivity in past or who have acute or chronic metabolic acidosis.

Metformin must be omitted before any radiologic investigation in which use of iodinated intravascular contrast agents is required.

Dosage

Metformin hydrochloride tablet is given in divided doses with maximum dose of 2500 mg per day. Initiation of metformin should be done at a lower dose for adjustment to gastrointestinal side effects. Metformin is initiated at 500 mg twice daily dose and increments of 500 mg per week can be done, according the blood sugar levels. In case, total dose is more than 2000 mg per day, drugs can be given in three divided doses.

Since there is lack of evidence regarding use of extended release form of metormin its use is not recommended in pregnancy.

Adverse Drug Reactions

- Metformin causes gastrointestinal intolerance.

- Metformin may lead to Vitamin B_{12} deficiency.
- Lactic acidosis is a rare but potentially fatal complication (approximately 0.03 cases/1000 patient-years) of metformin. Risk of lactic acidosis is increased in renal failure, impaired liver functions, in alcoholics and sepsis.

Drug Interactions

- Iodinated-contrast medium can increase the plasma concentration of metformin by decreasing its renal excretion and may lead to serious and potentially life-threatening interaction. Metformin must be withheld prior to administration of contrast medium.
- Ethanol should not be taken with metformin as it may cause potentially fatal drug interaction.
- Digoxin decreases the renal tubular excretion by competing with metformin.
- Ranitidine decreases renal clearance of metformin.
- Insulin has a synergistic glucose lowering effect with metformin so close monitoring is required.

Preparations

Metformin is available in tablet form in 250 mg, 500 mg, 850 mg, and 1000 mg strength.

Safety During Pregnancy

Metformin is FDA pregnancy category B drug.

OTHER DRUGS

Diabetes leads to maternal complications like pre-eclampsia, preterm labor, iatrogenic prematurity, etc. Management of each of them has been dealt elsewhere in the book. Antenatal corticosteroids interfere with blood sugar control so it has been discussed in detail here.

Corticosteroids

Antenatal corticosteroids lead to significant reduction in rates of neonatal death, RDS and intraventricular hemorrhage and are recommended between 24 and 34+6 weeks gestation, if there is risk of prematurity.

Dosage

- *Betamethasone*: Two doses of betamethasone, 12 mg each, should be given at an interval of 24 hours.
- *Dexamethasone*: Four doses of dexamethasone, 6 mg each, should be given at an interval of 12 hours.

Both are given intramuscularly.

The above regimen is most effective from 24 hours after initiation of therapy to 7 days. Antenatal corticosteroids administration has led to reduction in neonatal mortality, even if delivery occurs within 24 hours after initiation of therapy.

Administration of antenatal corticosteroids causes interference in carbohydrate metabolism, therefore leads to high false positive results of tests for diagnosis of diabetes in pregnancy and also it alters the blood sugar control. So any form of screening and diagnostic tests for diabetes in pregnancy should be avoided, as it will give a false positive result, when corticosteroid course is being given. According to RCOG green top guideline (2010), NICE guideline (2015) diabetes in pregnancy is not a contraindication for antenatal corticosteroids but because of their effect[15,5] on blood sugars, women receiving antenatal corticosteroids should be given insulin according to sliding scale.

KEY POINTS

- Control of blood sugar is crucial in preventing adverse outcome in mother and fetus.
- Insulin is preferred over oral hypoglycemic agents for management of diabetes in pregnancy.
- Use of Glyburide and metformin has not been found to be associated with any harm to the fetus. Also no adverse effects have been found in breastfed neonates of diabetic mothers on these drugs.

- Oral hypoglycemic agents have the advantage of being cheaper and oral route of administration.
- Antenatal corticosteroids are not contraindicated in diabetes.

REFERENCES

1. Pollex E, Moretti ME, Koren G, Feig DS. Safety of insulin glargine use in pregnancy: A systematic review and meta-analysis. Annals of Pharmacotherapy. 2011;45(1):9-16 [PubMed: 21205954].
2. Hod M, Mathiesen ER, Jovanovic L, Mc Cance DR, Ivanisevic M, Garcia SD, Brandsted L, Nazeri A, Damm P. A randomized trial comparing perinatal outcomes using insulin determir and neutral protamine Hagedorn in type 1 diabetes. J Matern Fetal Neonatal Med. 2014;27(1):7-13. Published online 2013 Jun 4. doi:10.3109/14767 058:2013.799650.
3. Jovanovic L, Druzin M, Peterson CM. Effect of euglycemia on the outcome of pregnancy in insulin dependent diabetic women as compared with normal control subjects. An J Med. 1981;71:921-7.
4. Langer O, Anyaegbunam A, Brustman L, Guidetti D, Levy J, Mazze R. Pregestational diabetes: Insulin requirements throughout pregnancy. Am J Obstet Gynecol. 1988;159(3):616-21.
5. Diabetes in pregnancy. National Institute for Health and clinical excellence (NICE) 2015.
6. The American College of Obstetricians and Gynecologists. Gestational Diabetes Mellitus. ACOG practice Bulletin No. 137, 2013.
7. Langer O, Conway DL, Berkus MD, Xenakis EM, Gonzales O. A comparison of glyburide and insulin in women with gestational diabetes mellitus. N Engl J Med. 2000;343(16):1134-8.
8. Zeng YC, Li MJ, Chen Y, Jiang L, Wang SM, Mo XL, Li BY. The use of glyburide in the management of gestational diabetes mellitus: A meta-analysis. Advances in Medical Sciences. 2014;59(1): 95-101 [Pub Med: 24797983].
9. Balsells M, Patterson AG, Sola I, Roque M, Gich I, Corcoy R. Glibenclamide, metformin, and insulin for the treatment of gestational diabetes: A systematic review and meta-analysis.BMJ. 2015;350. doi: http:/dx.doi.org/10.1136/bmj. h102.
10. Gardiner SJ, Kirkpatrick CM, Begg EJ, Zhang M, Moore MP, Saville DJ. Transfer of metformin into breast milk. Clin Pharmacol Ther. 2003; 73(1):71-7.
11. Rowan JA, Hague WM, Gao W, Battin MR, Moore MP. Metformin versus insulin for the treatment of gestational diabetes. N Engl J Med.2008; 358(19):2003-15. Doi: 10.1056/NEJMoa0707193.
12. Rowan JA, Rusch EC, Obolonkin V, Battin M, Wouldes T, Hague WM. Metformin in gestational diabetes: The offspring follow-up (MiG TOFU): body composition at 2 years of age. Diabetes Care. 2011;34(10):2278-84. Doi: 10.2337/ dc11-0660.
13. Gui J, Liu Q, Feng L. Metformin vs Insulin in the Management of Gestational Diabetes: A Meta-Analysis. In: Buzzetti R, (Ed). PLoS One. 2013; 8(5):e64585.doi: 10.137/journal.pone.0064585.
14. Zhuo Z, Wang A, Yu H. Effect of Metformin Intervention during Pregnancy on the Gestational Diabetes Mellitus in women with polycystic ovary syndrome: A Systematic Review and Meta-analysis. In: Marfella M (Ed). Journal of Diabetes Research. 2014.
15. Royal College of Obstetricians and Gynaecologists. Antenatal corticosteroids to reduce Neonatal Morbidity and Mortality. RCOG green Top Guideline No. 7,2010.

CHAPTER 20

Cardiovascular Disorders of Pregnancy

Latika Sahu, Vaishali Paliwal

INTRODUCTION

Cardiovascular disorders (CVD) of varying severity complicate one percent of pregnancies and contribute significantly to maternal morbidity and mortality rates.[1] Rheumatic heart disease and congenital heart diseases are the common pre-existing conditions and hypertension is the most common acquired condition. The incidence of maternal CVD appears to be growing, due to increasing maternal age, cardiovascular risk factors (e.g. obesity) and lifespan of patients with congenital as well as rheumatic heart disease. Studies suggest that pregnancy-related mortality has also increased over the last several decades, with deaths attributable to CVD also increasing.[2] It is of vital importance to manage the patients with CVD during pregnancy and the associated complications. The management of these patients requires a multidisciplinary approach with the involvement of obstetrician, cardiologists, anesthesiologists who are experienced in caring for these patients.

Hemodynamic changes in pregnancy begins with 5–8 weeks of gestation, peak in the late second trimester and continue until delivery and these can have a profound effect on the underlying heart disease. The cardiac output, heart rate and left ventricular stroke volume increases and the systemic and pulmonary vascular resistance decreases. Cardiac decompensation coincides with this peak in patients with pre-existing cardiovascular disease. Pregnancy induces hypercoagulable state and most commonly in the peripartum period. Studies show that pregnant women are three to four times more likely to have arterial thromboembolism and four to five times more likely to have venous thromboembolism as compared with women who are not pregnant.[3] The physiological changes of pregnancy can affect the pharmacokinetic properties of cardiovascular drugs in the mother. Motility in the GI tract decreased which may affect drug absorption. Acid secretion decreased and mucus production increased which increases gastric pH and may affect the degree of ionization and solubility of drugs. Increased metabolism of drugs in the gut wall, or more complete drug absorption leading to increased bioavailability may occur due to longer transit time through the GI tract. Drug transfer across the placenta and the pharmacokinetic properties of certain drugs may influence the rate of passage to the fetus and fetal drug concentrations. Some antiarrhythmic drugs can be administered to the mother (e.g. digoxin), and through placental transfer, can treat fetal tachyarrhythmias.

As soon as a cardiovascular disease patient becomes pregnant or newly diagnosed heart disease during pregnancy the type of cardiovascular lesion should be confirmed, drugs dosage and schedule are to be modified based on patients risk status and NYHA class. In this chapter we are discussing the drugs used for valvular heart diseases, congenital heart diseases, pulmonary hypertension, cardiomyopathies, heart failure, anticoagulation for surgically corrected heart diseases during and before pregnancy, infective endocarditis prophylaxis and treatment of arrhythmias.

Cardiovascular Drugs

The commonly used cardiovascular drugs during pregnancy are listed in **Table 20.1**.

Adenosine

Pharmacology: This is a purine nucleoside that formed from breakdown of adenosine triphosphate (ATP) and occurred naturally.

Mechanism of action: Adenosine can bind to purinogenic receptors of vascular smooth muscle and causes vasodilatation. Adenosine binds to type 1(A1) receptors coupled to G1 proteins in cardiac tissue, which opens potassium channels and inhibits calcium channels and hyperpolarize the cells. At sinoatrial (SA) node adenosine decreases its rate by inhibiting the pacemaker current, which decreases the slope of phase 4 of the pacemaker action potential. At atrioventricular (AV) node it decreases conduction velocity by inhibition of calcium channel. It inhibits the release of norepinephrine by acting on sympathetic nerves. Due to its electrical effect it reduces heart rate and conduction velocity at AV node and decreasing action potential of atrium fibers.[4]

Table 20.1 Cardiovascular drugs commonly used during pregnancy

Drugs	*Uses*
• Adenosine	• Arrhythmias
• Beta-blockers	• Hypertension, arrhythmias, mitral stenosis, cardiomyopathy
• Nitrates	• Hypertension, angina, heart failure
• Digoxin	• Arrhythmia, congestive heart failure (CHF)
• Diuretics	• Hypertension, CHF
• Diltiazem	• Hypertension
• Lidocaine	• Arrythmia, anesthesia
• Sildenafil	• Pulmonary arterial hypertension
• Warfarin	• Mechanical valve, deep vein thrombosis (DVT), atrial fibrillation (AF), Eisenmenger syndrome
• Unfractionated heparin	• Mechanical valve, DVT, AF, Eisenmenger syndrome
• Low molecular weight heparin	• Mechanical valve, DVT, AF, Eisenmenger syndrome

Pharmacokinetics: It has very short half-life of 10 seconds due to uptake into the RBCs. In the RBC, it is deaminated by adenosine deaminase into inosine then further breakdown to hypoxanthine, xanthine and uric acid. These products are excreted by kidneys. Adenosine kinase acted on adenosine and rephosphorylated it to AMP and maintain the adenine nucleotide pool in cells. Administration by rapid IV over 1-3 seconds.[5]

Dosage: 6–18 mg IV bolus.[6] It can be repeated if required.

Indications: As antiarrhythmic drug used specially for paroxysmal supraventricular tachycardia (PSVT) due to its AV node suppression effect. For acute episode it is used as bolus IV injection or IV infusion.

Adverse drug reaction: Patients can have flushing and headache due to vasodilatation. It can cause rapid arterial hypotension and AV block which is reversible after stopping the adenosine infusion. It is contraindicated in pre-existing 2nd or 3rd degree heart block. It may cause bronchospasm and cough, precipitate in asthmatics.[6,7]

It is a FDA Category C drug.

Beta-blockers: Metoprolol

Introduction: Beta-blockers bind to beta-adrenoceptors located in cardiac nodal tissue, the conducting system, and contracting myocytes. The heart has both β_1 and β_2

adrenoceptors. The predominant receptor type in number and function is β_1 beta-blockers by competing for the binding site prevent the normal ligand (norepinephrine or epinephrine) from binding to the beta-adrenoceptor.[8]

Pharmacology: It is a β_1 selective or cardioselective adrenergic receptor blocker but at higher plasma concentrations it also inhibits β_2 adrenoceptors in bronchial and vascular musculature.

Mechanism of action: It decreases contractility, relaxation rate and conduction velocity in heart. It decreases heart rate and cardiac output at rest. It reduces systolic blood pressure and heart rate upon exercise. It inhibits tachycardia induced by isoproterenol and reflex orthostatic tachycardia.

Pharmacokinetics: The oral bioavailability of immediate-release metoprolol is about 50% and the volume of distribution is 3.2–5.6 L/kg. About 10% of metoprolol bound to serum albumin. It crosses the placenta and blood-brain barrier. It is found in breast milk. It is metabolized by CYP2D6 in liver. The mean elimination half-life is 3–4 hours and it may be increased to 7–9 hours in poor CYP2D6 metabolizers. It is eliminated by kidney and excreted in urine. Mostly <5% of oral dose and <10% of intravenous dose are excreted as unchanged drug in the urine and approximately 95% of the dose can be recovered in urine.

Indications: Hypertension, AF rate control, SVT, heart failure, angina, myocardial infarction, arrhythmias, HCM, mitral stenosis, cardiomyopathy.[6,9]

Contraindications: Sinus bradycardia, greater than first degree heart block, sick sinus syndrome and peripheral arterial circulatory disorders.

Dosage: Intravenous used in SVT, AF rate control 5 mg over 3–5 min × 3 doses, 1.25–5 mg/6 hr. Tablets of 25 mg are available, 25–100 mg 6 hrly. Half-life 3–8 hr.[6] To be stored in 20–25°C. Start with 100 mg/day in single or divided doses with or immediately following meals. In hypertension the effect may take one week to manifest and increased dose up to 450 mg/day can be used.

Adverse drug reaction: CNS—Tiredness and dizziness occurs in 10% cases and depression in 5% cases. Other effects are mental confusion, short-term memory loss, headache and nightmare, insomnia. CVS—In 3% of cases shortness of breath and bradycardia occurred. It may cause in <1% cases, arterial insufficiency, palpitations, congestive heart failure, peripheral edema and hypotension. Respiratory—Broncho-spasm, wheezing and dyspnea seen in <1% cases. GI—Diarrhea seen in <5% cases, nausea, dry mouth, gastric pain, constipation reported in about 1% of cases. Hypersensitive reaction like pruritus or rash occurred in 5% cases.[7]

Drug interaction: Reserpine (Catecholamine depleting drugs), calcium channel blockers may have additive effect. Digoxin potentiates the action and increases the risk of bradycardia. CYP2D6 enzyme inhibitors (antidepressants) may increase the plasma concentration of Metoprolol. Concomitant use of hydralazine may increase the concentrations of metoprolol by inhibiting presystemic metabolism of metoprolol. It potentiate the action of alpha blockers like alpha methyldopa, vasoconstrictive action of ergot alkaloids.

Precaution: In geriatric patients due to less metabolism and in patients with hepatic or renal impairment caution should be taken. To be used with caution in diabetes patients using insulin.[8]

FDA category-C: It is secreted in breastmilk (<1 mg/L).

Nitrates/Nitroglycerin

In medical use it is commonly called as "glyceryl trinitrite" or "GTN". Used for the treatment of angina and heart failure.

Pharmacology: The GTN is a prodrug which must first be denitrated to produce the active metabolite nitric oxide (NO).

Mechanism of action: Nitrates produce NO by either reacting with sulfhydril group or with enzymes like glutathione S-transferases, cytochrome P450 (CYP), and xanthine oxidoreductase. NO is a potent activator of guanyl cyclase by heme-dependent mechanisms leading to cGMP formation which activates myosin light chain phosphatase.

Pharmacokinetics: Bioavailability <1%. Metabolized in liver, RBC and vascular wall. Half-life of GTN is 3 minutes. GTN is excreted in urine and bile. Duration of action in sublingual and spray route is 10 minutes. Transdermal patches 8–12 hr during intermittent therapy.

Dosage: Route of administration—Sublingual, spray, ointment, oral, IV, transdermal. Available in strength—0.2 mg/hr to 0.8 mg/hr NTG patches (transdermal). Sublingual tablets 0.3–0.6 mg up to 1.5 mg, spray 0.4 mg, ointment 2% 6 × 6 in, 15 × 15 cm, 7.5–40 mg. Effect lasts up to 7 hr. Oral sustained release 2.5–13 mg, duration of effect 4–8 hour. Intravenous 5–200 mcg/min, duration of effect 7–8 hour.[10]

Adverse drug reaction: Severe headache, severe hypotension, bradycardia. Together with sildenafil may cause severe hypotension, circulatory collapse and death.

It is a FDA pregnancy category C drug.

Digoxin

Introduction: It is extracted from foxglove plant *Digitalis lanata*.[11] This is mainly used for atrial fibrillation/flutter and heart failure.

Pharmacology: Digoxin is a purified cardiac glycoside.

Mechanism of action: It has ionotropic action and neurohormonal effects. It inhibits Na-K$^+$ATPase and activate the Na+-Ca$_{2+}$ membrane exchange pump and thereby increases myocardial contractility. Neurohormonal effects mediated by improved circulation which increases vagal tone and decreases sympathetic tone. This leads to prolonged refractory period and slowing of conduction through the atrioventricular node and thereby slowing the ventricular rate.[12] At lower serum digoxin levels neurohormonal effects are present and ionotropic effects are present at higher digoxin serum levels. Neurohormonal effects are the primary mechanism for the therapeutic actions in both heart failure and atrial fibrillation and Ionotropic effects are less important for therapeutic effects of digoxin.[13] This increases cardiac output in a hypodynamic heart without increasing oxygen consumption.[14] It has no prominent effect on the blood pressure and can be used safely in hypertensives. It has diuretic effect also and helps in gradual excretion of salt and water.[15]

Pharmacokinetics: Digoxin is usually given by oral route and intravenous route is also used in emergency. Half-life is about 36 hours in normal renal function and the dose is once daily 125–250 µg. T the half-life is longer in patients with decreased renal function, and dose should be reduced or change to other glycoside like digitoxin which has much longer elimination half-life (around 7 days). Excretion by kidney and involves P-glycoprotein which leads to significant clinical interactions with other drugs used in heart failure like spironolactone, verapamil and amiodarone.

Dosage

Oral: 0.125–0.5 mg/day, half-life 38–48 hour, IV 0.25 mg every 2 hr until 2 mg total maintenance 0.125–0.25 mg/day used in AF/AFL rate control.[6] Recommended effective plasma level for heart failure is 0.5–1.0 ng/mL and for atrial fibrillation is 1.0–2.0 ng/mL.[16]

Adverse drug reaction: Common adverse drug reactions include gastrointestinal symptoms like nausea, vomiting, anorexia, neurological symptoms like weakness, fatigue, confusion and cardiac symptoms like supraventricular/ventricular arrhythmias, first, second or third degree heart block, sinus bradycardia, etc. Rare adverse drug reactions like visual disturbances and cardiac arrhythmias are dose dependent.[12]

Some medical conditions like dehydration, renal impairment, unstable heart failure, hypokalemia-over diuresis, hypothyroidism, myocardial infarction, hypercalcemia can increase the risk of digoxin toxicity either due to increased digoxin concentration or sensitivity to digoxin.

If any toxicity develop the digoxin dose to be reduced or stopped temporarily depending on severity of symptom and symptomatic treatment of toxicity symptoms to be done.

Drug interaction: Quinidine, verapamil and amiodarone increases plasma levels of digoxin by displacing tissue binding sites and decreasing renal clearance. When used along with diuretics, it can cause increased K^+depletion resulting in tachyarrythmias.

It is a FDA Category C drug.

Diuretics

Furosemide

Introduction: The commonly used diuretics in cardiovascular disorder is Furosemide which is a loop diuretic.

Pharmacology: It acts in ascending limb of loop of Henle in kidney where it inhibits Na+-K+-2Cl- cotransport which causes a significant fraction of sodium reabsorption. So it causes increased loss of water, sodium, and potassium electrolytes.

Mechanism of cardiovascular effects: It effects on sodium and water balance, decreases blood volume and venous pressure leading to decrease in cardiac preload which is followed by decrease in ventricular stroke volume and cardiac output and then leads to a fall in arterial pressure.[17] It causes venodilatation which leads to lowering of venous pressure followed by reduction of capillary fluid filtration and promotes capillary fluid reabsorption and thereby reduces edema. On long-term use it results in decrease systemic vascular resistance that helps to sustain the reduction in arterial pressure. Due to its action on renal prostaglandin synthesis it causes increase in renal blood flow and redistribution of renal cortical blood flow there by increases GFR and helps in quick relief of LVF and pulmonary edema.[18]

Pharmacokinetics: The onset of action is 2–5 minutes in intravenous route, 10–20 minutes in intramuscular route and 20–40 minutes in oral route. It is rapidly absorbed but the bioavailability is 60%. In severe CHF, bioavailability may be markedly reduced necessitating IV administration. The duration of action lasts for 4–6 hours. It is highly bound to plasma proteins and partly conjugated with glucuronic acid and mainly excreted by glomerular filtration as well as tubular secretion in kidney. Plasma half-life averages 1–2 hours but is prolonged in pulmonary edema, renal and hepatic insufficiency.[19]

Therapeutic dose: It is prescribed in pregnant females in rheumatic heart disease, cardiomyopathies, cerebral edema, along with blood transfusion in severe anemia to prevent volume overload, hypertension with renal insufficiency and CHF, hypertensive emergencies and pulmonary edema.[20]

Dosage: Furosemide 20–80 mg divided in 6–12 hourly (PO/IM/IV).

Adverse drug reaction: Common Adverse drug reaction include hypokalemia, metabolic alkalosis, hypomagnesemia, hyperuricemia, dehydration, hypotension and dose related ototoxicity.

Drug interaction: Loss of potassium potentiate digitalis toxicity. NSAIDs reduces diuretic efficacy. Corticosteroids enhance hypokalemia. Amino glycosides enhance ototoxicity, nephrotoxicity.[21]

It is a FDA category C drug.

Spironolactone

Introduction: This is a potassium sparing diuretics. They do not produce hypokalemia.

Pharmacology: This is an aldosterone receptor antagonist acts at the distal segment of distal tubule.

Mechanism of action: It causes more sodium and water to pass into the collecting duct and then be excreted in urine. By inhibiting aldosterone-sensitive sodium reabsorption by this transporter, less potassium and hydrogen ion are exchanged for sodium and therefore less potassium and hydrogen excreted in the urine. This diuretic has relatively weak effects on overall sodium balance, so it is often used in conjunction with Frusemide/loop diuretics to prevent hypokalemia.[21]

Indications: Same as Frusemide and used in combination.

Dosage: 25-400 mg/day in 1-2 divided dosage.

Adverse drug reaction: Hypokalemia, metabolic acidosis, gynecomastia, gastritis and peptic ulcer.[21]

Drug interaction: ACE inhibitors potentiate hyperkalemia. NSAIDs reduces diuretic efficacy.

Diltiazem

Introduction: It blocks the L type calcium channels of the heart and causes direct depression of the SA node and AV conduction and blocks the entry of calcium into the cells.

Pharmacology: It is a calcium channel blocker.

Mechanism of action: It causes vascular smooth muscle relaxation and vasodilatation, decrease contractility of cardiac muscle, conduction velocity inside heart and heart rate. Diltiazem is able to reduce arterial pressure by having both cardiac depressant and vasodilator actions without producing the same degree of reflex cardiac stimulation caused by dihydropyridines.[22]

Pharmacokinetics: Absorption is 90–100%, peak at 3 hours. The oral bioavailability is 40–60% due to high first pass metabolism in liver. It is bound to plasma protein (80%). It is metabolized in liver and the active metabolites excreted in urine. The half-life is 2–6 hours.

Indications: Pulmonary/systemic hypertension. Angina and arrhythmias (PSVT and supraventricular), AF rate control.

Dosage: Available in 30 mg, 60 mg, 90 mg sustained release tablets, 30–60 mg/6 hourly, Half-life 3–4.5 hour. Can be taken once/twice/thrice daily. IV dosage 0.25 mg/kg over 3–5 min (max 20 kg), maintenance 5–15 mg/hr. (SVT, AF rate control).[6]

Adverse drug reaction: More common adverse drug reaction are body ache, dryness or soreness of the throat, congestion, cough, fever, hoarseness, runny nose, tender lymph node and voice changes. The less common effects are chest pain, diarrhea, difficult breathing, lightheaded, flushing, headache, joint pain and loss of appetite, nausea and vomiting.

Drug interaction: It should not be given with beta blockers, excessive cardiac depression may occur. It increases plasma digoxin level by decreasing its excretion, toxicity may develop.

Monitoring: By heart rate monitoring.

It is a FDA category C drug, compatible with breastfeeding.

Lidocaine Hydrochloride

Introduction: It is an antiarrhythmic drug used in ventricular arrhythmias.

Pharmacology: It is a membrane stabilizing antiarrhythmic agent.

Mechanism of action: It suppresses automaticity in His-Purkinje system and spontaneous depolarization of the ventricles during diastole and thereby controls arrhythmias.[23]

Pharmacokinetics: It absorbs from GI tract and passes into hepatic circulation. Only 35% of oral dose reaches systemic circulation unchanged. Onset of action in IV route 45–90 sec and in IM route 10 mins. Duration of action up to 10–20 min in IV route. Plasma concentration of 1–5 μg/mL are required to suppress ventricular arrhythmias, concentration of >5 μg/mL associated with toxicity. It crosses blood brain barrier and placenta. It secretes into milk. It binds to plasma proteins in 60-80% cases. It is metabolized in liver and excreted in urine. It has half-life of 1.5–2 hours.[24]

Dosage: IV/IM, preferred is IV, 1–3 mg/kg at 20–50 mg/min, maintenance 1–4 mg/min, used for VT.[6] Preparations available in 40, 100, 200 mg/mL. For ventricular arrhythmias-IV bolus dose administered at a rate of 25–50 mg/minute (0.5–0.7 mg/kg/min) and up to 1–1.5 mg/kg (50–100 mg/kg) administered as rapid IV injection. Can be repeated after 5–10 minutes if necessary, up to a total of 3 doses/up to 3 mg/kg. For cardiac arrest start at 1–1.5 mg/kg as rapid IV injection repeated at 5–10 minutes if necessary, up to a total of 3 doses/up to 3 mg/kg.[23]

If arrhythmias recur during maintenance infusion 0.5 mg/kg bolus dose administered and infusion rate increased to a maximum of 4 mg/minute.

Contraindications: Severe degree heart block and known hypersensitivity.

Precaution-constant ECG monitoring required. To discontinue infusion if cardiac depression occur.

Adverse drug reaction: Hypersensitivity reactions. Nervous system—muscle twitching or tremors, seizure, unconsciousness and coma (in high doses). Cardiovascular system-possibility of hypotension, arrhythmias, heart block, cardiovascular collapse and bradycardia. Respiratory system—respiratory depression in high doses. Possibility of local thrombophlebitis in prolonged IV infusions.[23]

It is FDA pregnancy category B drug. It is secreted in breast milk so to be used with caution.

Pulmonary Vasodilators

Sildenafil

Pharmacology: It is a selective inhibitor of phosphodiesterase type-5 (PDE5). PDE5 is known to enhance nitric oxide-mediated vasodilatation by inhibiting degradation of cyclic GMP in patients with/without heart failure.[25]

Mechanism of action: It lowers the pulmonary arterial pressure and has been shown to improve arterial oxygenation in pulmonary hypertension. It significantly increases exercise capacity. It improves symptoms of right sided heart failure by reducing workload of the right ventricle of the heart.

Pharmacokinetics: Oral bioavailability of sildenafil is 40% and peak blood levels are attained in 1–2 hour. It is metabolized by the CYP3A4 and an active metabolite is produced. The half-life is 4 hours.

Indications: Pulmonary hypertension in rheumatic heart disease and Eisenmenger's syndrome.

Contraindication: Severe hepatic/renal impairment, hypotension, recent stroke or heart attack. When taking nitric oxide donors like nitroglycerine and hereditary degenerative retinal disorder.

Dosage: 20 mg tds.

Adverse drug reaction: It can cause headache, flushing, nasal congestion, and impaired vision including photophobia or blurred vision and indigestion. Severe adverse drug reactions can occur rarely. Those are hypotension, myocardial infarction, ventricular arrhythmias, stroke, increased intraocular pressure and sudden hearing loss.[26]

Drug interaction: Protease inhibitors used in HIV can increases adverse drug reaction by inhibiting the metabolism of sildenafil. Those who are on protease inhibitor can reduce the sildenafil dose to 25 mg/48 hours. Erythromycin and cimetidine can lead to prolonged plasma half-life. If taken with alpha blocker may cause low blood pressure. Both should be taken at 4 hour interval.

It is a FDA category B, drug compatible with breastfeeding.

Anticoagulation in Pregnancy

There are many cardiovascular disease conditions require the initiation or maintenance of anticoagulation during pregnancy those include, patients using mechanical heart valves, acute deep vein thrombosis or thromboembolism or history of venous thromboembolism during pregnancy, atrial fibrillation. The three most common agents considered for use during pregnancy are warfarin, unfractionated heparin (UFH) and low-molecular-weight heparin (LMWH).

Warfarin

Introduction: In 1954, it was approved for use as a medication. Most widely prescribed anticoagulant. The name Warfarin was taken from its discovery the organization that funded the key research "WARF" (Wisconsin Alumni Research Foundation) and the ending-arin is due to link with coumarin.

Pharmacology: It is a synthetic derivative of dicoumarol, a 4-hydroxycoumarin derived mycotoxin anticoagulant.

Mechanism of action: Warfarin, produces anticoagulant effect by interfering with the cyclic interconversion of vitamin K and its 2, 3 epoxide (vitamin K epoxide). Vitamin K is a cofactor for the carboxylation of glutamate residues to γ-carboxy glutamate (Gla) on the N-terminal region of vitamin K-dependent proteins-coagulation factors II, VII, IX and X, that binds to $Ca^{2+}$and coagulation sequence to proceed. By inhibiting the vitamin K conversion cycle, warfarin induces hepatic production of partially decarboxylated proteins with reduced coagulant activity.[27,28] Carboxylation promotes binding of the vitamin K dependent coagulation factors to phospholipid surfaces, thereby accelerating blood coagulation.[29] The reduced form of vitamin K (vitamin KH_2) is required for γ carboxylation. Coumarins inhibits the enzyme vitamin K epoxide reductase and block the formation of vitamin KH_2, thereby limiting the γ carboxylation of the vitamin K dependent coagulant proteins. The anticoagulant effect of coumarins can be overcome by low doses of vitamin K which bypasses vitamin K epoxide reductase. Warfarin interferes with the carboxylation of Gla proteins synthesized in bone, which contribute to fetal bone abnormalities when used in pregnancy but it does not affect bone metabolism in children or adults.[30]

Pharmacokinetics: Warfarin is rapidly absorbed from the gastrointestinal tract. It has high bioavailability and reaches maximal blood concentrations 90 minutes after oral administration. It has half-life of 36–48 hours, bound to plasma albumin and accumulates in the liver. The genetic and environmental factors, including common mutations in the gene coding for cytochrome P450, the hepatic enzyme responsible for oxidative metabolism of the warfarin S-isomer influences the relationship between the dose and the response of warfarin. Many genetic polymorphisms in cytochrome P450 have been described that are associated with requirements of lower dose and higher complication rates (bleeding). It crosses placenta, can cause warfarin embryopathy in first trimester exposure patients and is secreted in the milk, however not enough to affect the infant.[31]

Dosage and monitoring: 4–5 mg, increase up to 10 mg/day. After beginning oral warfarin the anticoagulant effect observed within 2–7 days. Heparin should be given concurrently with warfarin for ≥4 days if a rapid effect is required. Average maintenance dose is 5 mg/day which usually results in an INR (patient prothrombin time/mean normal prothrombin time) of ≥2.0 after 4 or 5 days. Heparin can be stopped once the INR comes to therapeutic range for 2 days. For nonemergency situation (e.g. chronic atrial fibrillation) treatment can be started outpatient wise and satisfactory anticoagulation within 6 days can be achieved with a dose of 4–5 mg/day. In patients sensitive to warfarin, the elderly and in those at increased risk of bleeding should be treated with lower doses (<4–5 mg).

Monitoring of treatment with warfarin: Daily prothrombin time (PT) and INR to be done till the therapeutic range (INR 2–3) has been achieved and sustained for 2 consecutive days. After that PT and INR can be done 2–3 times weekly for 1–2 weeks and then less often as required to the stability of the results. Once the INR becomes stable, the frequency of testing can be as long as 4 weeks intervals. Frequent monitoring is resumed when dose adjustments are required—when there is change in diet of the patient, concurrent medication changes, poor compliance or alcohol intake by the patient.[31]

INR therapeutic range: The therapeutic range for INR is between 2 and 4. INR <2 may increase the risk of thromboembolism. The risk of bleeding increases when INR of the patient exceeds 4 and the risk rises sharply with INR values of >5. When INR is elevated, to lower it the first step is to stop warfarin; the second step is to administer vitamin K and the third and most rapidly effective step is to infuse fresh frozen plasma or prothrombin concentrate. After warfarin stopped INR comes back to 2–3 after 4–5 days but it can decline within 24 hr with vitamin K.[31]

Precaution during pregnancy: During the first trimester of pregnancy, warfarin therapy should be avoided. And in some special circumstances it is avoided throughout pregnancy. In women with mechanical prosthetic heart valves warfarin is recommended in second and third trimesters of pregnancy and to be converted to heparin/ LMWH at 38 weeks and elective induction to be planned at 40 weeks of pregnancy. Lesser dose of heparin required to prevent maternal thromboembolism also might outweigh the risk of warfarin embryopathy during first trimester. If administer to nursing mother it does not affect feeding infant.

Adverse drug reactions

- *Bleeding due to high INR values*: In a clinical situation when INR is above therapeutic range but <5, with no significant bleeding and if patient does not require rapid reversal for surgical intervention, then the dose of warfarin can be reduced or the next dose can be omitted and to be resumed (at a lower dose) when INR becomes normal. If INR is between 5–9 and the patient is not bleeding and has no risk factor that predispose to bleeding, the next ½ doses of warfarin omitted and reinitiated after INR falls at a lower dose. Vitamin K 1–2.5 mg orally given if the patient is high-risk for bleeding. If rapid reversal is required in case of urgent surgery or dental extraction oral vitamin K 2–5 mg and may repeat dose vitamin K 1/2 mg if INR remains high after 24 hours. If INR is >9 and clinically there is no significant bleeding, oral vitamin K 3–5 mg can be given and may repeat if necessary. If INR is >20 and rapid reversal is required because of serious bleeding, vitamin K should be given as slow intravenous infusion in a dose of 10 mg, supplemented with transfusion of fresh plasma or prothrombin complex concentrate. Additional dose of vitamin K may be necessary every 12 hours. After administration of high dose of vitamin K, if warfarin is to be resumed, additional heparin should be given until there is reversal of vitamin K effects and response to warfarin of the patient is seen.[31]
- Other adverse drug reactions include alopecia, cutaneous necrosis, dermatitis and diarrhea. Extensive thrombosis of venules and capillaries within subcutaneous fat can lead to skin necrosis (rare) which is observed on third to eighth day of therapy. This may be associated with warfarin induced protein C or S deficiency but exact pathogenesis not known. With this complication warfarin is contraindicated and heparin to be given. As heparin at long-term can cause osteoporosis restart of warfarin can be done with lower dose of 2 mg with heparin and gradually increase in several weeks.
- *Teratogenicity with warfarin*: Two types of birth defect can occur if exposed during developmental period. If exposed between 6th and 9th week the fetus is at risk of warfarin embryopathy. This is characterized by nasal and midface hypoplasia, and stippled vertebral and femoral epiphyses and vitamin K dependent clotting factors are not demonstrable in the embryo.[32] Warfarin derivatives exert their teratogenic effect by inhibiting post-translational carboxylation of coagulation proteins. The risk of embryopathy is dose dependent >5 mg daily throughout first trimester. During second and third trimesters, the defects associated with fetal exposure to warfarin may cause hemorrhage leading to disharmonic growth and deformation from scarring in any organs. Defect may lead to agenesis of corpus callosum, Dandy Walker malformation, and midline cerebellar atrophy, microphthalmia, optic atrophy and blindness, developmental

delay and mental retardation. It may cause miscarriage, stillbirths also.[33]

Drug interactions: Some commonly used drugs enhance the anticoagulant effect of warfarin. Broad spectrum antibiotics (Ceftriaxone and Cefoperazone) and sulfonamides inhibit gut flora and reduce vitamin K production, aspirin, indomethacin, phenytoin, amiodarone and metronidazole inhibit warfarin metabolism. Phenylbutazone, sulfinpyrazone, metronidazole and trimethoprim-sulfamethoxazole potentiate its effect by inhibiting clearance of S-warfarin. Amiodarone inhibit the metabolic clearance and potentiate the action of warfarin. Anticoagulant effect of warfarin is inhibited by barbiturates, rifampicin and carbamazepine by increasing hepatic clearance. In patients consuming green vegetables or vitamin K containing supplements like weight reducing diet and in patients receiving intravenous vitamin K supplements can reduce the anticoagulant response to warfarin.

It is a FDA category X drug.

Unfractionated Heparin

Introduction: McLean in 1916 discovered Heparin.[34] Brinkhous and associates demonstrated that heparin requires a plasma cofactor for its anticoagulant activity more than 20 years later, and that was named antithrombin III by Abildgaard in 1968 but now referred as antithrombin (AT).[35] Rosenberg Lindahl, and others in 1970s, elucidated the mechanism for Heparin/AT interaction. The active center serine of thrombin and other coagulation enzymes is inhibited by an arginine reactive center on the AT molecule and that heparin binds to lysine sites on AT, producing a conformational change at the arginine reactive center that converts AT from a slow, progressive thrombin inhibitor to a very rapid inhibitor. AT binds covalently to the active serine center of coagulation enzyme, and then heparin dissociates from the ternary complex and can be reutilized. Later on it was discovered that heparin binds to and potentiate the activity of AT through a glucosamine unit contained within a pentasaccharide unit.[36]

Pharmacology: The molecular size (3000–30000 Da), anticoagulant activity (only 1/3rd have this function) and pharmacokinetic properties (depends on chain length) of heparin is heterogeneous. High molecular weight species of heparin cleared from circulation early than low molecular weight species. This is responsible for the difference in the relationship between plasma heparin concentration (measured in antifactor Xa units) and the activated thromboplastin times (aPTT).

Mechanism of action: After administration of heparin one third of its dose binds to AT which is responsible for the anticoagulant action and the remaining two third has minimal therapeutic action. The heparin AT complex inactivates a number of coagulation enzymes, including thrombin factor IIa and factors Xa, IXa, Xia and XIIa.[36] Thrombin and factor Xa are the most responsive to inhibition. By inactivating thrombin, heparin prevents fibrin formation as well as inhibits thrombin-induced activation factor V and factor VIII.

Heparin prolongs bleeding time in human. Interaction of heparin with platelets and endothelial cells may contribute to heparin induced bleeding by a mechanism independent of its anticoagulant effect. Heparin increases vessel wall permeability, suppresses the proliferation of vascular smooth muscle cells and suppresses osteoblast formation and activates osteoclasts, effects that promote bone loss.[37]

At low concentrations of heparin, factor Xa mediated conversion of prothrombin to thrombin is selectively affected. In higher doses, it prevents platelet aggregation.[38]

Pharmacokinetics: Heparin is a large molecule so not absorbed orally. It is given continuous IV infusion and subcutaneous (SC) injection. On SC injection, the anticoagulant effect may delay for 1–2 hours. In blood-stream it binds to number of plasma proteins, endothelial cells and macrophages. After binding to endothelial cell receptors and macrophages heparin is depolymerized and cleared from circulation. Heparin does not cross blood brain barrier or placenta. It is metabolized in liver by heparinase enzyme and excreted through urine.[39] The half-life of heparin is dose-dependent and can be prolonged to 1–4 hours at doses of more than 100 U/Kg.

Dosage: Therapeutic dose of heparin is 10000–35000 U/SC/24 hour. Prophylactic dose of heparin is 5000–10000 U Sc/8–12 hour. For women with mechanical prosthetic valves, heparin should be started with daily dose of 35000 U. Monitoring with patients on heparin should be performed with either activated partial thromboplastin time or heparin assays at least twice weekly. Higher heparin doses may be required in third trimester because of an increase in heparin-binding proteins.

Adverse drug reaction: Bleeding can occur if over dosage and manifest as hematuria. The antidote is protamine sulfate can be given on a weight by weight basis for the treatment of heparin induced bleeding. With proper monitoring, this can be prevented. Heparin may induce thrombocytopenia which may lead to thromboembolic events.[40] Caution-with aspirin and other antiplatelet agent. Contraindication of use are bleeding disorder, history of heparin induced thrombocytopenia, severe hypertension, ocular and neurosurgery, subacute bacterial endocarditis (risk of embolism), tuberculosis (risk of hemoptysis, cirrhosis and renal failure.

Monitoring: Activated partial thromboplastin time is used to monitor the therapeutic levels. It is kept 1.5–2.5 times the patient's pretreatment levels.

It is compatible with breastfeeding (ACOG 2011).

Low Molecular Weight Heparins

Introduction: The LMWHs are developed for clinical use because of LMWH has reduced antifactor IIa activity relative to antifactor Xa activity and superior pharmacokinetic properties in comparison to UFH.[41]

Pharmacology: LMWH are formed from Heparin by reducing the molecular size while still inhibiting the factor Xa. LMWH has mean molecular weight of 4500–5000 Da.

Mechanism of action: LMWH produce their anticoagulant effect by activating AT due to their pentasaccharide sequence found in <1/3rd of molecules. They selectively inhibit factor Xa with little effect on factor IIa by bringing only a conformational change in antithrombin III. As a result they have less effect on aPTT, lesser antiplatelet action and thus less interference with hemostasis.

Pharmacokinetics: LMWH has a longer plasma half-life (because of less binding to macrophages and endothelial cells) and better bioavailability at low doses than heparin and have more predictable dose response (because of reduced binding to plasma protein). They have subcutaneous bioavailability of 70–90% with minimum variability in response. They have a longer half-life of 4–6 hour so once daily dose is feasible. LMWH cleared through kidney and biological half-life prolonged in renal failure patients.

Dosage: One mg/kg body weight, twice daily. For patients with mechanical prosthetic valve LMWH should be given subcutaneously at a dose of 100 anti-Xa U/kg twice daily. The dose is adjusted to maintain the anti-Xa level between 0.5 and 1.0 U/mL, 4–6 hour after injection.

Adverse drug reaction: LMWH has reduced binding capacity to platelet so less chance of heparin induced thrombocytopenia and it has less binding to osteoblasts leading to less bone loss. It is compatible with breastfeeding.

Monitoring: aPTT is not prolonged so lab monitoring is not needed.

Preparations: Enoxaparin available in 20 mg and 40 mg prefilled syringe.

Use in mechanical valves: For anticoagulation for mechanical valves, LMWH is definitely inadequate and has high associated maternal mortality rate. Even full anticoagulation with unfractionated heparin or LMWH is associated with valvular thrombosis.

Options of anticoagulation use in pregnancy in women with prosthetic valves: Regimes recommended by the American College of Chest Physicians for anticoagulation in pregnancy with prosthetic valves—*any one of the following* (William 24th edition).

- Adjusted LMWH throughout pregnancy twice daily. The doses should be adjusted to achieve the peak anti-Xa level 4 hours after subcutaneous injection
- Adjusted UFH throughout pregnancy every 12 hours. Dose adjusted to maintain aPTT at least twice control or attain an antiXa level of 0.35–0.70 U/mL.
- LMWH or UFH till 13 weeks, then warfarin substitution, and at 38 weeks of pregnancy LMWH or UFH resumed and planned labor induction at 40 weeks or until close to delivery.
- In very high-risk women, warfarin throughout the pregnancy and substitution with LMWH or UFH close to delivery, at 38 weeks of pregnancy and planned labor induction at 40 weeks. In addition, low dose aspirin 75–100 mg daily should be given.

Heparin/LMWH should be discontinued 12 hours before planned induction of labor. Heparin/LMWH should be started postpartum and overlapped with warfarin for 4–5 days.[42]

It is a FDA category B drug.

Antibiotic Prophylaxis

Patients with heart disease who are at highest risk of developing infective endocarditic (IE) include—a prosthetic heart valve, valve repair with prosthetic material, a prior history of IE, and many congenital cyanotic heart diseases like single ventricle state, transposition of the great arteries and tetralogy of Fallot even if the abnormalities repaired, valvulopathy after heart transplantation.[43] These patients must require IE prophylaxis prior to certain procedures during pregnancy like-undergoing dental procedure that involve manipulation of the tissue of the gums, the peripheral region of the teeth or perforation of the lining membranes of the gums such as tooth extractions, dental scaling or drainage of a dental abscess. Any oral or upper respiratory tract procedure also requires IE prophylaxis.

Antibiotics Recommendations by American Heart Association

Single dose of antibiotics to all highest risk patient is necessary. All heart disease patients who are of moderate and low risk for infective endocarditis do not require any antibiotic prophylaxis. Usually penicillin is given. People who are allergic to penicillin can be treated one hour before the procedure with an alternate antibiotic. Patients those are unable to take oral medication can be treated with an antibiotic injection 30 min before the procedure. Antibiotic prophylaxis is not recommended by AHA for any genitourinary or gastrointestinal procedures.

A pregnant patient who has at high-risk for IE does not usually need antibiotic prophylaxis before a normal vaginal delivery or cesarean section in the absence of pelvic infection. Antibiotics may be recommended before labor or cesarean section for complications related to Group B *Streptococcus* like PROM and PPROM, etc.

ACOG 2011 recommendation[44] of antibiotic prophylaxis for infective endocarditis in high-risk women.

Standard (IV): Ampicillin 2 g or cefazolin or ceftriaxone 1 g penicillin allergic (IV): cefazolin or ceftriaxone 1 g or clindamycin 600 mg. Oral amoxycillin 2 g. Azithromycin 500 mg PO, Cephalexin 500 mg PO.[2] These drugs are administered as close to 30–60 minutes before anticipated delivery time as is feasible.

REFERENCES

1 Cunningham GF, Leveno KJ, Bloom SL, Spongy CY, Dashe JS, Hoffman BL, Casey BM, et al. Cardiovascular disorders. William's Obstetrics 24th edn. McGraw-Hills, New York. 2014;49.pp. 973-99.

2. Berg CJ, Callaghan WM, Syversion C, Henderson Z. Pregnancy related mortality in the united states, 1998-2005. Obstet Gynecol. 2010;116:1302-9.
3. Weiss BM, von Segesser LK, Alon E, Seifert B, Turina MI. Outcome of cardiovascular surgery and pregnancy a systematic review of the period 1984-1996. Am J Obstet Gynecol. 1998;179:1643-53.
4. Lerman BB, Belardinelli L. Cardiac electrophysiology of adenosine: Basic and clinical concept. Circulation. 1991;83:1499-509.
5. Roden DM, Echt DS, Lee JT, Murray KT. Clinical pharmacology of antiarrythmic agents. In: Josephson ME, ed. Sudden Cardiac Death. Blackwell Scientific, London. 1993.pp.182-5.
6. Loscalzo J, Libby P, Ebstein J. Disorder of cardiovascular system. Longo DL, Kasper DL, Jameson Jl, Fauci AS, Hauser SL, Loscalzo J (Eds) In: Harrison's Principle of Internal Medicine, 18th edn. McGraw Hill, New York. 2012;10. pp.1883-4.
7. Roden DM. Risks and benefits of antiarrhythmic therapy. N Engl J Med. 1994;331:785-91.
8. Richard EK. Cardiovascular pharmacology concepts Beta-blockers.updated 13.3.2013. Available at *www.cvpharmacology.com/betablockers.*
9. MERIT-HF Study group. Effect of metoprolol CR/XL in chronic heart failure: Metoprolol CR/XL Randomized Intervention Trial in Congestive Heart Failure (MERIT-HF). Lancet. 1999;353:2001-7.
10. Loscalzo J, Libby P, Ebstein J. Disorder of cardiovascular system In: Longo DL, Kasper DL, Jameson Jl, F auci AS, Hauser SL, Loscalzo J (Eds). Harrison's Principle of Internal Medicine. 18th edn. McGraw-Hill, New York. 2012;10. pp.2008-10.
11. Hollman A. Digoxin comes from Digitalis lanata. BMJ. 1996;312(7035):912.
12. Auman J, Didemenico R, Galanter W. Mechanisms, manifestations and management of digoxin toxicity in the modern Era. Am J Cardiovasc Drugs. 2006;6:77-86.
13. Barclay M, Begg E. The practice of digoxin therapeutic drug monitoring. NZMJ. 2003; 116(1187).
14. Bristow MR, Linas S, Port DJ. Drugs in the treatment of heart failure. In: Zipes Plibby P, (Eds). Braunwald's Heart Disease: A Textbook of Cardiovascular Medicine, 7th edn. Elsevier Saunders, Philadelphia. 2005.pp.569-601.
15. Eichhorn EJ, Gheorghiade M. Digoxin-New perspective of an old drug. N Engl J Med. 2002;347:1394-5.
16. Hunt SA, Abraham WT, Chin MH, et al. ACC/AHA 2005 guideline update for the diagnosis and management of chronic heartfailure in the adult: a report of the American College of Cardiology/American Heart Association Task Force on Practice Guidelines (writing committee to update the 2001 guidelines for the evaluation and Management of Heart Failure): Developed in collaboration with the American College of Chest Physicians and the International Society for Heart and Lung Transplantation:endorsed by the Heart Rhythm Society. Circulation. 2005; 112(12):e154-235.
17. Bristow MR, Linas S, Port DJ. Drugs in the treatment of heart failure. In: Zipes P, Libby P, (Eds). Braunwald's Heart Disease: A Textbook of cardiovascular medicine, 7th edn. Elsevier Saunders, Philadelphia. 2005.pp.569-601.
18. Dresser MJ, Leabman MK, Giacomini KM. Transporters involved in the elimination of drugs in the kidney: Organic anion transporters and organic cation transporters. J Pharm Sci. 2001;90:397-421.
19. Barter DC. Clinical pharmacology of loop diuretics. Drugs. 41:14-22.
20. Barter DC. Diuretic therapy. N Engl J Med. 1998;339:387-95.
21. Richard EK. Cardiovascular pharmacology concepts Diuretics. Updated 29.10.2012. Available at *www.cvpharmacology.com/diuretics.*
22. Richard EK. Cardiovascular pharmacology concepts calcium channel blockers. updated 22.3.2015. Available at *www.cvpharmacology.com/CCBs.*
23. The American Heart Association. Guidelines 2005 for cardiopulmonary resuscitation and emergency cardiovascular care. Circulation. 2005;112(Suppl 1):1V1-211.
24. AHFS Drug information 2007. McEvoy GK ed. Lidocaine Hydrochloride. Bethesda. MD: American Society of Health System Pharmacists. 2007. pp. 1599-602.
25. Semigran MJ. Type 5 phosphodiesterase inhibition: the focus shift to the heart. Circulation. 2005;112(17):2589-91.
26. Viagra Prescribing information. Pfizer. October 2007. Retrieved 2012.
27. Choonara IA, Malia RG, Haynes BP, et al. The relationship between inhibition of vitamin K-epoxide reductase and reduction of clotting

factor activity with warfarin. Br J Clin Pharmacol. 1988;25;1-7.
28. Mutucumarana VP, Acher F, Straight DL, et al. A conserved region of human vitamin K-dependent carboxylase between residues 398 and 404 is important for its interaction with glutamate substrate. J Biolchem. 2003;278:(46)488-93.
29. Borowsski M, Furie BC, Bauminger S, et al. Prothrombin requires two sequential metal dependent conformational transitions to bind phospholipids: confirmation specific antibodies directed against the phospholipid binding site on prothrombin J Biol Chem. 1986;261:(14)969-75.
30. Hauschka PV, Lian JB, Cole DEC, et al. Osteocalcin and matrix Gla protein vitamin K dependent protein in bone. Phys Rev. 1989; 990-1047.
31. Hirsh J, Fuster V, Ansell J, Halperin JL. American Heart Association/American College of Cardiology Foundation guide to warfarin therapy. Circulation. 2003;107:1692-711.
32. Scaefer C, Hanneman D, Meister R, et al. Vitamin K antagonists and pregnancy outcome-A multi-center prospective study. Thromb Haemost. 2006;95(6):949.
33. Cunningham GF, Leveno KJ, Bloom SL, Spongy CY, DasheJs, Hoffman BL, Casey BM, et al. Teratology, teratogen, and fetotoxic agent. Williams 24th edn. McGraw-Hills, New York. 2014;12.pp.240-58.
34. Mc Lean J. The thromboplastic action of cephalin. Am J Physiol. 1916;41:250-7.
35. Abildgaard U. Highly purified antithrombin 3 with heparin cofactor activity prepared by disc electrophoresis. Scand J Clin Lab Invest. 1968;21:89-91.
36. Olson ST, Chuang YJ. Heparin activates antithrombin anticoagulant function by generating new interaction sites (exosites) for blood clotting proteinases. Trends Cardiovasc Med. 2002;12:331-8.
37. Rosenberg RD, Bauer KA. The heparin antithrombin system: a natural anticoagulant mechanism. In: Colman RW, Hirsh J, Marder VJ, Salzman EW, (Eds). Hemostasis and thrombosis:Basic principles and clinical practice. 3rd edn. Philadelphia, Pa: JB Lippincott Co. 1994. pp. 837-60.
38. Shantsila E, Lip GY, Chong BH. Heparin-induced thrombocytopenia. A contemporary clinical approach to diagnosis and management. Chest. 2009;135:1651-64.
39. Sugahara K, Kitagawa H. Heparin and heparan sulphate biosynthesis. IUBMB Life, 2002;54:163-75.
40. Bhandari M, Hirsh J, Weitz JI, et al. The effects of standard and low molecular weight heparin on bone nodule formation in vitro. Thromb Haemost. 1998;80:413-7.
41. Weitz JI. Low molecular weight heparins. N Engl J Med. 1997;337:688-98.
42. Bates SM, Greer IA, Middleldorp S, et al. VTE, thrombophilia, antithrombotic therapy, and pregnancy. Chest. 2012;141:e691S.
43. Wilson W, Taubert KA, Gewitz M, et al. Prevention of infective endocarditis. Guidelines from the American Heart association. Circulation. 2007;116:1736.
44. American College of Obstetrician and Gynaecologist: use of prophylactic antibiotics in labor and delivery. Practice Bulletin No 120, June 2011a.

CHAPTER 21

Thyroid Disorders in Pregnancy

Ashok Kumar, Gunjan Bhatnagar, Deepika S Sharma, Madhur Kumar

Thyroid is the one of the most common endocrine disorders affecting women of reproductive age, second only to diabetes mellitus.[1] The incidence of hypothyroidism during pregnancy is 0.3–0.5% for overt and 2–3% for subclinical hypothyroidism.[2] Hyperthyroidism is less common than hypothyroidism (0.2% during pregnancy).[3]

All are associated with adverse pregnancy outcomes and should be promptly treated. Also, preconceptional optimization of thyroid status of affected women should be stressed upon.

DRUGS USED IN THYROID DISORDERS

An outline of various drugs used in thyroid disorders:

Hypothyroidism Levothyroxine
Hyperthyroidism Antithyroid agents
Thionamides - Methimazole
Carbimazole
Propylthiouracil(PTU)
Nonselective beta blockers
Propranolol
Glucocorticoids
Digitalis glycosides - Digitalis

Used only in cases of thyroid storm (a medical emergency which manifests as an acute, life-threatening, hypermetabolic state due to excessive release of thyroid hormones in patients with thyrotoxicosis).

Hypothyroidism

Levothyroxine

Levothyroxine sodium tablets, contain synthetic crystalline L 3,3',5,5' tetraiodothyronine sodium salt [Levothyroxine (T4) sodium], chemically similar to thyroxine (T_4).

Pharmacology

Absorption: When orally administered, 40–80% is bioavailable. Concurrent intake of food, caffeine, iron and calcium supplements decrease the absorption,[4] therefore should be ingested in the morning at least 60 minutes before eating.[4]

Metabolism and excretion: Slowly eliminated. Metabolized mainly through sequential deiodination and primarily eliminated by the kidneys. About 20% eliminated in stool. Narrow therapeutic range, may lead to deviations from euthyroidism when switching from one brand to another.[5]

Mechanism of Action

Levothyroxine mimics the action of thyroxine (T4) which is converted in the body to its active form, L-triiodothyronine (T3). T4 and T3 bind to thyroid receptors in the cell nucleus and cause metabolic effects by controlling DNA transcription and protein synthesis.

Indications: Used in subclinical hypothyroidism, overt hypothyroidism, myxedema coma.

Contraindications

- Hypersensitivity
- Acute myocardial infarction
- Uncorrected adrenal insufficiency.

Dosage: The recommended initial dose is 12.5–25 mcg/day. Dose titration is done by increase of 25 mcg/day every 2–4 weeks, with clinical and laboratory monitoring, until the TSH level is normalized.

Patients who are known hypothyroid must increase their dose by 25% (9 tablets instead of 7 per week) as soon as pregnancy is confirmed due to increased requirement in pregnancy.[6] After delivery, thyroxine dose must be reduced to prepregnancy dose or TSH must be measured 6 weeks postpartum.[7]

Adverse drug reactions

Minor: Fatigue, fever, hyperhidrosis, anxiety, emotional lability, flushing.

Major: Palpitations, arrhythmia, decreased bone mineral density, menstrual irregularities

Drug interactions: Reduction in the dose of oral anticoagulants and increase in digitalis may be required. There should be a difference of at least four hours between ferrous sulfate and thyroxine dosages.

Monitoring: Goal of therapy is to maintain serum TSH <2.5 mIU/L. Serum TSH measured every four to six weeks until 20 weeks gestation and on a stable medication dose, then again at 24 to 28 weeks and 32 to 34 weeks gestation.

Safety during pregnancy and lactation: It is safe during pregnancy and lactation and is FDA category A drug.

Hyperthyroidism

Propylthiouracil (PTU)

Preferred agent of choice during first trimester and in women with methimazole allergy.[8] PTU is shifted over to methimazole in the second trimester because the probability of developing methimazole embryopathy diminishes in second trimester and risk of hepatotoxicity associated with PTU is high.

Pharmacology

It is rapidly absorbed and 50–80% is bioavailable (large first pass effect). It is metabolized in liver and excreted by kidneys. It crosses placental barrier and secreted in breast milk (however less readily than methimazole).

It acts by blocking oxidation of I_2 in thyroid gland inhibiting thyroid hormone synthesis. It also blocks type1 deiodinase[9] Inhibiting T_4 to T_3 conversion (advantage over other drugs). Because of this property it is also used in thyroid storm.

Indications: It is used in hyperthyroidism of any etiology e.g. Grave's disease, solitary toxic adenoma, nodular goiter. It is rarely used in transient hyperthyroidism as in gestational trophoblastic disease, hyperemesis gravidarum and gestational transient thyrotoxicosis.

Contraindication: Hypersensitivity to the drug is only contraindication.

Dosage: 300–450 mg/day orally divided three times a day initially (up to 800–900 mg/day).

Maintainence: 100–150 mg/day three times a day(lowest possible dose is given to keep FT_4 near the upper normal range to prevent fetal hypothyroidism and fetal goiter).

Thyrotoxic crisis: A loading dose of 300–600 mg is given orally or via nasogastric tube or as suppository by rectum followed by 150–300 mg every 6 hours.

Adverse drug reactions: Overall 3–12%.

Minor: Nausea, vomiting, epigastric distress.

Major: Liver injury, liver failure.

- Agranulocytosis (most serious 0.3–0.6%). Idiosyncratic reaction, symptoms like sore throat, fever, ulcers, etc. must be reported immediately.
- Drug fever
- Lupus like syndrome
- Hypoprothombinemia and bleeding
- Vasculitis.

Drug interactions: Reduced dose of oral anticoagulants (e.g. warfarin) due to inhibition of vitamin K activity and of beta blockers, digitalis and theophylline due to slowing of their metabolism may be required.

Monitoring: Serum TSH and FT_4 measured every two weeks till dose is stabilized.

FT_4 and FT_4I is a better indicator of control of hyperthyroidism as compared to FT_3, FT_3I and TSH because normalization of FT_4 and FT_4I precedes over them.

Safety during pregnancy and lactation: Drug of choice in lactation. Only 0.077% ingested dose is secreted in milk. However, mothers are cautioned to take no more than 150–200 mg a day in divided doses, each dose after feeding.

It is a FDA Category D drug.

Methimazole

The main concern with the use of methimazole in pregnancy is its reported association with birth defects—'methimazole embryopathy.'[10] Characterized by aplasia cutis, craniofacial malformations (facial dysmorphism, choanal atresia), gastrointestinal malformations (esophageal atresia with or without trachea-esophageal fistula) and umblical abnormalities. So, its use is avoided in the first trimester **(Table 21.1)**.

Pharmacology

Bioavailability is 80–95%,it is well absorbed.

It is metabolized by liver and eliminated by kidneys. Half life 4–6 hours (less frequent dosing can be done for noncompliant patients).

Less protein bound than PTU-so increased placental and breast milk transfer.

Mechanism of Action

Acts by blocking oxidation of I_2 in thyroid gland, thus inhibiting thyroid hormone synthesis.

Indication: Hyperthyroidism in 2nd and 3rd trimester of pregnancy, e.g. Grave's disease, solitary toxic adenoma, nodular goiter.

Contraindication: Hypersensitivity.

Dosage: Lowest possible dose required so that FT_4 remains near the upper normal range. This is done to prevent fetal hypothyroidism and fetal goiter.

Mild: 15 mg/day PO q8h

Moderate: 30–40 mg/day

Severe: 60 mg/day

Maintainence: 5–15 mg/day.

Adverse drug reactions

Minor: Skin rash, urticarial, nausea, vomiting.

Major

- Agranulocytosis
- Alopecia
- Aplastic anemia
- Dermatologic disorders (rash, pruritic skin)
- Hepatotoxicity.

Drug interaction: Reduced dose of warfarin, beta blockers, digitalis and theophylline may be required.

Monitoring: Serum TSH and FT_4 measured every two weeks till patient is on a stable medication dose.

FT_4 and FT_4I is a better indicator of control of hyperthyroidism as compared to FT_3, FT_3I and TSH because normalization of FT_4 and FT_4I precedes FT_4, FT_3I and TSH.

It is a FDA Category D drug.

Compatible with breastfeeding. Drug should be taken after feeds to minimize transfer to breast milk.

Carbimazole

Carbimazole is a prodrug as after administration it is converted in the body the active form -methimazole.

Preparation

Neomercazole.

Dosage: Equivalent doses of carbimazole to methimazole are 0.6 to 1.0. Treatment is generally started at a high dose of 15–40 mg, continued till the patient has normal thyroid function and then reduced to a maintenance dose of 5–15 mg. Interindividual variability leads to considerable difference in absorption of methimazole and carbimazole , which is more often observed with methimazole than with carbimazole.

Lugol's iodine and iodide: Not considered as a first line therapy. Only used as an adjuvant therapy with other hyperthyroidism medications. Prolonged use of iodide products may lead to fetal hypothyroidism via transplacental passage; so, iodide use should be limited to less than 2 weeks.

Pharmacology and mechanism of action: Temporary inhibition of iodine organification in the thyroid gland results from administration of pharmacologic amounts of iodine—a phenomenon called the Wolff-Chaikoff effect. They are given 1-3 hours after antithyroid drugs to avoid build up of hormones stored within gland. Iodide decreases serum T4 and T3 levels by 30–50% in 10 days.

Indications
- Preoperative treatment of patients with hyperthyroidism.
- Thyroid storm.

Contraindication: Hypersensitivity.

Dosage: In thyroid storm-Lugol's solution 30–60 drops daily in divided doses or saturated solution of potassium iodides 3 drops orally thrice a day are given for a few days. If it is not tolerated by mouth then intravenous solution of sodium iodides 0.5 g is given every 12 hours.

Prior to thyroidectomy-approximately 250 mg of potassium iodide three times a day for ten days before surgery, usually administered concurrently with an antithyroid agent.[11]

Adverse drug reactions

Side effects
- Diarrhea, nausea, vomiting
- Stomach pain
- Allergic reactions, specifically angioedema
- Arthralgia
- Eosinophilia
- Swelling of lymph nodes
- Urticaria

It is a FDA Category D drug.

It should be avoided in pregnancy and breastfeeding. Excreted in breast milk.

Breastfeeding—may lead to skin rash and thyroid problems in breastfed babies.

Use of radioactive iodine is contraindicated in pregnancy.

Table 21.1: Differences between propylthiouracil and methimazole

Propylthiouracil	*Methimazole*
1. Decreases synthesis and release of thyroid hormones and inhibits peripheral conversion of T_4 to T_3 2. Serum t1/2–1 hour 3. Dosage 50–200 mg daily 4. Amount of drug secreted in breast milk is very little. 5. *Complications:* Hepatocellular damage 6. Given in first trimester as risk of methimazole embryopathy is high in first trimester	1. Decreases synthesis and release of thyroid hormones 2. Serum t1/2–6 hours 3. Dosage 10–60 mg 12 hourly 4. Higher concentration of drug is secreted in breast milk 5. *Complications:* Cholestasis, aplasia cutis congenita 6. Given in second and third trimester as risk of hepatotoxicity with PTU is higher than the risk of teratogenicity after first trimester

Beta Blockers

Nonselective beta blockers such as propranolol, are preferred because they have more effect on hypermetabolism, which occurs during states of hyperthyroidism.

Pharmacology: Rapidly and completely absorbed but variable bioavailability due to extensive first pass metabolism. Hepatic impairment increases bioavailability. Coadministration with food enhances bioavailability.

Metabolism and Elimination: Metabolized by hepatic P450 enzymes CYP2D6 and CYP1A2. About 96–99% excreted by kidneys.

Mechanism of Action: Nonselective beta adrenergic receptor blocker; competitive beta1 and beta2 receptor inhibition results in slowing of heart rate, decreased myocardial contractility and myocardial oxygen demand, and lowering of blood pressure. Class 2 antidysrhythmic.

Indications

- Symptomatic relief of the adrenergic symptoms of hyperthyroidism such as tremor, palpitations, heat intolerance, and nervousness
- Thyroid storm.

Contraindications

- Reversible airways diseases example asthma.
- Bradycardia (<60 beats/minute)
- *Sick sinus syndrome:* Patients may demonstrate an inappropriately slow heart rate accompanied by symptoms such as dizziness or syncope.
- Atrioventricular block—may be asymptomatic, but in some patients, irregularities of the heartbeat, presyncope, or syncope may occur; may manifest as bradycardia (especially Mobitz II) and/or irregularity of heart rate (especially Mobitz I [Wenckebach])
- Shock
- Severe hypotension.

Dosage: Initiated at 10–20 mg every six hours, progressively increased until symptoms are controlled. 80–320 mg per day suffices in most cases.

Monitoring: Monitoring of blood pressure is important.

Drug interaction: Concomitant use with digitalis increase the risk of bradycardia. Reduced dose of warfarin and theophyllin may be required.

Adverse drug reactions

Minor: Nausea, vomiting, fatigue, pruritis.

Major: Bronchospasm, hyperkalemia, pulmonary edema, hyperlipidemia, hypotension, bradycardia, hyperglycemia.

It is a FDA Category C drug.

Long-term treatment with propanolol is not recommended because of potential neonatal morbidity. There is 24.4% incidence of spontaneous abortion in patients using beta blockers with antithyroid drugs compared to 5.5% in patients using antithyroid drugs alone. No special precautions are needed for breastfeeding mothers and is considered safe.

FDA recommendations regarding use of antithyroid agents:[12] The FDA recommends the following criteria be considered for prescribing PTU:

- Reserve PTU use during first trimester of pregnancy, or in patients who are allergic to or intolerant of methimazole.
- Closely monitor PTU therapy for signs and symptoms of liver injury, especially during the first 6 months after initiation of therapy.
- For suspected liver injury, promptly discontinue PTU therapy and evaluate for evidence of liver injury and provide supportive care.
- Counsel patients to promptly contact their health care provider for the following signs or symptoms: fatigue, weakness, vague abdominal pain, loss of appetite, itching, easy bruising, or yellowing of the eyes or skin.

The American Thyroid Association Taskforce Recommendations on Thyroid Disease during Pregnancy and Postpartum:[13] Following are its recommendations:

- The recommended treatment of maternal hypothyroidism is with administration of oral LT4. It is strongly recommended not to use other thyroid preparations such as T3 or desiccated thyroid. **Level A- US PREVENTIVE SERVICES TASK FORCE USPSTF**

- The goal of LT4 treatment is to normalize maternal serum TSH values within the trimester-specific pregnancy reference range (first trimester, 0.1–2.5 mIU/L; second trimester, 0.2–3.0 mIU/L; third trimester, 0.3–3.0 mIU/L). **Level A-USPSTF**
- Treated hypothyroid patients who are newly pregnant should independently increase their dose of LT by ~25%–30% upon a missed menstrual cycle or positive home pregnancy test and notify their caregiver promptly. **Level B-USPSTF**
- Radioactive iodine (RAI) scanning or radioiodine uptake determination should not be performed in pregnancy. **Level D-USPSTF**
- Antithyroid drugs are not recommended for the management of gestational hyperthyroidism. **Level D-USPSTF**
- Propylthiouracil (PTU) is preferred for the treatment of hyperthyroidism in the first trimester. Patients on methimazole (MMI) should be switched to PTU if pregnancy is confirmed in the first trimester. Following the first trimester, consideration should be given to switching to MMI. **Level I-USPSTF**
- Cordocentesis should be used in extremely rare circumstances and performed in an appropriate setting. It may occasionally be of use when fetal goiter is detected in women taking antithyroid drugs to help determine whether the fetus is hyperthyroid or hypothyroid. **Level I-USPSTF**

REFERENCES

1. Reid SM, Middleton P, Cossich MC, et al. Interventions for clinical and subclinical hypothyroidism in pregnancy. Cochrane Database Syst Rev. 2010;(7):CD007752.
2. Abalovich M, Amino N, Barbour LA, Cobin RH, Degroot LJ, Glinoer D, et al. Management of thyroid dysfunction during pregnancy and postpartum: an Endocrine Society Clinical Practice Guideline. Journal of Clinical Endocrinology and Metabolism. 2007;92(8 suppl):S1-47.
3. Weetman A. Graves' disease. N Engl J Med. 2000;343:1236-48.
4. Liwanpo L, Hershman JM. Conditions and drugs interfering with thyroxine absorption. Best Practice and Research Clinical Endocrinology and Metabolism. 2009;23:781-92.
5. Hennessey JV. Generic vs name brand L-thyroxine products: interchangeable or still not? J Clin Endocrinol Metab. 2013;98(2):511-4.
6. Yassa L, Marqusee E, Fawcett R, et al. Thyroid hormone early adjustment in pregnancy (the THERAPY) trial. J Clin Endocrinol Metab. 2010;95:3234-41.
7. Weetman AP, McGregor AM. Autoimmune thyroid disease: Further development is an understanding. Endocrinol Rev. 1994;15:788-830.
8. Stagnaro-Green A, Abalovich M, Alexander E, et al. American Thyroid Association Taskforce on Thyroid Disease During Pregnancy and Postpartum. Guidelines of the American Thyroid Association for the diagnosis and management of thyroid disease during pregnancy and postpartum. Thyroid. 2011;21(10):1081-125.
9. Wing DA, Millar LK, Koonings PP, et al. A comparison of propylthiouracil versus methimazole in treatment of hyperthyroidism in pregnancy. Am J Obstet Gynecol. 1994;170:90-5.
10. Di Gianantonio E, Schaefer C, Mastroiacovo PP, et al. Adverse effects of prenatal methimazole exposure. Teratology. 2001;64(5):262-6.
11. Feek C, Sawers J, Irvine J, Beckett G, Ratcliffe W, Toft A. Combination of potassium iodide and propranolol in preparation of patients with Graves' disease for thyroid surgery. N Eng J Med. 1980;302:883-5.
12. FDA MedWatch safety alerts for human medical products.Propylthiouracil (PTU). Accessed: June 3,2009. US food and drug administration.
13. Alex Stagnaro-Green, Marcos Abalovich, Erik Alexander, Fereidoun Azizi, Jorge Mestman, Roberto Negro, et al. The American Thyroid Association Taskforce on Thyroid Disease During Pregnancy and Postpartum, Thyroid. 2011;21(10):1081-125.

CHAPTER 22

Gastrointestinal and Hepatic Disorders of Pregnancy

Chetna Arvind Sethi

Gastrointestinal (GI) symptoms occur quite frequently in pregnant women and require early attention so as to ascertain the well-being of the developing fetus as well as to reduce maternal complications.[1-3] The common GI disorders and drugs used are enlisted in the **Table 22.1**.

Table 22.1: Drugs used in common gastrointestinal and hepatic disorders of pregnancy

Condition	*Drug*
Nausea and vomiting during pregnancy Hyperemesis gravidarum	Doxylamine succinate Pyridoxine hydrochloride
	Metoclopramide 5-HT_3 receptor antagonist—ondansetron, granisetron, dolasetron and palonosetron
Heartburn in pregnancy	Antacids
	Sucralfate`
	H_2-receptor antagonists—ranitidine, famotidine, roxatidine
	Proton pump inhibitors (PPI)* omeprazole, pantoprazole, rabeprazole, esomeprazole and lansoprazole.
Constipation	Lactulose
	Bisacodyl
Diarrhea: Watery (no outbreak) Outbreak of watery diarrhea Bloody diarrhea	ORS Azithromycin 1 g single dose OR erythromycin 500 mg thrice daily for 3 days Ciprofloxacin 500 mg twice daily for 3 days, if amebic dysentery suspected metronidazole 500 mg thrice a day for 7–10 days
Intrahepatic cholestasis of pregnancy	Ursodeoxycholic acid

*All PPIs are category B except omeprazole which is category C

Nausea and Vomiting During Pregnancy

The most common GI symptom during pregnancy is nausea and it is complained by almost 90% of the pregnant women. Vomiting is additionally associated with nausea in about half of the pregnancies. This self-limiting problem usually presents as "morning sickness" in the first trimester and disappears by the fourth month of pregnancy.

However more severe form of vomiting during pregnancy designated as hyperemesis gravidarum occurs in 2% of pregnancies. It requires urgent medical care especially in view of complications including hypokalemia, acid/ base disturbances and ketosis. In addition these patients require antiemetics and sedatives.

Doxylamine Succinate

Pharmacology: It is a first generation H1 antagonist antihistamine. Its bioavailability after oral administration is 24.7%. It is metabolized in liver and has a half-life of 10–12 hours with peak action at 2–4 hours and excreted in urine as its metabolite.

Indications of use: It is used in combination with pyridoxine in controlling nausea and vomiting in pregnancy.

Contraindications: Hypersensitivity to the drug and acute asthma.

Dosage: 20 mg orally at bed time. If required 5-10 mg more is given in the morning and afternoon.

Adverse effects: It is a potent anticholinergic and has side effects including dry mouth, ataxia, urinary retention, drowsiness and psychosis.

Drug interaction: Generally does not have interaction with the commonly used drugs in obstetrics and gynecology.

Preparation: Available as a combination with pyridoxine.

- *Doxinate, nosic*: 10 mg of pyridoxine with 10 mg of doxylamine tablet.

Safety during pregnancy and lactation: It is category A drug and in combination with pyridoxine is recommended for use in pregnancy.

Pyridoxine Hydrochloride

Pharmacology: Pyridoxine hydrochloride is a vitamin B_6 analog. Mainly absorbed in jejunum and further metabolized in the liver. It is highly protein bound, primarily to albumin. Its active metabolite pyridoxine pyridoxal 5′ phosphate accounts for atleast 60% of the circulating vitamin. Excreted mainly in the urine.

Indications of use: It is used in combination with doxylamine in morning sickness.

Also used in vitamin B_6 deficiency states and along with INH.

Contraindication: No known contraindication.

Dosage: For nausea vomiting of pregnancy the dose is 20 mg at bed time and additional 10 mg before breakfast and lunch may be added.

Adverse effect: Occasional numbness, tingling and drowsiness.

Drug Reaction

INH: Produces a state of pyridoxine deficiency by inhibiting generation of active metabolite pyridoxal phosphate and enhances its excretion due to formation of hydrazone.

Oral contraceptives reduce pyridoxal phosphate levels.

Pyridoxine promotes formation of dopamine from L-Dopa in peripheral tissues and reduces its brain availability, thus abolishing its therapeutic effect.

Preparation

- *Pyridoxine*: 10 mg tablet, 50 mg/2 mL injection.
- *Benadon*: 40 mg tablet.
- *Pyricontin*: 100 mg tablet.

Doxinate, nosic: 10 mg of pyridoxine with 10 mg of doxylamine tablet.

Safety during pregnancy: Safety has been proven and is a category A drug. FDA approved in 2013, April.

Metoclopramide

Pharmacology: Metoclopramide has complex mechanisms of action. It acts as HT_4-receptor agonist, vagal and central 5-HT_3-antagonist, dopamine receptor antagonist and sensitizes muscarinic receptors on smooth muscle. It is an oldest prokinetic agents. It acts increasing lower esophageal sphincter tone along with stimulation of antral and small intestinal contractions. It does not have a significant effect on large-bowel motility. Oral metoclopramide is rapidly absorbed, undergoes conjugation in the liver, and is mainly excreted in the urine. It also crosses placenta and is secreted in breast milk. Its peak concentration being achieved in 1 hour and pharmacological action lasts for 1–2 hours.

Indications of use: Metoclopramide has been used in pregnant patients having symptoms due to gastroparesis including hyperemesis. It may be used to ameliorate vomiting during labor. It also has role preoperatively in patients undergoing emergency cesarean section, who are not nil per oral. In these cases it helps to prevent vomiting intraoperatively and therefore prevents Madelson's syndrome.

Contraindications: It is contraindicated in elpilepsy, pheochromocytoma and in newborns.

Dosage

Hyperemesis: 10 mg orally thrice a day, 30 minutes before each meal till symptomatic improvement. It's action starts within 30–60 minutes after an oral dose. If patient unable to take orally then 10 mg 8 hourly IV or IM till patient starts accepting orally.

Before cesarean section 10 mg IV or IM.

Adverse effects: The extrapyramidal effects, such as dystonias (usually occurring after I/V administration) are the major side effects. Tardive dyskinesia and Parkinsonian-like symptoms also can occur on long-term use.

Drug interaction: It hastens absorption of many drugs like aspirin, diazepam, etc. by speeding gastric emptying time. But reduces absorption of digoxin and cimetidine by decreasing time for absorption in the stomach.

Preparation

- *Perinorm*: 10 mg tablets, 10 mg per 2 mL injections, 5 mg/5 mL syrup.
- *Reglan*: 10 mg tablet, 10 mg/2 mL injection, and 5 mg/5 mL syrup form.

Safety during pregnancy and lactation: It has been shown to cross placenta but has not been documented to have teratogenic effects. Though secreted in milk in small amounts can cause loose stools and dystonia in suckling infant.

It is a FDA category B drug.

5-HT_3-Receptor Antagonists

This group of drugs includes ondansetron, granisetron, dolasetron and palonosetron.

Pharmacology: The antiemetic effect of these drugs persists longer than the drug being present in circulation, suggesting their continuous interaction at the receptor level. In fact, all of these drugs are sufficient even in single daily doses.

After being well absorbed from the GI tract, it undergoes extensive metabolism in the liver by CYP pathways, followed by its glucuronide or sulfate conjugation. Plasma clearance of these drugs reduces in patients with hepatic dysfunction, thus requiring adjustment in the dosage in this subset of patients. Although clearance of ondansetron is also reduced in elderly patients, no adjustment in dosage for age is required.

Indications of use: All three agents are equally efficacious.

They are effective against hyperemesis gravidarum, and to some extent in postoperative nausea. These agents are most effective in the treatment of chemotherapy-induced nausea as well as in treatment of nausea secondary to irradiation of upper abdomen.

Contraindications: Hypersensitivity. These are to be used cautiously in those with renal impairment.

Dosage

- The most commonly used 5-HT_3 receptor antagonist is ondansetron.
- In emesis in pregnancy is 4–8 mg orally 3 times a day.
- *In hyperemesis*: 4–8 mg IM or IV 8 hourly
- *For pre- and postoperative nausea and vomiting as in cesarean section*: 4–8 mg I/V given before induction and repeated 8 hourly till oral allowance.

Adverse effects: These drugs are in general very well tolerated, with the most common adverse effects being diarrhea or constipation, light-headedness and headache occurring only in a small number of cases. These agents, as a class have been shown on experimental basis to induce clinically significant ECG changes.

Drug interaction: No significant drug interactions have been noted.

Preparations

- Ondansetron-Emset, Ondem, Emsetron—4 mg, 8 mg tablet, 2 mL and 4 mL ampules containing 2 mg/mL for injections.

Safety during pregnancy and lactation: These are FDA category B drugs.

Heartburn in Pregnancy

It is a common problem during pregnancy and occurs due to progressive decrease in pressure of lower esophageal sphincter (LES). Patients usually do well with simple lifestyle changes.[4]

Nonsystemic drug therapy which includes antacids and sucralfate should be given first to those pregnant women who do not improve with lifestyle modifications. If patient does not respond to these medications then H_2 receptor antagonists (*ranitidine, famotidine,* and *roxatidine*) may be used. If the patient still does not respond then proton pump inhibitors (PPIs) can be used.

Antacids

Pharmacology: Combination of magnesium hydroxide (rapid action) and aluminum hydroxide (slow action) provide a relatively sustained neutralizing capacity and are the preferred antacids. In gastric acid, magaldrate (hydroxyl magnesium aluminate complex) gets rapidly converted to hydroxides of magnesium and aluminum which lead to a sustained antacid effect. Because they stay locally due poor absorption.

Antacids get cleared from the empty stomach in about 30 minutes. However, the presence of food elevates gastric pH to about 5 for about an hour and thus prolongs the neutralizing effects of antacids. Antacids vary in the extent to which they are absorbed, and hence in their systemic effects. In general, most antacids can elevate urinary pH by about one pH unit. Antacids containing aluminum, magnesium and calcium ions are absorbed less completely than the ones that contain sodium bicarbonate.

Indications of use: These are used in the treatment of gastroesophageal reflux disease and peptic ulcer disease mainly for pain relief. Also used for nonulcer dyspepsia and heart burn, commonly seen in pregnancy.

Contraindications: Hemorrhoids, intestinal obstruction, renal disease, CHF, diarrhea, aluminum poisoning.

Dosage: Dosage for antacids is expressed in terms of mEq of acid neutralized. For uncomplicated ulcers antacids are generally given orally 1 and 3 hours following meals and at bedtime. This regimen provides about 120 mEq of an magaldrate per dose, and may be almost as effective as conventional dosing with an H_2-receptor antagonist.

For pain relief in ulcers and GERD—40-80 mEq acid neutralizing capacity is given for 1-2 weeks.

For healing of ulcers 80-160 mEq is given for 4-6 weeks.

For severe symptoms or uncontrolled reflux, antacids can be given as often as every 30-60 minutes.

Adverse effects: Commonly encountered side effects include belching, nausea, abdominal distention, and flatulence.

Milk-alkali syndrome (alkalosis, hypercalcemia, and renal insufficiency) occurred frequently in the past, following administration of large doses of $NaHCO_3$ and $CaCO_3$ with milk or cream. This syndrome is rare today and generally results from the chronic ingestion of large quantities of Calcium carbonate when taken with milk. Patients may be asymptomatic or may present with the insidious onset of hypercalcemia, reduced secretion of parathyroid hormone, precipitation of calcium salts in the kidney, ultimately renal insufficiency.

With preserved renal function, the modest accumulations of aluminum, calcium and magnesium do not pose a problem however with renal insufficiency; absorbed aluminum contributes to proximal myopathy, osteoporosis and encephalopathy.

Drug interaction: Antacids may affect a number of drugs by altering gastric and urinary pH. They can affect concentrations of imidazole antifungals, thyroid hormones and allopurinol in the body by altering their rates of dissolution and absorption resultant bioavailability as well as their renal clearance. Aluminum and magnesium containing antacids also have tendency to chelate other drugs present in the GI tract resulting in formation of insoluble complexes that pass through the GI tract without absorption. Most of these interactions are avoidable by taking antacids at a gap of two hours before or after ingestion of other such drugs.

Preparations: Usually antacids are administered in suspension form because it gets uniformly distributed.

- *Milk of magnesia*: Magnesium hydroxide 0.4 g/5 mL (5 mL neutralizes 12 mEq).
- *Aludrox*: Aluminium hydroxide 0.84 g per tablet, 0.6 g/10 mL suspension (5 mL neutralizes 1 mEq only).
- *Stacid*: 400 mg Magaldrate (hydrated complex of hydroxyl-magnesium aluminate) tablet, 400 mg per 5 mL suspension (1 g neutralizes 28 mEq).

Antacid Combinations

- *Ulgel*: 400 mg Magaldrate with 20 mg Simethicone per tablet or 5 mL suspension.
- *Digene gel*: Magnesium hydroxide 185 mg, aluminum hydroxide 830 mg, sodium carboxymethylcellulose 100 mg, methylpolysiloxane 25 mg per 10 mL suspension.
- *Gelusil*: Dried aluminum hydroxide gel 250 mg, Magnesium trisilicate 500 mg per tablet.
- *Mucaine gel*: Aluminum hydroxide gel 290 mg, Magnesium hydroxide 98 mg, Oxthazaine 10 mg per 5 mL suspension.

Safety during pregnancy and lactation: Antacids are safe and effective for the treatment of heartburn of pregnancy. Sodium bicarbonate containing antacids are not recommended to be used as they lead to fluid overload and metabolic alkalosis in both the fetus and mother. Antacids do not get concentrated in breast milk and are thus safe during lactation. These are FDA category B drugs.

Sucralfate

Pharmacology: Sucralfate consists of aluminum hydroxide added to the octasulfate of sucrose. In an acid environment, it undergoes extensive cross-linking and turns into a viscous and sticky polymer that adheres to ulcer craters and epithelial cells. This action lasts for up to 6 hours after a single dose. It had added effect of cytoprotection and promotion of healing of gastric ulcer by stimulating the local prostaglandin production and epidermal growth factors.

Indications of use: It is used in pregnant patients with chronic gastritis, duodenal and gastric ulcer.

Sucralfate offers an advantage over other drugs for the prophylaxis of stress ulcers in critically ill patients.

Its unique mechanism of action makes it suitable for use in a lot of other conditions associated with mucosal inflammation or ulceration that is not responsive to acid suppression, like radiation and aphthous ulcers as well as and bile reflux gastropathy.

Sucralfate rectal enema also is useful for solitary rectal ulcers and radiation proctitis.

Contraindications: There are no known contraindications.

Dosage: It is used in the usual dosage of 1 g 1 hour before each meal and at bedtime. It should be taken empty stomach because it requires acid medium for its activation and action. Therefore should be taken one hour before meals and antacid use within one hour should be avoided.

Adverse effects: Constipation occurs in about 2% of the cases and is the most common side effect of sucralfate. Because of its aluminum containing composition, it is better avoided in patients with chronic renal failure as some aluminum can be absorbed and can lead to aluminum overload. Likewise, in some patients the sticky viscous gel produced by sucralfate may also result in the development of gastroliths. Patients with underlying gastroparesis are particularly prone to it.

Drug interaction: Due to formation of a viscous layer in the stomach, sucralfate inhibits absorption of the other drugs including phenytoin, digoxin, cimetidine, ketoconazole and fluoroquinolone antibiotics. It should therefore be taken at a gap of at least 2 hours after the administration of other drugs.

The aluminum-containing antacids should not be combined with sucralfate especially in presence of chronic renal disease.

Preparations

- *Ulcerfate, Sucrace*: 1 gm tablets.
- *Sparacid*: 1 g/10 mL suspension.

Safety during pregnancy and lactation: Sucralfate, with virtually no absorption, it is safe during pregnancy and lactation. It is a FDA category B drug.

H2-Receptor Antagonists

Pharmacology: H_2-receptor antagonists reduce acid production by reversibly competing with histamine for binding to H_2-receptors on the basolateral membrane of gastric parietal cells.

H_2-receptor antagonists available for use are cimetidine, ranitidine, famotidine, and roxatidine. These drugs are not as potent as PPI but still lead to suppression of 24-hour gastric acid secretion by about two thirds. The drugs inhibit basal acid secretion and these accounts for their higher efficacy in suppressing nocturnal acid secretion.

These are rapidly absorbed after oral administration, with peak serum concentrations being achieved within 1–3 hours. Therapeutic levels are also achieved rapidly after intravenous dosing and are maintained for 4–12 hours depending on the drug used. Only a small amount of drug is protein-bound and a small amount is metabolized in the liver. However liver disease does not warrant any adjustment of the dose. These drugs are excreted through the kidney and it is important to reduce doses in patients with compromised renal function.

Indications of use: It is used in pregnancy mainly for treatment of gastric and duodenal ulcers, uncomplicated GERD and for prevention of stress ulcers.

Dosage

- *Ranitidine*: 150–300 mg thrice a day or at bedtime orally, 50 mg I/M or slow I/V injection every 6–8 hours.
- *Famotidine*: 20 mg BD, 40 mg bedtime orally or 20 mg I/V 12 hourly.

- *Roxatidine*: 75 mg twice daily, 150 mg at bedtime.
- Total duration of therapy for ulcer healing is 6–8 weeks.

Cimetidine is usually not an agent of choice during pregnancy.

Adverse effects: Generally these drugs are well tolerated, with only minor effects including diarrhea, headache, drowsiness, fatigue, muscular pain, and constipation. Less common side effects occur primarily in elderly patients with IV administration include headaches, hallucinations, slurred speech, confusion and delirium.

These drugs can cause galactorrhea in women. H_2-receptor antagonists have also been associated with various blood dyscrasias, including thrombocytopenia in several reports.

Drug interactions: Occur mainly with cimetidine, and its use has decreased markedly. Cimetidine inhibits CYPs and thus can lead to increase in the levels of a variety of drugs that are metabolized by these enzymes. Ranitidine also interacts with hepatic CYPs, but with an affinity of only one tenth that of cimetidine. Famotidine is even safer in this regard, with no significant drug interactions mediated by inhibiting hepatic CYPs.

Preparations

- *Ranitidine*: Rantac, Histac, Aciloc, Zinetac—150 mg, 300 mg tablets, 50 mg/2 mL injections.
- *Famotidine*: Famtac, Famocid, Topcid-20 mg, 40 mg tablets, 20 mg/2 mL injections
- *Roxatidine*: Rotane, Zorpex—75 mg, 150 mg SR tablets.

Safety during pregnancy and lactation: These drugs cross the placenta and have been shown to be excreted in breast milk in pregnancy cautious use has been suggested, although no major teratogenic effects have been reported with these agents. These are FDA category B drugs. Ranitidine and famotidine have been suggested to be safe during lactation.

Proton Pump Inhibitors

The various proton pump inhibitors (PPIs) which are in clinical use are omeprazole, pantoprazole, rabeprazole, esomeprazole and lansoprazole.

Pharmacology: These are the most potent suppressors of gastric acid secretion and can reduce the acid production by up to 95% daily. All drugs of this class have equivalent efficacy at comparable doses as they have similar pharmacological properties. They act by irreversible blockade of hydrogen-potassium ATPase of the gastric parietal cells. This pump is the terminal stages in gastric acid secretion, hence an ideal target for inhibiting acid secretion. These drugs are absorbed rapidly and are highly protein bound. These are extensively metabolized by hepatic CYPs and have a short half-life of 60–90 minutes in plasma but have a sustained effect at the site of action for about 24 hours.

Indications of use: Proton pump inhibitors are used principally for the treatment of gastroesophageal reflux disease (GERD), including erosive esophagitis as well as for the healing of gastric and duodenal ulcers. These are also used in treatment of bleeding peptic ulcers and for prophylaxis of aspiration pneumonitis.

Contraindication: Dose reduction is recommended in patients with severe hepatic disease as the clearance of esomeprazole and lansoprazole in hepatic disease is reduced significantly.

Dosage

- *Omeprazole*: 20–40 mg once a day orally.
- *Pantoprazole*: 40 mg once a day orally.
- *Rabeprazole*: 20 mg once a day orally.
- *Esomeprazole*: 20–40 mg once a day orally.
- *Lansoprazole*: 5–30 mg once a day orally.
- Total duration of treatment for healing of ulcers is generally 4–8 weeks.

High dose intravenous therapy (pantoprazole 40–120 mg per day; rabeprazole 40–80 mg per day) for 72 hours followed by oral therapy is given for bleeding peptic ulcers. Pantaprazole 40 mg intravenously once daily for 7 days followed by oral is given for erosive gastritis with GERD.

Adverse effects: Remarkably few adverse effects have been seen with these drugs. Nausea, abdominal pain, constipation, flatulence and diarrhea are the most common side effects noted. Some of the rare side effects reported are subacute myopathy, arthralgia, headaches and skin rashes.

Hypergastrinemia occurs more frequently and is reported to be more severe with proton pump inhibitors than with H_2-receptor antagonists and thus on the discontinuation of therapy may predispose to rebound hypersecretion of gastric acid and also may promote the development of gastrointestinal tumors. These findings have raized concerns regarding their use in humans. These have never the less been in use for over two decades with no major safety issues.

Drug interactions: Because of their metabolism through the CYP pathways these have been seen to interact with warfarin, diazepam and phenytoin. They inhibit oxidation of these drugs hence increase their levels. They are also known to increase absorption of digoxin leading to its increased levels. The drug interaction risk is maximum with omeprazole and esmoperazole, less with lansoprazole and the least with pantoprazole and rabeprazole.

Preparations

- *Omeprazole*: Omez, Ocid, Omizac, Protoloc-10, 20 mg capsules.
- *Pantoprazole*: Pantocid, Pantodac, Pantop–40 mg enteric coated tablet.
- *Injection*: Pantium 40 mg per vial for Intravenous use.
- *Rabeprazole*: Rablet, Razo, Rabeloc-10, 20 mg tablets, Happi—20 mg per vial injection.
- *Lansoprazole*: Lanzol, Lanzap, Lanpro–15, 30 mg capsules.
- *Esomeprazole*: Nexpro, Raciper, Izra-20, 40 mg tablets.

Safety during pregnancy and lactation: These have been found to be safe during pregnancy and are classified as category B except omeprazole which is a category C drug. Data regarding infant safety or PPI excretion in breast milk is lacking in lactating women. Hence these medications should be better avoided during breastfeeding.[5]

Constipation

Constipation and diarrhea occur at rates not higher than the general population. It is suggested that pathophysiology of alteration in bowel habits may be secondary to hormonal changes that occur during pregnancy.[6]

The management of constipation in pregnancy is similar to nonpregnant state. It is managed primarily by behavioral and dietary modification which includes increase in the intake of water and fiber. Pharmacologically bulk laxatives, psyllium and methylcellulose have been shown to be safe and effective in pregnancy also. Polyethylene glycol (PEG) and lactulose on the other hand act by stimulation of fluid accumulation in the intestine. It increases bowel frequency by acceleration of intestinal transit time and thus in patients with non-organic constipation, it improves defecation.

Hyperosmotic agents like saline and castor oil must be avoided as these may induce salt and water retention and induction of premature uterine contractions, respectively. On the contrary stimulant laxatives including anthraquinones, senna and cascara, are considered safe in pregnancy. These are however not recommended for regular use.

Lactulose

Pharmacology: It is a synthetic disaccharide of galactose and fructose. It remains unaffected by intestinal disaccharidases. It is hydrolyzed in the large intestine to short-chain fatty acids, which then draw water into the lumen of the gut osmotically and thus stimulate colonic propulsive motility.

Its effect is only seen after 24–48 hours of administration.

Indications of use: Lactulose is efficacious in the treatment of constipation in pregnancy.

It is also efficacious in idiopathic chronic constipation of elderly as well as the one resulting from opioids and *vincristine*. Hepatic encephalopathy is another indication for use of lactulose.

Dosage: 15–30 mL of 70% solution is given at night, and can be increased up to 60 mL per day in divided doses.

Adverse effects: Abdominal discomfort and flatulence occur relatively commonly in the first few days of treatment which usually subside with continued usage.

Drug interaction: Concomitant use of antacids is to be avoided.

Preparations

- Duphalac, Livo-luk-6.67 g/10 mL liquid.
- Lacscan, Mtlac-10 g/15 mL liquid.

Safety during pregnancy and lactation: It is a FDA category B drug.

Bisacodyl

Pharmacology

It gets activated in the intestine by deacylation. Its primary site of action is in colon. It causes irritation of the mucosa, produces mild inflammation and secretion.

The laxative effect of lactulose is seen after 6 hours of oral intake, as it requires activation following hydrolysis in the bowel by endogenous esterases. When taken at bedtime, it usually produces its effect the next morning. Suppositories, however work within 30–60 minutes as it reduces the transit time. On the other hand bisacodyl gets excreted mainly in the stool; however a minor 5% gets absorbed and is excreted in the urine as its glucuronide conjugate.

Indications of use: It is used in the treatment of constipation in pregnancy or otherwise.

Dosage: It is used as 10–15 mg of enteric-coated preparation daily and for rectal administration as a suppository.

Adverse effects: Over-dosage leads to catharsis and fluid and electrolyte deficits. Bisacodyl should not be used for more than 10 consecutive days due to its propensity to develop atonic colon.

Drug interaction: It is dispensed as enteric coated tablets. It should thus be swallowed without chewing/crushing so as to avoid drug activation in the stomach with resultant gastric irritation and cramping. Concomitant use of milk and antacids must also be avoided within one hour of ingestion of bisacodyl.

Preparations

- *Dulcolax*: 5 mg, 10 mg tablets, 5 mg suppository.
- *Conlax*: 5 mg, 10 mg suppository.

Safety during pregnancy and lactation: It is a FDA category B drug.

DIARRHEA

The causative factors for diarrhea during pregnancy are similar to that as in nonpregnant individuals.

Treatment of acute diarrheal episode is typically managed conservatively with oral rehydration and correction and maintenance of electrolyte balance. Patient should be given oral rehydration solution (ORS).

The WHO (2002) ORS-1 liter contains 13.5 gm of carbohydrate, 75 mEq sodium, 20 mEq potassium and 30 mEq base (HCO_3). This is available as dry powder and it is required to be dissolved in 1 liter of water.

The role of antimicrobials is limited to severe cases of bloody diarrhea and cases of diarrheal out breaks. In low resource countries, watery diarrhea does not require any antimicrobial treatment. The only exception is outbreak of cholera when antibiotic would reduce the duration of illness. Usually during cholera outbreak during pregnancy single dose of 1 g azithromycin or 500 mg 4 times a day of erythromycin for 3 days is effective.

In case of bloody diarrhea the most common cause is infection by *Shigella* and in these cases ciprofloxacin is considered the drug of choice. It is given in dose of 500 twice a day for 3 days. If stool examination reveals presence of *Entamoeba histolytica* then amebic dysentery is suspected and in these cases metronidazole 500 mg three times a day is given for 7-10 days.

Intrahepatic Cholestasis of Pregnancy

It is one of the most common causes of jaundice in pregnancy and a relatively benign condition that occurs during the third trimester and disappears soon after delivery.

The main feature of IHCP is disabling pruritus and therapy is directed towards resolution of pruritus in the mother as well as improving the fetal outcome. Cholestyramine, although used in the past has been discontinued as it was found to increase the risk of fetal hemorrhage and thus compromise the fetal outcome.

Ursodeoxycholic acid (UDCA) is considered to be the treatment of choice.

Ursodeoxycholic Acid

Pharmacology: It is a hydrophilic, dehydroxylated bile acid, formed by epimerization of the cheno-deoxycholic acid in the gut by intestinal bacteria. It constitutes up to 3% of the total bile acid pool. Upon oral administration, it alters the relative concentrations of bile acids and also reduces the cholesterol content of the bile and thus makes it less lithogenic. It is also considered to be cytoprotective for hepatocytes and is thus indicated for use in cholestatic liver diseases.

Majority of ursodeoxycholic acid is absorbed passively by diffusion, following oral administration. In the absence of liver disease, following absorption it is extracted by the liver to the tune of 50%. Then following conjugation with glycine or taurine it is secreted into bile. These conjugates then get absorbed in the ileum by both passive and active mechanisms. Nonabsorbed conjugates pass into the large intestine where they get 7-dehydroxylated resulting in lithocholic acid. These metabolites are poorly soluble and are thus excreted in the feces. It has a small volume of distribution since it is mostly distributed in the bile and small intestine.

Indications of use: It is the treatment of choice in intrahepatic cholestasis of pregnancy, in which its use is aimed at ameliorating maternal pruritis and improving fetal outcome.

Contraindications: In presence of radio-opaque stones or radioluscent bile pigment stones, in patients with compelling reasons for cholecystectomy.

Dosage: 13-15 mg/kg per day in two divided doses.

Adverse effects: Common side effects of Ursodeoxycholic acid include stomach upset or pain, nausea, diarrhea, constipation, dizziness, tired feeling, headache, hair loss, body aches, fever, chills, stuffy nose, flu like symptoms.

Drug interaction: Ursodeoxycholic acid may interact with cholestyramine, estrogens, or antacids that contain aluminum.

Preparation: UDCA, Udihep, Udiliv—150 mg, 300 mg tablets.

Safety during pregnancy and lactation: It is FDA category B drug that has been found to be safe for use after 1st trimester in randomized clinical trials. One gram given in three divided doses daily provides significant symptom relief.

REFERENCES

1. Thukral C, Wolf JL. Therapy Insight: drugs for gastrointestinal disorders in pregnant women. NCP Gastro and Hep. 2006;3:256-66.
2. Pregnancy in gastrointestinal diseases. Educational monograph by American College of Gastroenterology. 2009.
3. Jones D, Wilson J, Warnock NG, Alexander DJ. Abdominal pain in pregnancy. BMJ. 2012; 345:e6818.
4. Malfertheiner SF, Malfertheiner MV, Kropf S, Costa SD, Malfertheiner P. A prospective longitudinal cohort study: evolution of GERD symptoms during the course of pregnancy. BMC Gastroenterol. 2012;12:131.
5. Pasternak B, Hviid A. Use of proton-pump inhibitors in early pregnancy and the risk of birth defects. N Engl J Med. 2010; 363(22):2114-23.
6. Goodman & Gilman's: The Pharmacological Basis of Therapeutics, 12th edn, 2011.

CHAPTER 23

Respiratory Disorders

Poonam Kashyap, Mridul Daga

The various respiratory disorders in pregnancy are asthma, pneumonia, and tuberculosis. In this chapter we will deal with asthma and pneumonia while tuberculosis will be covered separately.

ASTHMA IN PREGNANCY

Asthma is a common disorder during pregnancy and the prevalence varies from 1% to 4%.[1] Drugs used in asthma during pregnancy are enlisted in **Table 23.1**.

Bronchodilators

When administered in therapeutic doses and by an appropriate route, bronchodilators relieve asthmatic symptoms and improve pulmonary functions by relaxing the bronchial smooth muscles. Since these agents provide

Table 23.1: Drugs used in asthma during pregnancy[2,3]

Bronchodilators	Beta 2 sympathomimetic (agonists)	*Short acting*: Salbutamol *Long acting*: Salmeterol, formoterol
Methylxanthines		Theophylline
Anticholinergics		Ipratropium, tiotropium
Leukotriene antagonist		Montelukast, Zafirlukast
		Leukotreine inhibitors: Zileuton
Mast cell stabilizer		Sodium cromoglycate, Ketotifen
Corticosteroids	Inhalational	Beclomethasone dipropionate, Budesonide, Fluticasone Propionate, Ciclesonide
	Systemic	Prednisolone, Methylprednisolone, Hydrocortisone
Anti-IgE antibody		Omalizumab

symptomatic relief but do not control disease process, these are often termed as relievers.[2]

Sympathomimetics

Inhaled beta-agonists are powerful bronchodilators that have been the mainstay of acute and chronic asthma for decades. Inhaled beta-agonists are used as need rather than on a regular schedule and are usually sufficient for the control of mild asthma. Terbutaline is the only inhaled beta-agonist rated as pregnancy category B drug by Food and Drug Administration.[1,2] Salbutamol and salmeterol are also widely used in pregnancy.

Salbutamol (Albuterol)

Pharmacology: It is a highly selective short acting beta 2-agonist.

It causes bronchodilation through beta-2 receptor stimulation. It increases cAMP formation in bronchial muscle cells and causes relaxation. In addition, increased cAMP formation in mast cells and other inflammatory cells leads to inhibition of release of mediators of immediate hypersensitivity from mast cells, basophils and other inflammatory cells.

Mostly given as inhalers, oral bioavailability is 50% as it undergoes presystemic metabolism in the gut.

Indications of use: Inhaled salbutamol and terbutaline are currently the most powerful drugs for quick reversal of bronchospasm but should not be used on a regular basis as chronic use does not reduce bronchial hyperactivity and may even worsen it.[3]

Oral therapy is useful for patients who cannot correctly use inhalers and also as an alternative or adjuvant drugs in severe asthma.[1,2]

Contraindications: It should be used cautiously in patients with hypertension, ischemic heart disease and patients on digitalis therapy. Beta-adrenergic agonists can produce significant cardiovascular effects measured by pulse rate, blood pressure, or electrocardiogram (ECG) changes, e.g. flattening of T waves, prolongation of the QTc interval, and ST segment depression.

Dosage: These can be administered either by inhalation or orally. However, selectivity of action is less when the drug is given orally. These can also be given by IV or IM route.

Inhalational: Mostly given through pressurized metered dose inhaler, it produces bronchodilation within 5 min and the action lasts for 2–4 hours. When inhaled, these drugs produce bronchodilation with minimal cardiac stimulation. 90 µg of drug is released per inhalation: Two inhalations are given every 4–6 hours and then for maintenance therapy 2 inhalations 4 times a day are sufficient.

Oral: 2–4 mg tablets and 8 mg extended release tablets are available. Usual dose is 8 mg every 12 hours. Maximum dose is 32 mg per day. Orally, it is used for the relief of bronchospasm in adults with reversible airway obstructive disease.

Parenteral: It is used in dose of 0.25–0.5 mg subcutaneously in case of severe asthma which does not respond to inhalational drugs.

Adverse effects: Muscle tremors are dose related effects. Palpitations restlessness, nervousness, throat irritation and ankle enema can occur.

Hypokalaemia is also a possible complication.

Tachyphylaxis, cardiac arrhythmias and paradoxical bronchoconstriction can sometimes occur.

Drug interaction: They should be used cautiously in patient already on digitalis drug therapy.

Monitoring: Usually not required.

Preparations: Asthalin-2,4 mg tab, 8 mg SR tablets, 2 mg per 5 mL syrup, 200 µg rota caps, 100 µg metered dose inhaler, respules (solution for inhalation via nebulizer) 2.5 mg asthalin per 2.5 mL solution in normal saline **(Figs 23.1A and B)**.

- *Ventorlin*: 100 µg metered dose inhaler
- *Derihaler*: 100 µg per metered dose inhaler.

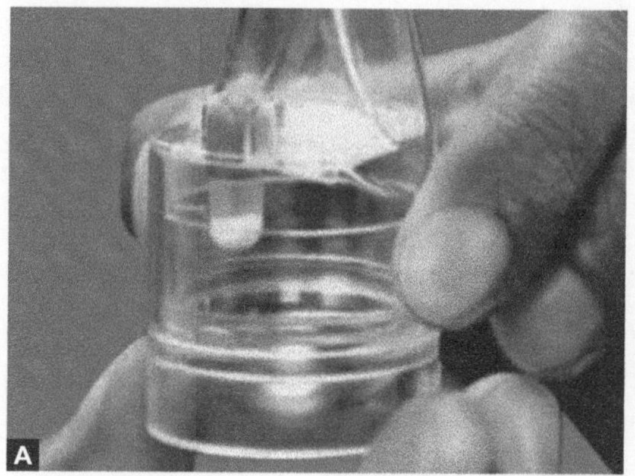

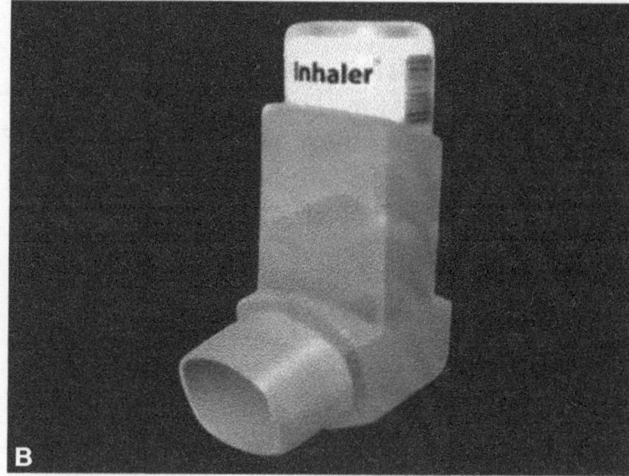

Figs 23.1A and B: (A) Rota-haler; (B) Inhaler

Safety during pregnancy and lactation: These are considered safe during pregnancy and lactation through inhalational route.

DCGI/FDA approval: Salbutamol is FDA category C drug.[4-9]

Salmeterol

Pharmacology: It is the first selective long acting beta 2-agonist. It is used on twice daily schedule because it has slower onset of action (15 to 30 min) and longer duration of action (>12 hours). It is more β2 selective and more lipophilic which accounts for its longer duration of action.

Indications of use

- It is used for prevention of exercise induced asthma.[9]
- It is used with the standard doses of inhaled corticosteroids. This provides more effective symptom control as compared to increasing the corticosteroid dosage.[9,10]
- It used for the long-term as the maintenance treatment of bronchospasm associated with chronic obstructive pulmonary disease (COPD). It is also used for long-term prevention of nocturnal symptoms.

Contraindications: It is not used to treat acute symptoms or acute exacerbations of asthma. Recent studies indicate that risk of life threatening asthma may be increased by regular use of these long acting beta 2-agonists. Therefore it should be used only in combination with inhaled steroids.[9]

Dosage: Inhalation of 50 μg salmeterol in combination with 250 μg fluticasone twice daily

In exercise induced bronchospasm one inhalation 30 minutes before exercise.

Adverse effects: It can cause tachycardia, tremors, hypokalemia and in larger doses may cause prolongation of QT interval.

Drug interaction: Simultaneous use with beta blockers may inhibit its bronchodilation effect and severe bronchospasm may get precipitated.

Monitoring: Patient should be monitored for any sign of worsening asthma and patients of hepatic impairment should be monitored closely.

Preparations

- *Seroflo 125 inhaler*: Contains fluticasone 125 μg and salmeterol 25 μg. Also combination with various strengths of fluticasone and salmeterol are available.
- *Combitide inhaler*: Available as different combinations of salmeterol 25 μg and varying strengths of fluticasone 50, 125 or 250 μg.

Safety in pregnancy and lactation: It is safe in pregnancy and lactation and is FDA category C drug.[7-9]

Formeterol

Pharmacology: It is long acting selective beta-2 agonist which acts for 12 hours when inhaled. In comparison to salmeterol, it has faster onset of action. It is used on a regular morning-evening schedule for round the clock bronchodilation.

Dose: 12 µg through inhalation twice a day.

Preparation

- *Foratec*: 12 µg rotacaps
- *Foradil*: Available as metered dose aerosol 12 µg of formoterol per inhalation.

Methylxanthines

Theophylline

Pharmacology: Theophylline benefits by causing bronchodilatation as well as by decreasing release of inflammatory mediators, promoting eosinophil apoptosis, and improved mucociliary clearance, stimulation of respiratory drive and by augmenting diaphragm contractility.

It is well absorbed orally; rectal absorption is erratic. It is distributed in all tissues, crosses placenta and is excreted in milk, 50% plasma protein bound and extensively metabolized in liver. Only 10% is excreted unchanged in urine. Its elimination varies considerably with age. At therapeutic concentrations the half-life in adults is 7–12 hours. Children eliminate it faster and elderly more slowly.

There are marked inter individual variations in plasma concentrations attained with the same dose. Theophylline metabolizing enzymes are saturable and, half-life is prolonged with higher doses as kinetics changes from first to zero order.

Factors which need dose reduction are age more than 60 years, pneumonia and liver failure.[2,3]

Indications of use: Because of narrow margin of safety and limited efficacy, its use has declined. Sustained release theophylline can be used in mild to moderate cases as a 3rd line or alternative/adjuvant drug, especially in patients with nocturnal asthma. It is more useful in COPD patients and is often added to other drugs and also used in pregnancy in those pregnant patients with moderate persistent asthma not controlled by inhaled steroids alone.[4,11]

Contraindications: Hypersensitivity, peptic ulcer, underlying seizure disorder.

Dosage: Loading dose of 4.6 mg/kg is administered intravenously over 30 minutes if the patient has not received theophylline in the previous 24 hours. Maintenance dose is 10 mg/kg per day orally and should not exceed 900 mg per day.

If the patient has received theophylline in 24 hours, then loading dose should not be given.

Adverse effects: Theophylline has narrow margin of safety.

Dose dependent toxicities occur. Headache, nervousness and nausea are early symptoms. High doses have been observed to cause tachycardia, jitteriness and vomiting in mothers and babies.

Drug interactions: Drugs which enhance theophylline metabolism primarily by inducing *CYP1A2* lower its efficacy like phenytoin, rifampicin, phenobarbitone, etc. Drugs which inhibit theophylline metabolism and increase its plasma level are erythromycin, ciprofloxacin and oral contraceptives. Theophylline enhances the effects of digitalis, oral anticoagulants, hypoglycemics and sympathomimetics. It decreases the effects of phenytoin and lithium.

Monitoring: Therapeutic drug monitoring is required as it has narrow margin of safety. The therapeutic serum concentration range for theophylline is 10–20 mcg/mL.

Preparations

- *Theobid*: 200 mg tablet
- *Deriphyllin*: 100 and 200 mg tab, Deriphyllin Retard 300 mg tablets
- Deriphyllin 2 mL injections.

Safety during pregnancy and lactation: The clearance of aminophylline and theophylline is increased in pregnancy but may be variable. There is no evidence of teratogenicity.[8,9]

It is a FDA category C drug.[4,8,9]

Anticholinergics

Ipratropium Bromide

Pharmacology: Ipratropium bromide is a quaternary derivative of N-isopropylatropine. It inhibits the augmentation of mucus secretion that occurs in asthma and may increase the mucociliary clearance of bronchial secretion. It has no effect on the late inflammatory phase of asthma. They cause bronchodilation by blocking M3 receptor mediated cholinergic constrictor tone.

Ipratropium is given by aerosol inhalation. As a quaternary nitrogen compound, it is highly polar and is not well absorbed into the circulation which limits its systemic effects. The maximum effects occur 30 minutes after inhalation and persist for 3–5 hours.

Ipratropium bromide is a short acting inhaled anticholinergic bronchodilator both are less efficacious than inhaled beta 2 sympathomimetics in bronchial asthma.

Uses: It is the bronchodilator of choice in COPD. The inhaled anticholinergics produce slower response than inhaled beta 2 sympathomimetics and are better suited for regular prophylactic use than for quick relief of breathlessness. Patients of asthmatic bronchitis, COPD and psychogenic asthma respond better to anticholinergics.[2,3]

Combination of ipratropium with beta-2 agonist produces more marked and longer lasting bronchodilation because the effects are additive. Anticholinergics are effective as adjunctive therapy in acute exacerbations of asthma.

Adverse effects: These are minimal in therapeutic doses except for dry mouth and bad taste.

Dosage: 500 μg every 6–8 hourly by nebulizer.

Contraindications: History of hypersensitivity to atropine or its derivatives.

Monitoring: No specific monitoring is required.

Preparations

- Ipravent containing 20 μg Ipratropium per metered dose
- Ipravent respules 2.5 mL containing 500 μg Ipratropium
- *Duolin rotacap*: 200μg Salbutamol + 40 μg Ipratropium per rota cap
- *Duolin inhaler*: 100 μg Salbutamol plus 20 μg Ipratropium per metered dose
- Duolin respules 2.5 mg Salbutamol + 500 μ Ipratropium in 2.5 mL solution.

Safety in pregnancy and lactation: Ipratropium is safe in pregnancy and lactation. It is FDA category B drug.[4,9]

Tiotropium Bromide

Pharmacology: Tiotropium bromide is longer acting than ipratropium bromide. It exhibits pharmacological effects through inhibition of M3 receptors at the smooth muscle causing bronchodilation.

Indications: It is used on long-term maintenance treatment of bronchospasm associated with chronic obstructive pulmonary disease, including chronic bronchitis and emphysema.

Contraindications: Hypersensitivity to atropine or any of its derivatives including ipratropium.

Dosage: Inhalation of one capsule of 18 μg once daily through an inhalational device.

Adverse effects: Dry mouth, abdominal pain, constipation, dyspepsia and vomiting can occur.

Preparations

- Tiovarotacap contain 18 μg of tiotropium,
- Tiovamultidose inhaler containing 9 μg tiotropium per dose.

Safety in pregnancy and lactation: Tiotropium is safe in pregnancy and lactation. It is FDA category C drug.[9]

Leukotriene Receptor Antagonists

Zafirlukast

It is well absorbed orally, highly plasma protein bound and metabolized by CYP2C9. Plasma half-life is 8–12 hours and the peak plasma concentrations are generally attained in 3 hours. The oral bioavailability may be decreased when taken with food.

Zafirlukast is a selective and competitive receptor antagonist of leukotriene D4 and E4 components of slow reacting substance of anaphylaxis. It also blocks cys LT1 receptor mediated bronchoconstriction, airway mucus secretion, increased vascular permeability and recruitment of eosinophils. It inhibits bronchoconstriction caused by several kinds of inhalational agents like sulphur dioxide and cold air. It is not a bronchodilator.

Indications of use: Zafirlukast is indicated for the chronic treatment of asthma regularly and prescribed even during symptom free periods. It is not indicated to treat acute episodes of asthma. The dose of other antiasthma medications need not be reduced or stopped.

Contraindications: Hypersensitivity to zafirlukast or any of its active ingredients.

Dosage: For adults and children above the age of 12 years—20 mg tablet orally twice daily.

For children less than 5 years—10 mg twice daily.

Adverse effects: Abdominal pain, serum transaminase elevation, asthenia and back pain can occur. Rise in serum transaminases is reversible on discontinuation of drug. Rarely cases of hepatic failure have been reported.

Hypersensitivity reactions including urticaria, angioedema, and rashes with or without blistering can occur.

In rare cases, patients on therapy may present with systemic eosinophilia.

Drug interaction: Aspirin may cause increase in mean plasma levels of zafirlukast. Erythromycin and theophylline result in decreased mean plasma levels of zafirlukast.

Monitoring: In patients who are on warfarin therapy, administration of zafirlukast results in increase in prothrombin time. Close monitoring of PT and dose adjustment is required in these cases.[10]

Preparations

- ***Zuvair tablet:*** 10, 20 mg.

Safety during pregnancy and lactation: There are no adequate and well-controlled trials in pregnant women and animal studies have shown maternal and fetal toxicity during pregnancy, it is used in pregnancy when clearly indicated.

Zafirlukast is excreted in breast milk. Because of the potential for tumorigenicity shown in mouse and rats, it is advised not to administer the drug during lactation.

It is FDA category B drug.[4,8,9]

Montelukast

It is rapidly absorbed following oral administration. The mean oral bioavailability is 64% and the peak plasma concentration is achieved in 3–4 hours. The oral bioavailability is not affected by food. It is 9% bound to plasma proteins. It is metabolized extensively by cytochrome P450 and excreted in urine.

Indications of use

- It is used for the prophylaxis and chronic treatment of asthma in adults.
- It is used for the treatment of allergic rhinitis in adults and children older than 2 years of age.
- It is used for the prevention of exercise induced bronchoconstriction.

Contraindications: Hypersensitivity to any component of this product.

Dosage: 10 mg orally once daily.

Adverse effects: Asthenia, fatigue, dizziness, headache, can occur. GI symptoms like abdominal pain, dyspepsia, gastroenteritis are other side effects. Rise in serum transaminases has also been seen.

Drug interactions: Montelukast plasma concentrations may be reduced with administration of cytochrome P450 enzyme inducers like phenobarbitone and rifampicin. Edema may increase if co-administered with prednisone.

Monitoring: No specific monitoring is required.

Preparations

- *Montair tablet*: 10 mg
- *Montek tablet*: 10 mg
- *Romilast tablet*: 10 mg.

Safety during pregnancy and lactation: Montelukast crosses placenta following overdosing in rats and rabbits. There are however no adequate and well controlled studies in humans. Therefore use during pregnancy when clearly indicated.

Studies in mice have shown that it is excreted in milk but in humans this is not established; therefore should be cautiously used in lactating women.

It is FDA category B drug.[4,8,9]

Leukotreine Inhibitors

Zileuton

Pharmacology: It is rapidly absorbed upon oral administration with a mean peak plasma concentration achieved in 1.7 hours. It is 93% bound to plasma proteins. It is metabolized in liver by enzymes and excreted in urine and feces.

Zileuton is a specific inhibitor of 5-lipoxygenase and thus inhibits leukotriene (LTB4, LTC4, LTD4, LTE4) formation and thus inhibiting augmentation and eosinophil migration, increased capillary permeability and smooth muscle contraction.

Indications of use: It is used for the prophylaxis and chronic treatment of asthma in adults and children above the age of 12 years.

Contraindications: Active liver disease or persistent rise in serum transaminases and history of allergy to zileuton.

Dosage: 600 mg extended release tablets twice daily, maximum dose 2400 mg per day.

Adverse effects: Nausea, nasopharyngeal pain, sinusitis can occur.

Drug interactions: It increases plasma concentration of propranolol, terfenadine and theophylline. It leads to increase in prothrombin time when co-administered with warfarin. Dose of warfarin needs to be adjusted and monitored.

Preparations: Zyflo CR-600 mg extended release tablet.

Safety in pregnancy and lactation: It is to be used during pregnancy only if the potential benefits outweighs the risk. Zileuton is excreted in rat milk but it is not known whether it is excreted in human milk. Therefore, its use in breast feeding is restricted.[9]

It is FDA category C drug.

Mast Cell Stabilizers

Cromolyn Sodium

Pharmacology: It is given by inhalation as aerosols or dry powder and also topically.

It is anti-inflammatory and blocks early and late reactions to the allergen. It interferes with chloride channel function, stabilises mast cell membranes and inhibits activation and release of mediators from epithelial cells and eosinophils. It also inhibits acute response to exercise, cold dry air, and SO_2. Cromolyn sodium is nonsteroidal anti-inflammatory agents that work by preventing mast cell degranulation.

Indications

- As prophylactic management of bronchial asthma. Cromolyn is given on a regular basis daily in patients with frequent symptomatology requiring a continuous medication regimen.
- To prevent acute bronchospasm induced by exercise, environmental pollutants and known antigens.
- To prevent and treat allergic rhinitis, caused by airborne pollens from trees or ragweed,

and by mould, animals and dust. To prevent and relieve nasal symptoms such as running nose, sneezing and allergic stuffy nose.

Contraindications: Hypersensitivity to cromolyn sodium.

Dosage: 20 mg administered by nebulization 4 times per day at regular intervals. Solution is administered from a power operated nebulizer having an adequate flow rate and equipped with a suitable face mask or mouth piece.

Adverse effects: Bronchospasm, throat irritation, and cough may occur in some patients especially with fine powder inhalation. Dizziness, headache, dysuria, urinary frequency and anaphylaxis are infrequent side effects.

Monitoring: No specific monitoring is required.

Preparations

- *Fintal inhaler*: 1 mg per puff.
- *Cromal inhaler*: 5 per puff in a metered dose inhaler.

Safety in pregnancy and lactation: There is no reported experience with nedocromil in human pregnancy. It is FDA category B drug.[4,8]

Inhaled Corticosteroids

Beclomethasone and Budesonide

Pharmacology: These are beclomethasone dipropionate, triamcinolone acetonide, budesonide, fluticasone, flunsolide and ciclesonide.

The peak effect is seen after 4–7 days of instituting inhaled steroids and benefit persists for a few weeks after discontinuation.

These are anti-inflammatory. They block late reaction to allergens and reduce airway hyper-responsiveness, inhibit cytokine production, adhesion protein activation and inflammatory cell migration and activation. They also reverse beta 2-receptor down regulation and inhibit microvascular leakage.

Indications of use

- They are indicated in all cases of persistent asthma when inhaled beta 2-agonists are required almost daily. Inhaled steroids suppress bronchial inflammation, increase peak expiratory flow rate, reduce dose of beta 2-agonist and prevent episode of acute asthma.
- In COPD patients, the airway inflammation is not very responsive to corticosteroids. Only high dose inhaled steroids are beneficial in advanced COPD with frequent exacerbations.

Contraindications: None for inhaled corticosteroids.

Adverse effects: Systemic effects of long-term inhaled glucocorticoids are clinically relevant in doses more than 600 µg per day. Hoarseness of voice, dysphonia, sore throat, asymptomatic or symptomatic oropharyngeal candidiasis are the most common side effects. These can be minimized by the use of spacer, gargling after every dose and local use of clotrimazole.[2]

Dosage of beclomethasone: Start with 100–200 µg twice daily, titrate dose upward every 3–5 days with maximum 400 µg four times a day.

Preparations of beclomethasone

- *Beclate inhaler*: 50 µg per metered dose
- *Beclate rotacaps*: 100, 200, 400 µg
- *Aerocort inhaler*: 50 µg beclomethasone and salbutamol 100 µg per metered aerosol dose
- *Aerocort rotacaps*: 100 µg beclomethasone and salbutamol 200 µg.

Dosage of budesonide: 200–400 µg twice to four times daily by inhalation.

Preparations of budesonide

- *Pulmicort inhaler*: 100, 200, 400 µg metered dose Budecort.
- *Rhinocort inhaler*: 50 µg per metered dose
- *Foracort rotacaps*: Budesonide 100/200 µg and formeterol 6 µg.

Safety in pregnancy and lactation: Inhaled steroids are safe in pregnancy. Beclomethasone is a category C drug. Budesonide is widely used in pregnancy and is category B drug and is a preferred drug in pregnancy.[7-9,14,15]

Fluticasone Propionate

This inhaled glucocorticoid has high potency; longer duration of action and negligible oral bioavailability. The swallowed dose after inhalation has little propensity to produce systemic effects. At high doses, systemic effects may be due to absorption through lungs.

Dosage: 50 μg by nasal spray, two puffs twice daily.

Preparations

- *Flohale inhaler*: 25, 50, 125 μg per metered dose
- *Flohale rotacaps*: 50, 100, 250 μg.

Safety in pregnancy and lactation: Although Fluticasone has not been studied in pregnancy, its minimal absorption and the safety of other drugs in this category makes its use in pregnancy generally justifiable.

Ciclesonide

This inhalational steroid utilizes a novel approach to improve topical: Systemic activity ratio. It is a prodrug that is cleaved by esterases in the bronchial epithelium to release the active moiety. Though it is absorbed from the lungs, oral bioavailability is < 1%. In the circulation it is extensively bound to plasma proteins, further minimizing exposure of tissue cells to the free and active drug.

Dosage: 80–160 μg by inhalation once daily preferably in the evening.

Preparation: Ciclez inhaler-80 μg, 160 μg per metered dose with HFA propellant.

Systemic Steroid Therapy

Prednisolone

Pharmacology: It is 4 times more potent than hydrocortisone, also more selective glucocorticoid, but fluid retention does occur with high doses. It has intermediate duration of action. It causes less pituitary—adrenal suppression when single morning dose or alternate day therapy is given.

It has anti-inflammatory action, blocks late reaction to allergen and reduce airway hyper responsiveness. It inhibits cytokine production, adhesion protein activation, and inflammatory cell migration and activation. It reverses beta 2-receptor down regulation and inhibits microvascular leakage. Glucocorticoids are not bronchodilators. They benefit by reducing bronchial hyperactivity, mucosal edema and by suppressing inflammatory response to antigen antibody reaction or other trigger stimuli.

They offer more complete and sustained symptomatic relief than bronchodilators, improve airflow, reduce asthma exacerbations, may influence airway remodelling and retard disease progression. They also increase smooth muscle responsiveness to beta 2-agonists and reverse refractoriness to these drugs.

Indications of use

- It is given in severe chronic asthma not controlled by bronchodilators and inhaled steroids and when there are frequent recurrences of increasing severity.
- Systemic steroids are given in status asthmaticus and acute exacerbations of asthma not responding to intensive bronchodilator therapy.
- In COPD a short course of oral steroid may benefit some patients.

Contraindications: Consideration should be given to co-existing conditions that could be worsened by systemic steroids such as herpes infection, *Varicella*, tuberculosis, hypertension, peptic ulcer, psychosis, epilepsy, congestive heart failure and renal failure.

Dosage: In the beginning prednisolone 20–60 mg orally daily started, after 1–2 weeks of good control dose reduction is done gradually and the patient shifted on inhaled steroid therapy.

Adverse effects: With short term use; reversible abnormalities in glucose metabolism, increased appetite, fluid retention, weight gain, mood alteration, hypertension, peptic ulcer, and rarely aseptic necrosis of femur.

With long-term use; adrenal axis suppression, growth suppression, dermal thinning, hypertension, diabetes, Cushing's syndrome, cataracts, muscle weakness and in rare instances impaired immune function.

Preparations

- *Wysolone tablets*: 10 mg
- *Deltacortril tablets*: 5 mg
- *Nucort tablets*: 5, 10 mg
- *Hostacortin tablets*: 5 mg.

Safety during pregnancy and lactation: Several case control studies have found a significant association with first trimester steroid use and oral clefts. However, this was not seen in cohort studies. But it is important to note that even if this association is real, the risk is still small. For every 1000 embryos exposed during the susceptible days of first trimester, probably no more than 3 will develop an oral cleft. The background risk in the general population is 1 per 1000. Therefore, the benefits of controlling a life-threatening disease makes steroid use, when indicated in the first trimester, still generally justifiable.

It is FDA category C drug.[9,12-15]

Methylprednisolone

It is slightly more potent and more selective than prednisolone.

Dosage

- 4–32 mg per day orally
- 0.5 g–1 g IV or IM injection.

Preparations

- *Acto-pred*: 4 mg tablet, 500 mg and 1 gm for injection
- *Cecort*: 40 mg per mL injection
- *Depomax-s*: 40 mg for injection
- *Solu-medrol*: 40, 125, 500 mg, 1 g powder for IV and IM use.

Hydrocortisone

It acts rapidly but has short duration of action. In addition to primary glucocorticoid, it has significant mineralocorticoid activity as well.

Dosage: 100 mg IV in status asthmaticus.

Preparations

- *Efcorlin injection*: 100 mg, 200 mg, 400 mg per vial
- *Wycort*: 25 mg per mL–5 mL injection available
- *Primacort*: 200 mg per vial.

Monoclonal Antibody

Omalizumab

Pharmacology: Omalizumab is a recombinant DNA derived humanized IgG monoclonal antibody that binds to human IgE. It inhibits the binding of IgE to the high affinity IgE receptors on the surface of basophils and mast cells.

After subcutaneous administration, it has an average bioavailability of 62%. Following a single subcutaneous administration, it is absorbed slowly reaching peak plasma concentration in 7–8 days. It is eliminated by liver reticuloendothelial system and endothelial cells.

Indications of use: It used for adults and adolescents above 12 years of age with moderate and severe persistent asthma who have a positive skin test or *in vitro* reactivity to perennial aeroallergens and whose symptoms are inadequately controlled with inhaled steroids.

Contraindications: Severe hypersensitivity reaction to omalizumab.

Dosage: Usual dose is 300 mg subcutaneously every 4 weeks.

Adverse effects: Common side effects are injection site reaction, viral infection, upper respiratory infection, sinusitis headache and pharyngitis.

Serious side effects are anaphylaxis and malignancies. Anaphylaxis can occur in 0.1% of the users.

Drug interaction: None known.

Preparation: Xolair injection–150 mg per mL in a prefilled syringe.

Flow chart 23.1: Management of asthma during pregnancy[16,17]

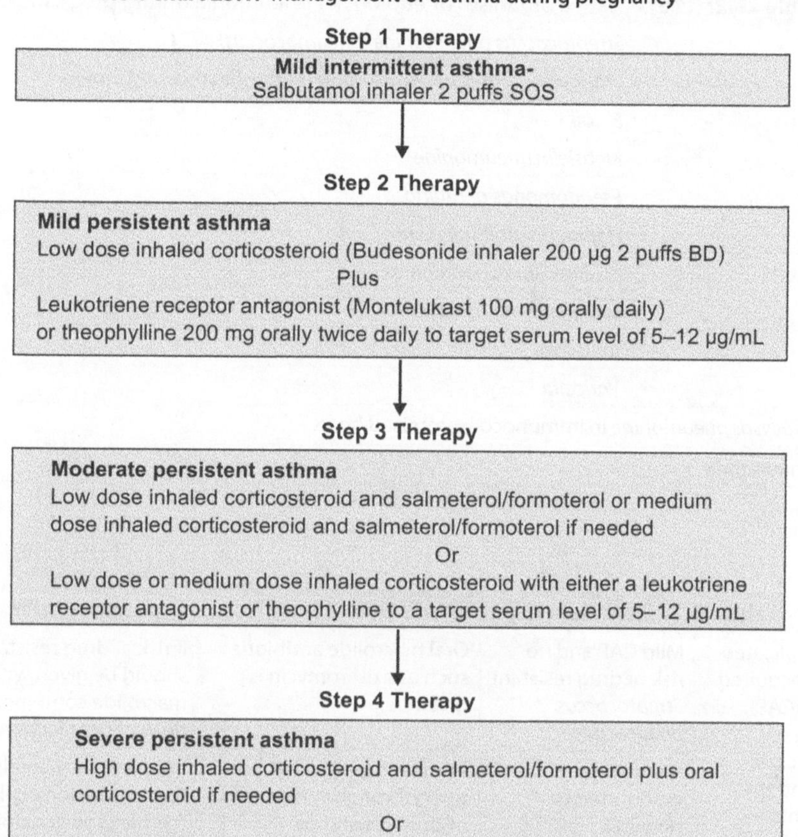

Safety in pregnancy and lactation: IgG molecules are known to cross the placental barrier. Because animal production studies are not always predictive of human response, use omalizumab in pregnancy only if indicated.

The potential for omalizumab absorption or harm to a breast feeding infant is not known but the potential of adverse effects is low, therefore exercise caution when used during lactation.

It is FDA category B drug.[9]

Approach to a pregnant patient with asthma is shown in **Flow chart 23.1**.

PNEUMONIAS IN PREGNANCY

Treatment of pneumonia during pregnancy is requires knowledge about the possible causative organisms and the antibiotic preferences as most of the time treatment is based on clinical judgement **(Table 23.2)**. Pneumonia is a life-threatening complication during pregnancy and though infrequent it is the most common nonobsteric infection and third most common nonobstetric cause of maternal mortality.[18]

Therapy for Pneumonia During Pregnancy

The general principles of management of pneumonia during pregnancy are same as during nonpregnant state. The only concern is safety of antibiotics during pregnancy and lactation and choosing such antibiotics which

Table 23.2: The causative organism or etiology of pneumonia during pregnancy[18,19]

Bacterial	*Streptococcus pneumoniae (Pneumococcus)*
	Staphylococcus aureus including methicillin resistant strains
	E. coli
	Klebsiella pneumoniae
	Pseudomonas aeruginosa
	Haemophilus influenzae
Atypical bacteria	*Mycoplasma pneumoniae*
	Legionella pnemophila
Viral	Influenza
	Varicella
Fungi: Pneumocystis pneumoniae in immunocompromised hosts	
Aspiration pneumonia	

Table 23.3: Treatment of pneumonia during pregnancy and puerperium[18,22]

In an uncomplicated community acquired pneumonia (CAP), cover for the *Pneumococcus, H. influenzae* and the atypical agents	Mild CAP and no risk of drug resistant *Streptococcus pneumoniae*	Oral macrolide antibiotic such as azithromycin is given	If risk of drug resistance, therapy should be given with a high dose macrolide combined with high dose of beta lactam (amoxicillin)
	If the patient is admitted to hospital	Intravenous azithromycin or erythromycin if no risks of drug resistance	Intravenous macrolide and 3rd generation cephalosporin (ceftriaxone or cefotaxime)
	ICU admitted patient with severe CAP	Intravenous macrolide and 3rd generation cephalosporin (ceftriaxone or cefotaxime)	If risk of *Pseudomonas* infection then antipseudomonal beta lactam (ceftazidime, imipenam, piperacillin) with an aminoglycosides and a macrolide given intravenously
Bacterial pneumonia associated with influenza outbreaks	It should include coverage for the *Pneumococcus, Staphylococcus aureus* and gram–negative bacteria. Antibiotics against *methicillin-resistant Staphylococcus aureus* (MRSA) should be considered in patients with severe CAP after influenza. However, although the safety of vancomycin and linezolid in pregnancy is not established, benefits of these drugs in patients with severe pneumonia probably outweigh the risks of the drugs, and patients should be counseled accordingly.		
Nosocomial infection	Treatment should cover include gram–negative bacteria and anaerobes		
Aspiration pneumonia	Treatment should cover gram negative bacteria and anaerobes		

are safe for the fetus and the breastfeeding baby **(Table 23.3)**.

There are reports of increasing antibiotic resistance of common bacterial pathogens to common first line antibiotics. Ampicillin was previously the drug of choice for therapy of uncomplicated community acquired pneumonia. However, cephalosporins are now recommended because of increasing drug resistance. Current guidelines recommend that patients should not receive empiric therapy with a beta lactam (penicillin or cephalosporins) alone and that all patients be treated for atypical pathogens and *Pneumococcus*.[19-21]

Supportive Care

Supportive therapy of the pregnant patient with pneumonia is similar to the nongravid state; hydration, antipyretic therapy, and supplemental oxygen remain key. The oxygen saturation should be maintained more than 94%. Preterm labor is a known complication of systemic infections, which should be suspected and addressed based on gestational age, fetal maturity, and maternal and fetal wellbeing.[23]

REFERENCES

1. Hardy-Fairbanks AJ, Baker ER. Asthma in pregnancy: pathophysiology, diagnosis and management. Obstet Gynecol Clin North Am. 2010;37(2):159-72.
2. Tripathi KD. Drugs used in Bronchial asthma. Essentials of Medical Pharmacology, 7th edn. Jaypee Brothers Medical Publishers (P) Ltd. New Delhi. 2013.pp.221-38.
3. Grahamme-Smith DG, JK Aronson. Drug treatment of Bronchial asthma. Oxford Textbook of Clinical Pharmacology and Drug Therapy, 3rd edn. OUP Oxford UK. 2002.pp.632-49.
4. National Asthma Education and Prevention Program expert panel report. Managing asthma during pregnancy: recommendations for pharmacologic treatment-2004 update. J Allergy Clin Immunol. 2005;115:34-46.
5. Dombrowski M, Schatz M. Asthma in pregnancy: ACOG practice bulletin. Obstet Gynecol. 2008;111:457-64.
6. Rayburn WF, Atkinson BD, Gilbert K, Turnbull GL. Short-term effects of inhaled albuterol on maternal and fetal circulations. Am J Obstet Gynecol. 1994;171(3):770-3.
7. Bracken MD, Triche EW, Belandger K, et al. Asthma symptoms, severity, and drug therapy: A prospective study of effects on 2205 pregnancies. Obstet Gynecol. 2003;102:739-52.
8. Boothby LA, Doering PL. FDA labeling system for drugs in pregnancy. Ann Pharmacother. 2001; 35(11):1485-9.
9. Erwin K, Cathy AM, et al. Respiratory agents. Drug Facts and Comparisons. edn Wolters Kluwer Health USA. 2010.pp.947-74.
10. Brunton LL, Lazo JS, Parker KL, eds. Goodman and Gilman's The Pharmacological Basis of Therapeutics. 10th ed. New York, NY: McGraw-Hill. 2001.
11. Dombrowski MP, Schatz M, Wise R, Thom EA, Landon M, Mabie W, Newman RB, McNellis D, Hauth JC, Lindheimer M, et al. Randomized trial of inhaled beclomethasone dipropionate versus theophylline for moderate asthma during pregnancy. Am J Obstet Gynecol. 2004;190(3):737-44.
12. Briggs GG, Freeman RK, Yaffe. Drugs in pregnancy and lactation: A Reference Guide to Fetal and Neonatal Risks. 8th edn. Philadelphia, PA: Wolters Kluwer Health/Lippincott Williams and Wilkins. 2008.
13. Schatz M, Dombrowski MP, Wise R, et al. The relationship of asthma medication use to perinatal outcomes. J Allergy Clin Immunol. 2004;113(6):1040-5.
14. Blais L, Beauchesne MF, Rey E, et al. Use of inhaled corticosteroids during the first trimester of pregnancy and the risk of congenital malformations among women with asthma. Thorax. 2007;62(4):320-8.
15. Kallen B, Rydhstroem H, Aberg A. Congenital malformations after the use of inhaled budesonide in early pregnancy. Obstet Gynecol. 1999;93(3):392-5.
16. EPR—Update 2002. NAEPP Expert Panel Report: Guidelines for the Diagnosis and Treatment of Asthma—Update on Selected Topics 2002. NIH Publication No. 02-5074. Bethesda, MD: U.S. Department of Health and Human Services; National Institutes of Health; National Heart, Lung, and Blood Institute, 2003. Available from URL: *http://www.nhlbi. nih.gov/guidelines/asthma/asthupdt. htm*. Accessed July 8, 2004.

17. GINA Report, Global Strategy for Asthma Management and Prevention. *http://www.ginathma.com/2007/Guidelines Resources.*
18. Patrick SR, Kirk DR. Pneumonia during pregnancy. Obstetrics and Gynecology Clinics of North America. 2001;28(3):553-69.
19. Shariatzadeh MR, Marie TJ. Pneumonia during pregnancy. Am J Med. 2006;119(10):872-6.
20. Goodnight WH, Soper DE. Pneumonia in pregnancy. Crit Care Med. 2005;33(10):390-7.
21. Berkowitz K, LaSala A. Risk factors associated with the increasing prevalence of pneumonia during pregnancy. Am J Obstet Gynecol. 1990;163(3):981-5.
22. Yost NP, Bloom SL, Richey SD, Ramin SM, Cunningham FG. An appraisal of treatment guidelines for antepartum community-acquired pneumonia. Am J Obstet Gynecol. 2000;183(1):131-5.
23. Munn MB, Groome LJ, Atterbury JL, Baker SL, Hoff C. Pneumonia as a complication of pregnancy. J Matern Fetal Med. 1999;8(4):151-4.

CHAPTER 24

Neurological and Psychiatric Disorders of Pregnancy

Pushpa Mishra

Neurological disorders are quite common in women during their childbearing age. There are several neurological diseases that are seen often in pregnant women. These disorders further go on to be a major cause of maternal morbidity and mortality. Many neurological diseases are chronic and when women become pregnant with these diseases, outcomes are usually successful with few risks.[1,2]

Some of the most commonly encountered neurological diseases during pregnancy are headache, seizure disorder, and psychiatric disorders.[1]

HEADACHE

Headache is the most common neurological disease during pregnancy. The most common type of headache is tension type (69%) followed by migraine (16%). In cases of headache secondary to some systemic illness, treatment of the cause is important.

Tension headache mostly responds to rest and anti-inflammatory medications or mild tranquilizers, i.e. aspirin, ibuprofen, alprazolam (one or two doses).[3]

Migraine headache is a benign and recurring syndrome of headache with many accompanying symptoms such as nausea, vomiting, photophobia, visual disturbances, vertigo, etc. It is often triggered by certain stimulatory factors.

Drugs which are used in the treatment of migraine are enlisted in **Table 24.1**.

Mostly, symptoms respond to potent analgesics, but in severe cases it should be treated aggressively with IV fluids and parenteral antiemetic and opioids.

In first and second trimester treatment should be started with paracetamol and low dose caffeine combination. Pregnant women should not use more than 200 mg daily dose

Table 24.1: Drug treatment of migraine[4]

Treatment of acute attack of migraine	
Nonsteroidal anti-inflammatory drugs (NSAIDs)	Naproxen
	Ibuprofen
5 HT Receptor agonist	Ergotamine
	Sumatriptan
Dopamine receptor antagonist	Metoclopramide
	Chlorpromazine
	Chlorperazine
Prevention of migraine attack	
Beta blocker	Propranolol
Tricyclic antidepressants	Amitriptyline

of caffeine, as it may cause increased risk of spontaneous abortion. High dose of caffeine (>300 mg/day) can increase the risk of preterm labor and fetal growth retardation. Caffeine is excreted in breast milk; infants become restless and jittery if nursing mother consumes more than 300 mg of caffeine but no long-term adverse effect.

Drugs Used in Headache

Naproxen[4-6]

Pharmacology: It is a nonsteroidal anti-inflammatory drug (NSAID), an inhibitor of COX-1 and COX-2 as other NSAIDs, and a member of profen family.[4-6]

Indications of use: Used as analgesic in migraine and dysmenorrhea, as anti-inflammatory and analgesic in arthritis.

Contraindications: Hypersensitivity to naproxen, asthma, severe acid peptic disease, urticaria, etc.

Dosage: 220 mg–275 mg orally, maximum up to 1400 mg per day.

Adverse effects: Gastrointestinal (GI) side effects similar to other NSAID like nausea, heartburn, stomach ulcers, hematemesis, constipation and diarrhea, etc.

Drug interaction: Not significant.

Monitoring: It should not be taken empty stomach, nor should be combined with antacids.

Preparations
- *Artagen*: 250 mg tablets
- *Napris*: 250 and 500 mg tablets
- *Headset*: Tablet containing sumatriptan 35 mg plus 500 mg naproxen
- *Napra D*: Tablet combination of 250 or 500 mg naproxen with domperidone 10 mg.

Safety during pregnancy and lactation: As with other NSAIDs it is not teratogenic but it has a potential risk of causing premature closure of ductus arteriosus and oligohydramnios in late 3rd trimester. Its use is also associated with abortions and preterm births. It should be avoided in 3rd trimester of pregnancy. It is considered safe in breastfeeding.

FDA has approved it as over the counter drug for dysmenorrhea.

Ibuprofen

It has similar profile as naproxen.

Dosages: 200–400 mg tablets given 3–4 times a day.

Preparations
- *Brufen*: 400 mg tablets
- *Ibuprofen*: 400: 400 mg tablets
- *Ibugesic*: 200 mg tablets
- *Emflam*: 400 mg tablets
- *Combiflam*: Combination of 200 mg ibuprofen and 500 mg paracetamol.

Ergotamine

Pharmacology: It is an ergopeptine and belongs to ergot alkaloids. In migraine, it acts as a vasoconstrictor. It causes constriction of intracranial, extracerebral blood vessels through the 5-HT_{1B} and by inhibiting trigeminal neurotransmission by 5-HT_{1D} receptors.

Indications: Acute attack of migraine. Previously it has been used in postpartum hemorrhage.

Contraindications: Pregnancy, atherosclerosis, vascular diseases, coronary artery disease, liver and renal disorder, etc.

Dosage: 1–2 mg orally or sublingually at the onset of the symptoms and then 1–2 mg 4 times a day.

Adverse effects: Thrombosis, gangrene.

Preparations
- *Cafergot, ergomer*: 2 mg sublingual tablets.
- *Ercaf, wigraine*: Combination of 1 mg ergotamine and 100 mg caffeine.

Safety during pregnancy and lactation: Small, infrequent doses of ergotamine used for migraine headaches do not appear to be fetotoxic or teratogenic, but idiosyncratic responses may occur that endanger the fetus. Larger doses or frequent use, however, may cause fetal toxicity or teratogenicity that is probably due to maternal and/or fetal vascular disruption. Because the risk has not been adequately defined, and also due to the oxytocic properties of the agent, ergotamine should be avoided during pregnancy.

It is excreted in breast milk and it is a member of the same family as bromocriptine but it does not suppress the lactation, however it is better to avoid in lactation.

FDA approves it as prescription drug for migraine as second-line treatment.

Sumatriptan[4,5,7]

Pharmacology: It is a 5-$HT_{1B/1D}$ receptor agonist and a synthetic analog of naturally occurring neuroactive alkaloid dimethyltryptamine.[4,5,7]

Indications of use: Acute migraine. Cluster headache.

Contraindications: Ischemic heart disease, previous MI, uncontrolled hypertension.

Dosage: It can be given by SC injection, orally or by nasal spray.

- 4 or 6 mg SC, if no relief can repeat in 1 hour, maximum dose is two 6 mg injection in 24 hours.
- 50–100 mg orally, maximum dose of 200 mg per day in divided doses.
- 5-20 mg intranasal spray, should not exceed more than 40 mg/day.

Adverse effects: Drowsiness, paresthesia and cold sensations. Rarely vertigo, fatigue and malaise.

Preparations

- *Imitrex injection*: 0.5 mL vial containing 6 or 4 mg sumatriptan succinate for SC injection.
- *Imitrex, imigran*: 50 and 100 mg tablets.
- *Treximet*: Combination of sumatriptan 85 mg and naproxen 500 mg tablet.
- *Imitrex nasal spray*: 5 and 20 mg per spray.

Safety during pregnancy and lactation: Although, this caused toxicity and malformation in animals but sumatriptan does not cause any major teratogenic risk in humans and there is minimal risk of preterm labor. It is excreted in the milk, but no significant adverse effect on nursing infant.

FDA approves all forms of preparations and its combination with naproxen for migraine.

SEIZURE DISORDERS

After headache, seizure disorder is the most common neurological disorder which complicates the pregnancy. One out of two hundred pregnancies are associated with seizure disorder. These disorders themselves are not associated with any abnormal fetal development but anticonvulsant medications are teratogenic in nature.

Preconception Counseling

Most of the anticonvulsants are teratogens and women with epilepsy, who are planning for pregnancy, should be counseled and explained. Folic acid 0.4 mg/day should be started at least one month prior and dose should be increased to 4 mg/day once the woman conceives. Treatment with single drug and minimum dose should be considered to reduce fetal teratogenicity.[1,2]

Epilepsy during pregnancy: Seizure frequency increases in up to 30% of epileptic pregnant women due to physiological and psychological changes. In these women increase in dose or addition of another antiepileptic (with low teratogenic effects) should be considered.

Antiepileptic Drugs

All antiepileptic drugs (AEDs) have teratogenic effect. The safest drug during pregnancy is carbamazepine, however, that too affects 1% fetuses with spina bifida. Mothers on various AEDs, single drug or multiple, have 6–8% risk of fetal malformation.

Some level of cognitive dysfunction is observed in the babies of mothers on AEDs and it is more with valproate. Various antiepileptic drugs used during pregnancy are given in **Table 24.2.**

Phenytoin

Pharmaoclogy: It is a hydantoin derivative which causes voltage dependent blockage of voltage gated sodium channels. Being a membrane stabilizer, phenytoin is an important antiarrhythmic drug too.

Indications of use

- Tonic-clonic seizure, focal-onset seizure, seizure during surgery, status epilepticus, absence seizure. It is used in combination with other anticonvulsants.
- To prevent seizure in pre- and postsurgery neurosurgical cases.
- Arrhythmias—ventricular, atrial tachycardia and other abnormal cardiac rhythms.
- Digoxin toxicity.
- Trigeminal neuralgia.

Table 24.2: Various anti-epileptics used during pregnancy[1-5,8]

Class	*Drug*
Sodium channel blocker	Carbamazepine Phenytoin
Sodium and T type calcium channel blocker and blockade of GABA transaminase	Valproic acid
Sodium channel and high voltage dependent calcium channel blocker	Lamotrigine
High affinity for synaptic vesicle protein	Levetiracetam
T type calcium channel blocker	Ethosuximide
GABA analog	Gabapentin
benzodiazepine	Lorazepam

Contraindications: Hypersensitivity sinus bradycardia and heart blocks, etc.

Dosage: For control of seizures initial loading dose: 10–15 mg/kg or 800 mg IV slowly. Maintenance dose: 100 mg IV every 6–8 hours. Then orally 100 mg 3–4 times a day is started.

Adverse effects: Dizziness, confusion, gum hyperplasia, osteomalacia, skin rash, facial coarsening. Very low blood pressure, arrhythmias can be caused with rapid IV infusion of the drug.

Drug interaction: Drugs which increase concentration of phenytoin include-amiodaron, fluconazole, diazepam, fluoxetine, omeprazole, nifedipine. Drugs which decrease its level are folic acid, rifampicin sucralfate, theophylline etc.

Preparations

- *Dilantin*: 100 mg tablets and injection as 2 mL ampoules containing 50 mg/mL.
- *Epilan*: 100 mg tablets.
- *Epilan C*: Combination of 100 mg phenytoin and 30 mg phenobarbital.

Safety during pregnancy: Though it is category D drug for pregnancy but mostly used during pregnancy in conditions when maternal benefits outweigh the fetal risks.

It causes fetal hydantoin syndrome characterized by craniofacial anomalies, fingernail hypoplasia, growth deficiency, developmental delay, cardiac anomalies, oral clefts, etc. Approximately 5–11% of fetuses are affected.

Folic acid 4–5 mg should be given daily throughout pregnancy. Timely fetal screening by AFP, level II USG scan and echocardiography is mandatory.

Data on breastfeed is limited but considered to be safe.

Carbamazepine

It is considered to be the safest antiepileptic drug during pregnancy.

Pharmacology: It is a sodium channel blocker agent, therefore, reduces the propagation of an abnormal impulse in the brain.

Indications: Tonic-clonic seizure, focal-onset seizure, trigeminal neuralgia and as mood stabilizer.

Contraindications: Absence seizure (Petit mal seizure).

Dosage: 600–1800 mg/day orally in 2–3 divided doses.

Adverse effects: Dizziness, vertigo, ataxia, leukopenia, gastrointestinal irritation, aplastic anemia, hyponatremia, etc.

Drug interactions: If the patient is on oral contraceptive pills (OCPs), he/she should be warned that carbamazepine decreases efficacy of OCPs and she should use alternative contraceptive method. Whereas it increases plasma concentration of propoxyphene.

It enhances clearance of doxycycline, reduces tolerance to alcohol. When combined with lithium can be fatal due to neurotoxicity.

Monitoring: Patient should be observed for any evidence of side effects.

Preparation

- *Tegretol*: 100 and 200 mg tablets
- *Carbatol*: 100 and 200 mg tablets
- *Carbatol CR*: 200 and 400 mg tablets
- *Antilep*: 100, 200 mg tablets
- *Antilep CR*: 200, 300 and 400 mg tablets.

Safety during pregnancy and breastfeeding: Spina bifida is seen in 1% of the pregnancies, this risk is further reduced if patient takes folic acid regularly.

It is excreted in breast milk but no risk to infant.

FDA Category D.

Valproic Acid

Pharmacology: Its mechanism of action is sodium channel blockade, blockade of GABA transaminase and action at T type calcium channels.

Indications of use

- Tonic-clonic seizure
- Absence and atypical absence seizure
- Myoclonic, focal onset, atonic seizure
- Mood stabilizer.

Contraindications: Hypersensitivity acute or chronic liver disease, pancreatitis and porphyria, etc.

Dosage: Initial dose is 10–15 mg/kg/day orally or IV infusion in divided doses. Then according to response it is increased by 5–10 mg/kg/day.

Maximum dose is 60 mg/kg/day or 750–2000 mg per day orally in divided doses.

Adverse effects: Ataxia, sedation, tremors, hepatotoxicity, gastrointestinal irritation, hyponatremia, thrombocytopenia, etc.

Drug interaction: It increases CNS toxicity of alcohol, effects of anticoagulants leading to prolonged bleeding time, worsen CNS toxicity with benzodiazepines, may increase toxicity of ethosuximide, primidone and zidovudine. Cimetidine, aspirin and erythromycin increase valproate toxicity by inhibiting its metabolism.

Monitoring: Patient is monitored with platelet count and liver function test. Also monitored for any seizures or worsening depression.

Preparations

- *Encorate chrono*: 200,300 and 500 mg controlled release tablets
- *Monova*: 200, 300 mg tablets
- *Torvate*: 200, 300, 500, 750, and 1000 mg tablets
- *Valporate chrono*: 200,300 and 500 mg controlled release tablets.

Safety during pregnancy and lactation: Babies are affected with neural tube defects, clefts, cardiac anomalies and associated developmental delays. Major malformations occur in 9% fetuses if exposed in first trimester which included 4% neural tube defects. Babies with valproic acid exposure are reported to have low IQ than with other anticonvulsants.

It is FDA Category D.

Valproate syndrome: Babies, exposed to the drug *in utero* have characteristic features like triangle-shaped forehead, epicanthic folds, flat nasal bridge, broad nasal root, shallow philtrum and vermillion borders.

It is given to pregnant patients only when benefit outweigh the risk to the fetus but fetal screening should always be done in such cases.

In mothers on valproate who are breast-feeding, it is advised to monitor baby for hepatotoxicity.

Lamotrigine

It blocks sodium channel as well as high voltage dependent calcium channel.

Indications of use: Focal-onset, tonic-clonic, atypical absence, myoclonic seizures, Lennox-Gastaut syndrome. Other uses include peripheral neuropathy, trigeminal neuralgia and certain headaches.

Contraindications: Hypersensitivity to drug.

Dosage: Start as 200 mg orally twice daily, increase at weekly interval by 200 mg per day till optimal response is obtained. Maintenance dose is 800 -1200 mg per day and maximum dose is 166 mg per day.

Adverse effects: Dizziness, diplopia, sedation, ataxia, headache, skin rash, Stevens-Johnson syndrome, etc.

Drug interaction: When used with OCs, ethinyl estradiol decreases serum levels of lamotrigine and effectiveness of the drugs may decrease.

Valproate may increase its side effects.

Carbamazepine may decrease it effectiveness.

Preparations

- *Laetec-DT*: 5,25,50,100 mg DT tablets
- *Lamidus*: 25,50,100 mg DT tablets
- *Epitic*: 25,50,100 mg tablets
- *Epitic DT*: 25,50,100 mg DT tablets

Safety during pregnancy and lactation: More studies are required to established safety but lower risk of teratogenicity is observed. Oral clefts are seen recently in 1 to 4% of cases.

No adverse effect seen in infants of lactating mothers, though caution is advised.

FDA Category C.

Levetiracetam

It has high affinity for a synaptic vesicle protein.

Indication: Focal-onset seizure.

Contraindication: Hypersensitivity.

Dosage: 1000 mg orally daily in 2 divided doses. Depending on response 1000 mg per day is added every 2 weeks with a maximum of 3000 mg daily.

Adverse effects: Sedation, fatigue, incoordination, mood changes, anemia, leukopenia. Serious skin reaction like toxic epidermal necrolysis have been reported.

Drug interaction: There is no interaction with following drugs which commonly interact with each other namely phenytoin, phenobarbital, primidone, carbamazepine, valproic acid, lamotrigine, gabapentin, oral contraceptives warfarin and digoxin.

Preparations

- *Keppra*: 250, 500 and 1000 mg tablets. 300 mL syrup containing 100 mg levetiracetam per mL.
- *Levecetam*: 250, 500 mg tablets
- *Levera*: 250, 500 mg tablets. 100 mL syrup containing 100 mg levetircetam per mL.
- *Torleva*: 250, 500, 750 and 1000 mg tablets. 5 mL vial containing 500 mg levetiracetam for injection.

Safety during pregnancy and lactation: Theoretically, bone abnormalities are suspected but no definite evidence is there. Folic acid should be added with screening of the fetus. It has no adverse effect seen in infant.

FDA Category D.

Ethosuximide

It reduces propagation of impulse in brain by inhibiting T type calcium channel blocker.

Indication: It is first choice drug to treat absence seizure (petit mal seizure).

Contraindication: Hypersensitivity to drug, blood dyscrasias.

Dosage: 750–1250 mg/day orally in divided doses.

Adverse effects: Ataxia, lethargy, headache, gastrointestinal irritation, skin rash, bone marrow suppression.

Drug interaction: It interacts with other anti-epileptics phenytoin and valproate.

Preparation

- *Zarontin*: 50 mg/5 mL syrup
- *Ethosuximide*: 250 mg/5 mL syrup.

Safety during pregnancy and lactation: It is safer, regarding teratogenic potential, so should be considered drug of choice for absence seizures.

It is safe for infants who are on breastfeeding.
FDA Category C.
FDA approval is there for petit mal seizure.

Gabapentin

It is an analog of GABA.

Indications: Focal-onset seizure, postherpetic neuralgia , cluster headache.

Contraindications: Liver and kidney dys-functions.

Dosage: 900-2400 mg/day, oral.

Adverse effects: Sedation, dizziness, ataxia, fatigue, gastrointestinal irritation, weight gain, edema.

Drug interaction: It interacts with phenytoin, carbamazepine, sodium valproate.

Preparations

- *Neuropin*: 400 mg capsule
- *Templer*: 400 mg tablet
- *Zepentine*: 400 mg capsule
- *Zintigo*: 400 mg tablet

Safety during pregnancy and breast-feeding: Due to limited human data safety is not established but no definite pattern of birth defect is observed.

Limited data on safety during breastfeeding but safe.

FDA approval for petit mal seizure and neuropathic pain.

Lorazepam

It is a benzodiazepine, has short half-life.

Indications: Anxiety, agitation, insomnia, status epilepticus.

Contraindications: Hypersensitivity to drug, severe respiratory depression, acute narcotic intoxication, ataxia, sleep apnea and myas-thenia gravis.

Dosage: 1 mg orally 2–3 times a day initially, increased gradually to 2–3 times a day.

2 mg or 0.044 mg per kg body weight, whichever is less maybe given initially.

Adverse effects: Sedation, low blood pressure, confusion, ataxia, long-term effect is depressed cognitive function and abnormal memory.

Tolerance and dependence may occur in patients on lorazepam.

Preparation

- *Lorazepam*: 1 mg tablets
- *Ativan*: 1, 2 mg tablets
- *Lopez*: 2 mL injection
- *Loripam SL*: 1, 2 mg sublingual tablets.

Safety during pregnancy and lactation: It is a category D drug, causes fetal cardiac and facial abnormality if given antenatally. It can cause floppy infant syndrome. Regular lorazepam in 3rd trimester carries risk of benzodiazepine withdrawal syndrome in neonates. Lorazepam also causes neonatal jaundice.

It is excreted in milk so it should be used with caution.

Neonate of epileptic mothers should be given vitamin K, 1 mg IM to prevent coagulopathy, just after birth.

FDA Category D.

Treatment of Status Epilepticus (SE)

It is defined as continuous or recurrent seizures lasting more than 30 minutes without full recovery of consciousness in between. It needs prompt medical and ICU management.

Status epilepticus (SE) is usually generalized tonic-clonic seizures and its tonic phase affects the maternal and fetal oxygenation. Metabolic acidosis occurs in clonic phase, therefore, more than 30 minutes SE results in irreversible neuronal injury. SE can cause preterm labor, PROM, abruptio placentae and even IUD. Drugs treatment of SE is given in **Flow chart 24.1**.

PSYCHIATRIC DISEASES

Psychiatric illnesses are quite common in pregnancy due to stressful condition as well as in postpartum stage. Though pregnancy in psychiatric patients has been associated with less prenatal care, substance abuse, poor obstetric and fetal outcomes. There is a high-risk of postpartum psychiatric illness.

Flow chart 24.1: Drug treatment of status epilepticus

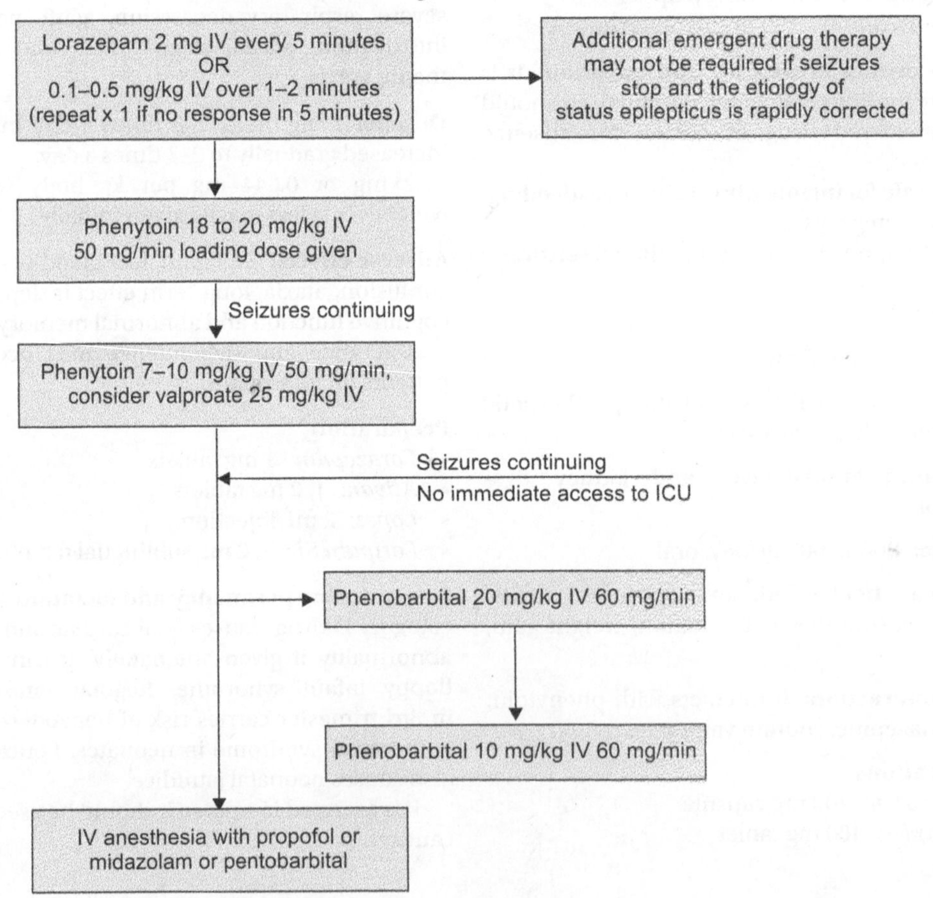

All postpartum mothers should be screened within two weeks of childbirth using Edinburgh postnatal depression scale (EPDS) for any subclinical depression.

Drugs Used in Psychiatric Diseases

Various drugs used in these disorders are given in **Tables 24.3** and **24.4.**

Benzodiazepines[1,3-5]

These are the group of the drugs which increases the effect of neurotransmitter gamma-aminobutyric acid (GABA).

Indications: Anxiety, panic disorder, seizures (status epilepticus), muscle relaxant, alcohol withdrawal symptoms premedication for general anesthesia.

Contraindications: Sensitivity to drug, myasthenia gravis, severe sleep apnea, bronchial asthma, acute respiratory diseases.

Dosage

- *Alprazolam*: 0.25–0.5 mg orally administered 3 times a day.
- *Diazepam*: 2–10 mg orally 2–4 times a day. For control of acute agitation can be given as 0.02–0.08 mg/kg IV over 2–5 minutes. Then maintenance dose: 0.2–0.4 mg/kg/hour by continuous IV infusion.
- *Lorazepam*: 1 mg orally 2–3 times a day initially, increased gradually to 2–3 times a day.
- *Clonazepam*: Started as 0.25 mg orally twice a day, maximum 4 mg per day.

Adverse effects: Drowsiness, dizziness, lightheadedness, fatigue, dry mouth, constipation, dependency, tolerance.

Drug withdrawal symptoms may occur. If taken in high doses, it should be tapered. Withdrawal symptoms are malaise, weakness, insomnia, dizziness, light headedness, tachycardia.

Table 24.3: Psychiatric disorders and their common treatments[1-4]

Psychiatric disorders	*Class of drug(s)*
Major depression, postpartum depression	SSRIs, in severe cases TCAs and MAOIs used
Schizophrenia, postpartum psychosis	Typical antipsychotics, sometimes atypical antipsychotics
Anxiety and panic disorders	Antidepressants (SSRIs are first choice of drug treatment), benzodiazepines
Bipolar disorder	Mood stabilizers

Abbreviations: SSRIs, selective serotonin reuptake inhibitor; TCAs, tricyclic antidepressants; MAOIs, monoamine oxidase inhibitors

Table 24.4: Drugs used in psychiatric disorders[1,4,5]

Class	*Drug(s)*
Benzodiazepines	Clonazepam, alprazolam, chlordiazepoxide, lorazepam, diazepam
Selective serotonin reuptake inhibitors (SSRIs)	Fluoxetine, sertraline, paroxetine, fluvoxamine
Tricyclic antidepressants (TCAs)	Amitriptyline, nortriptyline, imipramine doxepin
Serotonin-norepinephrine reuptake inhibitors	Venlafaxine, duloxetine
Mixed action drugs	Bupropion, amoxapine
MAO inhibitors (MAOIs)	Phenelzine, isocarboxazide
Antipsychotic agents	• *Low potency*: Chlorpromazine, thioridazine • *Mid potency*: Trifluoperazine, loxapine • *High potency*: Haloperidol, thiothixene clozapine, risperidone, olanzapine
Mood stabilizers	Lithium salts, carbmazepine, valproate

Preparations

- Alprazolam preparations
  - Alprax—0.25, 0.5 mg tablets
  - Bioclock—0.25, 0.5 mg tablets
- Diazepam preparations
  - Valium—5,10 mg tablets
  - Alzepam—5,10 mg tablets
- Lorazepam preparations
  - Lorazepam—1 mg tablets
  - Ativan-1, 2 mg tablets
  - Lopez-2 mL injection
- Clonazepam preparations
  - Adnil-0.5 mg tablets
  - Clonapax MD-0.5, 1 mg tablets

Benzodiazepines are given as short-term treatment for initial management (2–4 weeks) or as second-line treatment in treatment for panic disorder. Lorazepam is the first-line treatment for status epilepticus whereas chlordiazepoxide is a better drug for alcohol withdrawal.

Safety during pregnancy and lactation: No teratogenicity is seen but when pregnant woman takes in later half of pregnancy, neonates have abnormal neurobehavior. If exposed in late third trimester, risk of withdrawal symptoms is there in neonates.

Breastfeeding feeding should be with caution, withdrawal symptoms can be there such as irritability, crying, sleep disorder which subsides within two weeks.

Selective Serotonin Reuptake Inhibitors[1-5]

Selective serotonin reuptake inhibitors (SSRIs) are group of drugs which specifically inhibit serotonin uptake, 300–3000 greater selectivity for serotonin than norepinephrine.

Indications of use: Major depression, post-partum depression, obsessive-compulsive disorder (only fluvoxamine is approved for this use), panic disorder, generalized anxiety disorder, social anxiety disorder and Bulimia Nervosa (fluoxetins is approved for this use).

Contraindications: Sensitivity to drug or previous use of MAOIs.

Dosage

Fluoxetine: 20 mg orally once a day, maximum 80 mg daily.

Sertralin: 50 mg orally once a day, maximum 200 mg daily.

Adverse effects: Headache, sweating, anxiety and agitation, nausea, vomiting, diarrhea, weakness and fatigue, sexual dysfunction, sleep disturbances, etc.

Drug interactions: Fluoxetine and paroxetine are potent inhibitors of cytochrome p450, therefore, causes delayed elimination of TCAs, neuroleptic drugs and some antiarrhythmic drugs.

Preparations

Fluoxetine preparations:

- *Prodep:* 10,20,60 mg capsule, 20 mg/5 mL syrup
- *Persona:* 20 mg capsule

Sertraline preparations:

- *Seron:* 25, 50 mg tablets
- *Depser:* 25, 100 mg tablets

Serotonin syndrome: All SSRIs can cause this due to overdose. Symptoms are hyperthermia, muscle rigidity, sweating, myoclonus and changes in mental status.

Drug discontinuation syndrome: Fluoxetine has the lowest risk of causing this syndrome. Symptoms include headache, malaise, flu-like symptoms, nervousness and changes in sleep pattern.

Safety during pregnancy and lactation: No definite evidence of fetal malformation is observed but possible link with heart defect is there. Neonatal withdrawal syndrome is possible. Paroxetine is best avoided in pregnancy as it is associated with VSD in fetus (1 in 200). Echo should be done to rule out persistent pulmonary hypertension in infants, exposed to SSRIs *in utero* after 20 weeks. In third trimester risk of low birth weight, preterm labor is there.

Fluoxetine gets excreted in milk more than other SSRIs, so other drugs from the group should be chosen. Neonatal adverse effects include transient irritability, sleep disturbances and colic.

Tricyclic Antidepressants[1-5]

This group of drugs block norepinephrine and serotonin reuptake into the presynaptic nerve terminals. It is a mood elevator.

Indications of use: Major depression, panic disorder, bed wetting (imipramine <6 years), migraine and chronic pain syndrome (amitriptyline).

Dosage
- *Amitriptyline*: 75 mg orally daily in divided doses maximum 150 mg daily.
- *Imipramine*: 75 mg orally daily in divided doses maximum 150 mg daily.

Adverse effects: Anticholinergic effects like dry mouth, tachycardia, constipation, urinary retention, blurred vision are seen. Patients may have sweating, tremor, postural hypertension, cardiac conduction delay, sedation, weight gain.

TCAs should be given with caution in a known bipolar disorder person, as it may cause a manic episode.

Drug interaction: With alcohol, it can cause toxic sedation. If taken with MAOs inhibitors, patient may have hypertension, hyperpyrexia, convulsions and coma.

Preparations

Amitriptyline
- *Amiline:* 10,25,75 mg tablets
- *Dep:* 10,25,50,75 mg tablets

Imipramine
- *Depsonil:* 25 mg tablets
- *Antidep:* 25, 75 mg tablets

Safety during pregnancy and lactation: Though no teratogenicity is observed but these are used less frequently. Babies should be observed for long-term behavioral abnormality if exposed during breastfeeding.

Serotonin-Norepinephrine Reuptake Inhibitors (Duloxetine)[3-5]

Indications: Major depression, anxiety disorders, urinary incontinence and neuropathic pain.

Contraindications: Hypersensitivity, use of MAOIs, narrow angle glaucoma.

Dosage: 20 mg orally twice daily maximum dose 120 mg daily.

Adverse effects: Nausea, dizziness, dry mouth, headaches, increased blood pressure, anxiety and insomnia; nausea, dizziness, headache, insomnia, constipation, sexual dysfunction.

Discontinuation syndrome: On abrupt stoppage of drug, dysphoric mood, irritability, agitation, dizziness, paresthesia, emotional lability, insomnia and seizure can occur, therefore, gradual reduction of dose is advisable.

Preparations
- *Combac*: 20 mg tablets
- *Dulan*: 20, 30 mg capsules
- *Sympta*: 20, 30, 40, 60 mg tablets

Safety during pregnancy and lactation: No adequate evidence and studies. The effect on infant is unknown, if breastfed, infant should be monitored for drowsiness, motor and social milestones.

FDA Category C.

Mixed Action Drugs-Amoxapine[1,3-5]

Indications: Major depression, schizophrenia.

Contraindications: Hypersensitivity to drug, severe CVS disease, MI, narrow angle glaucoma.

Dosage: 50 mg orally two or three times a day, maximum 600 mg daily.

Adverse effect: Jitteriness, flushing, seizures in at risk parents, increased blood pressure, anorexia, tachycardia, psychosis (effects of bupropion); sexual dysfunction (effect of amoxapine), dry mouth, constipation, sedation.

Drug interactions: When drug is given with MAOIs, it prolongs the QT interval.

Preparations

- *Amolife*: 50, 100 mg tablets
- *Demolox*: 50, 100 mg tablets

Safety during pregnancy and lactation: It is a category C drug, potential risk of teratogenicity and toxicity is there but not seen in limited data. No information available about the safety. Caution is advised.

FDA Category C.

Monoamine Oxidase Inhibitor-Phenelzine

It is a nonselective and irreversible monoamine oxidase inhibitor (MAOI) of the hydrazine class.

Indications: Major depression unresponsive to other treatment, bipolar depression, low psychomotor activity, atypical depression (labile depression), dysthymia, bulimia.

Dosage: 30–90 mg/day.

Adverse effects: Insomnia, hypotension, weight gain, hypertensive crisis, toxic reactions with SSRIs, narcotics.

Drug interaction: May cause serotonin syndrome due to increase serotonin activity.

Preparations: Nardil, Nardelzin—15 mg tablets.

Safety during pregnancy and lactation: Limited data is there but teratogenicity is not seen. Baby can have dizziness, drowsiness, sleep disturbances, tremors, twitchings, hyperreflexia. If baby is symptomatic, breastfeeding should be discontinued. Most babies recover within two weeks.

Chlorpromazine

It is a low potency antipsychotic agent.

It is a dopamine antagonist, typical antipsychotic agent.[1-5]

Indications: Acute and chronic psychosis, schizophrenia, mania, porphyria, severe nausea, vomiting, severe hiccups and rarely for migraine.

Contraindications: Hypersensitivity to the drugs, severe CNS disease, hepatic failure, bone marrow suppression, coma and pheochromocytoma.

Dosage: 10–25 mg orally 3 times a day, maximum 200 mg daily.

Adverse effects: Anticholinergic effects, photosensitivity, cholestasis, QT prolongation, tardive dyskinesia and EPS.

Withdrawal syndrome: These drugs should not be discontinued abruptly to avoid these unpleasant symptoms. So, doses should be reduced gradually.

Drug interaction: Food, alcohol, benzodiazepines and antacids decrease its absorption and lithium, barbiturates and TCAs increase its clearance, so bioavailability of the drug decreases. Ciprofloxacin and fluvoxamine increase adverse effects of the drug due to decreased clearance. It causes increase in CNS depression and respiratory depression when used with benzodiazepines, barbiturates, opioids and lithium.

Preparations

- *Thorazine, largactil*: 25, 100 mg tablets.

Safety during pregnancy and lactation: Teratogenicity is uncommon in women on typical antipsychotics though chlorpromazine may cause extra pyramidal symptoms in neonate of the mother on antipsychotics, it recovers within few weeks.

If low dose single drug therapy is taken then benefit of the breastfeeding outweigh the risk of the drug. FDA category not classified.

Trifluoperazine

It is a mid potency antipsychotic agents.

Indication: Schizophrenia, severe nausea/vomiting, severe anxiety.

Dosage: 2–5 mg twice a day orally, maximum 20 mg a day.

Adverse effects: Fewer anticholinergic side effects, fewer EPSEs than with higher potency; frequent EPSEs with loxapine, neuroleptic malignant syndrome.

Preparations: Espazine 5 mg tablets.

Haloperidol

It is a high potency antipsychotic agents.

Indication: Schizophrenia, acute psychosis, mania, delirium, Tourette syndrome (tics) and others.

Dosage: 0.5 mg orally 2–3 times daily. maximum 3 mg per day.

Adverse effects: No antichlorigenic side effects, EPSEs often prominent; frequent EPSEs with Thiothixene.

Preparations
- *Halodil*: 0.25,0.5,1.5, 10 mg tablets
- *Serenace*: 0.25,0.5,1.5, 10 mg tablets

Safety during pregnancy and breastfeeding considerations are same as in other typical antipsychotics.

It is indicated in severe debilitating psychotic illnesses, so maternal benefit outweighs the fetal risk. Risk of NTD is observed in limited data so folic acid should be added and fetal screening should be done.

In third trimester, maternal intake of drug can cause risk to neonate extra pyramidal symptoms due to drug withdrawal. During breastfeeding caution should be practiced.

FDA Category C.

Clozapine

It is a high potency antipsychotic agents.

Indications: Schizophrenia not responding to other drugs, sometimes bipolar disorder and borderline personality disorder.

Adverse effects: Agranulocytosis (1%), weight gain, seizures, drooling, hypothermia (Clozapine); orthostasis (Risperidone); weight gain (olanzapine), myocarditis, hyperglycemia.

Dosage: Started with 12.5 mg orally once a day, this is gradually increased to twice daily. Then daily increments of up to 25.50 mg per day to a target dose of 300–450 mg per day.

Drug interaction: Carbamazepine decreases plasma levels, however, fluvoxamine, ciprofloxacin increase its plasma level, when used with benzodiazepines, it can cause cardiac and respiratory arrest, even death.

Preparations: 30 pine, Ek 10z. Lo_3 a pin -25,50,100 mg tablets.

Safety during pregnancy and lactation: It is same as with the typical antipsychotic drugs. It is excreted in the human milk in large amounts. If possible, breastfeeding should be avoided in women taking clozapine.

FDA approves it to decrease suicides in schizophrenic patients.

Lithium[1-5]

Lithium compounds are used as mood stabilizing drugs.

Indications: Bipolar disorder, particularly acute condition. More effective in mania.

Contraindication: Pregnancy, lactation, chronic heart failure, kidney disease, severe infections psoriasis.

Dosage: 300 to 600 mg orally 3 times a day, maximum 1800 to 2400 mg a day.

Adverse effects: Leukocytosis, polyuria, polydipsia, nausea, vomiting, headache, EPS side effects, euthyroid goiter, hypothyroidism.

Drug interactions: Its bioavailability increases with loop diuretics, NSAID, ACE inhibitors.

Preparations
- *Lithium*: 300, 400 mg tablets.
- *Alkalith CR*: 450 mg tablets.

Safety during pregnancy and lactation: Lithium is a category D drug associated with multiple fetal anomalies. It should only be given in pregnancy when there are no alternatives as Lithium Baby syndrome is a well-known entity.

Lithium toxicity in neonate of mothers on lithium, includes cyanosis, ECG changes, hypotonia. Lithium is excreted and accumulated in the human milk. It is better to avoid.

Majority of above drugs are pregnancy category C and D, but all are used in pregnancy and lactation in the wake of the severity of the diseases and their consequences. Pregnant mothers and their relatives should be counseled and informed regarding this and minimum therapeutic doses should be prescribed.

REFERENCES

1. Cunningham, Lenovo, Bloom, Spong, Dashe, Hoffman, Casey, Sheffield. Williams Obstetrics, 24th edition. USA, McGrawHill, 2014;246-247, 250-251, 1187-1212
2. James DK, Steer PJ, Weiner CP, et al. High Risk Pregnancy Management, 4th edition, Indian edition, Elsevier, 2011; 584-586, 861-891, 997-1009.
3. Briggs GG, Freeman RK. Drugs in Pregnancy and Lactation, 10th edition.
4. Longo, Fauci, Kasper, Hauser, Jameson, Loscalzo. Harrison Principles. Internal Medicine, 18th edition.
5. Whalen K, Finkel R, Panavelil TA. Lippincott Pharmacology, 5th Edition.
6. Reza Nakhai - Pour MD PhD, Hamid. "Use of nonaspirin nonsteroidal anti-inflammatory drugs during pregnancy and the risk of spontaneous abortion." Canadian Medical Association Journal. Retreived 7 September 2011.
7. Soldin OP, Dahlin J, O'Mara DM. Triptans in pregnancy. The Drug Monit 2008;30. Pages 5-9.
8. Holmes LB, Hernandez-Diaz S. Newer anticonvulsants: lamotrigine, topiramate and Gabapentin. Birth Defects Res A Clin Mol Teratol 2006;76:318.

Section VI

FAMILY PLANNING DRUGS

CHAPTERS

CHAPTER 25

Medical Termination of Pregnancy

Rachna Sharma, Ojaswini Sharma

INTRODUCTION

Drugs Used in Medical Abortion

The common drugs used in first and second trimester medical termination of pregnancy (MTP) by medical method is mifepristone and misoprostol. Use of prostaglandin F2 alpha has declined and taken over by mifepristone and misoprostol. For second trimester termination of pregnancy, use of ethacridine lactate is still the safest method **(Table 25.1)**.

Table 25.1 Drugs used in termination of first and second trimester termination of pregnancy

Medical termination of preganancy	*Drugs*
First trimester termination	Mifepristone and misoprostol combination
	Misoprostol alone
Second trimester termination	Ethacridine lactate
	Mifepristone and misoprostol combination
	Misoprostol alone
	Intramuscular prostaglandin F2 alpha
	Concentrated oxytocin infusion

For second trimester medical abortion prostaglandin F2 alpha had been used by intra-amniotic and extra-amniotic instillation. Hyperosmolar urea had been used by amnioinfusion. However, we do not use them as these procedures are invasive and more effective and safer methods are available. We will not describe them in this chapter.

Mifepristone and Misoprostol for Medical Termination of Pregnancy

Combination of mifepristone and misoprostol has been in use since 2000. It has been very effective in medical abortion and since then there have been several studies which have tried different regimen at different gestations. **Table 25.2** summarizes the salient features of these two important medicines.

Indications of use: The combination of two drugs is used for termination of first and second trimester termination of pregnancy.

- The combination is approved for medical abortion only up to 63 days of gestation by government of India, WHO (2012), RCOG (2011). Its use in pregnancy more than 63 days is an off label use based on the available clinical evidences.
- Medical abortion at 9–12 weeks of pregnancy.
- Medical abortion over 12 weeks of pregnancy.

Table 25.2 Salient features of mifepristone and misoprostol

Drug	*Mifepristone (RU-486)*	*Misoprostol*
Properties	Mifepristone is a synthetic steroidal anti-progestogen and antiglucocorticoid drug.	It is a synthetic prostaglandin E1 compound.
Mechanism of action	Blocks progesterone receptors resulting in endometrial decidual degeneration, this leads to detachment of trophoblast and decreased syncytiotrophoblast production of hCG. This in turn causes decreased synthesis of progesterone from corpus luteum. This decrease in progesterone causes cervical softening and dilatation, release of prostaglandins and increase in myometrium sensitivity to prostaglandins.	It binds to myometrial cells causing strong uterine contraction, cervical softening and dilatation which leads to expulsion of conceptus from the uterus.
Contraindications	• Allergy to compounds of mifepristone and misoprostol • Patient on anticoagulants, e.g. warfarin, heparin or corticosteroids • Presence of intrauterine device (IUD) • Ectopic pregnancy • Adrenal gland problems—chronic adrenal failure or Addison disease • Bleeding disorders, e.g. porphyria • Undiagnosed abdominal mass • Unable to come for follow-up as prescribed by the doctor or in case of emergency.	
Adverse effects	Nausea, vomiting, diarrhea, backache, uterine cramps, dizziness, joint pain, fever with chills, etc.	Nausea, headache and dizziness, abdominal pain, gastrointestinal side effects, vomiting, heavy bleeding per vagina.
Drug interactions	Interaction of various drugs may increase the risk of side effects including excessive bleeding. In some cases, other drugs may reduce the effectiveness of mifepristone. These drugs are: • Anticoagulants, e.g. warfarin or corticosteroids, e.g. hydrocortisone • Azole antifungals, e.g. ketoconazole • Certain anticonvulsants, e.g. carbamazepine, phenobarbital • Antitubercular drugs • Antithyroid drugs	Some medicines may interact with misoprostol. However, no specific interactions are known.

Dosage: Mifepristone and misoprostol are given in combination for medical abortion. The regimen varies with the period of gestation; these are given in **Table 25.3.**[1-3]

If mifepristone is not available misoprostol alone is also effective, misoprostol alone regimens are given in **Table 25.4**.

Misoprostol can be used in treatment of incomplete abortion at less than 13 weeks of gestation. The regimen for the same is given in **Table 25.5**.

Monitoring: Clinical examination is performed. Ultrasonography should be performed if exact period of amenorrhea is not known or ectopic pregnancy needs to be ruled out.

Hemoglobin should be checked to rule out anemia.

Patient is observed for 3–4 hours after administration of misoprostol for any excessive bleeding. Expulsion of products of conception occurs in 95% of the patients. The patient returns back on day 10–14 to confirm if abortion

Table 25.3 Mifepristone and misoprostol combination regimens for medical abortion

Gestational age	*Dosage*	
	Mifepristone	*Misoprostol*
Up to 9 weeks (63 days)	200 mg orally	24–48 later, 800 mcg intravaginally or sublingually. It can be taken orally as 400 mcg if gestation is less than 7 weeks
Between 9 and12 weeks	200 mg orally	36–48 later, 800 mcg inserted vaginally then 400 mcg vaginally or orally 3 hourly for maximum of 5 doses of misoprostol can be given*
Between 12 and 20 weeks	200 mg orally	36–48 later, 800 mcg inserted vaginally then 400 mcg vaginally or orally 3 hourly for maximum of 5 doses of misoprostol can be given*

*These regimens need to be given under observation in a health care facility.

Table 25.4 Misoprostol alone regimens for medical abortion*

Gestational age	*Dosage of misoprostol*
Up to 9–12 weeks	800 mcg vaginally or SL, followed repeat dose of 800 mcg at 3–12 hours interval, maximum 3 doses can be given
Between 12 and 20 weeks	400 mcg vaginally or SL, every 3 hourly, up to maximum of 5 doses

*These regimens need to be given under observation in a health care facility.

is complete and if it is not, surgical evacuation is done for completion of abortion.

Preparations: Combination of mifepristone and misoprostol.

- Combipack (1+4) approved by Government of India for MTP up to 63 days, contains 1 tablet 200 mg mifepristone and 4 tablets of 200 mcg mifepristone.
- I-pill, Pregwin kit, Pregnokit, MTP kit, Mifekit—all preparations contain 200 mg mifepristone tablet and misoprostol 200 mcg, 4 vaginal tablets.

Mifepristone preparations.

- Abo pill tab, Mifeprin tab, Termipril tab, MT pill tab-200 mg tablet.

Misoprostol preparations.

- *Zitotec*: 100, 200 mcg tablets

Table 25.5 Misoprostol for treatment of incomplete abortion at < 13 weeks of gestation

Dose of misoprostol	*Route of administration*
600 mcg	Orally
400 mcg	Sublingually

- *Prestakind*: 200 mcg tablets
- *Misoprost*: 25, 100, 200, 600 mcg tablets
- *Cytolog*: 25, 200 mcg tablets.

Safety during pregnancy and lactation: If pregnancy continues due to failure, surgical abortion is required because of potential for teratogenicity.

Ethacridine Lactate

Extra-amniotic instillation of ethacridine lactate had been used for second trimester termination of pregnancy for decades. Its use dates way back in 1940s. However, it has been studied only after 1969. It has been recognized as a safe, effective and cheap method of second trimester termination. It can even be used in patients with cesarean section, the cases in which use of prostaglandins is contraindicated, though it has to be used with caution. It has been found to be successful in up to 80–95% in various studies.[4–8]

Pharmacology: It is acridine derivative and also has antibacterial activity. It has been even used as an antiseptic solution. Though it is effective but, its mechanism of action is still not clear. It is proposed that its presence in extra-amniotic space brings about separation of placenta and membranes which causes secretion of prostaglandins. Presence of intracervical catheter itself has mechanical action and stimulates prostaglandin secretion. It also has been found to have oxytocic properties. 0.1% solution is found to be safe even if it is injected intravenously, therefore its intravasation from extra-amniotic space is safe.

Indications of use: Second trimester medical abortion.

Contraindications: Hypersensitivity, pregnancy.

Dosage and procedure of instillation: In primigravida no 14 Foley's catheter and in multigravida no 16 Foley's catheter is used. It is inserted through the cervix and the tip is inserted beyond internal os in the extra-amniotic space. The bulb is inflated with 5–10 cc of normal saline. Now 0.1% solution of ethacridine lactate is instilled through catheter slowly. Total volume of drug is calculated as 10 mL per gestational week up to maximum of 200 mL.

The Foley's catheter can be left *in situ* for 12–24 hours, can be removed early if contractions start. After 24 hours, the catheter is removed and oxytocin infusion can be started.

Adverse drug reactions: Hypersensitivity. Rarely cause uterine rupture, cervical injuries, coagulation defects, bone marrow depression.

Drug interactions: Activity is enhanced by alkaline solutions.

Monitoring: Coagulation profile, CBC, KFT and LFT should be monitored. Patient's vital monitoring should be done during the procedure. After abortion, the cervical exploration should be done to rule out any cervical injury.

Preparations: Emecredil, Aborcin, Abortil injection—available in 50 mL bottles containing 1 mg ethacridine lactate per mL.

Vecredil injections—available in 100 mL bottles containing 1 mg ethacridine lactate per mL.

Safety during pregnancy: Contraindicated.

Prostaglandin F2 Alpha

This is not a popular method of second trimester medical abortion because safer methods (ethacridine lactate) are available and due to its side effects.

It is used in failed second trimester abortion with conventional methods (ethacridine lactate and oxytocin). IM injection of 250 mcg, repeated every 2–4 hours. Maximum dose of 2500 mcg can be given (10 injections).[9]

Concentrated Oxytocin Infusion

This method of second trimester medical abortion requires high doses of oxytocin because uterus is comparatively very less sensitive to oxytocin before 20 weeks of gestation. The induction to delivery interval is also high. Therefore, this is also not a popular method of medical abortion.

50 IU of oxytocin in 500 mL of normal saline or 5% dextrose is given over 3 hours. This is followed by 1 hour rest. Then 100 IU of oxytocin in 500 mL of NS is given over 3 hours and then 1 hour of rest. Like this escalating dose of oxytocin given with 3 hour of oxytocin infusion and 1 hour of rest till oxytocin concentration of 300 IU is reached.

REFERENCES

1. WHO safe abortion guidance: Updates and recommendations. *URL file:///C:/Users/LENOVO/Downloads/WHOUPDE13.pdf* accessed on 20th Septmber 2015.
2. Induced Abortion Guidelines. SOGC clinical practice guidelines. No 184, November 2006.
3. Grossman D. Medical methods for first trimester abortion. RHL practical aspects by. WHO reproductive health library. *http://apps.who.int/rhl/fertility/abortion/dgguide/en/*accessed on 20th September 2015.

4. Zhuang Y, Chen X, Huang L. Mifepristone may shorten the induction-to-abortion time for termination of second-trimester pregnancies by ethacridine lactate. Contraception. 2012; 85(2):211-4.
5. Berg C, Ludwig M, Sturm N, Diedrich K, Gembruch U, Geipel A. Intraamniotic ethacridine lactate instillation versus vaginal PGE1 in second trimester termination of pregnancy. Eur J Obstet Gynecol Reprod Biol. 2006;126(2):193-6.
6. Purandare VN, Mhatre V, Krishna UR, Gogate SG, Gupta KC, Sheth UK, Khatu A. The place of ethacridine lactate for mid-trimester MTP (Multicentric study). J Postgrad Med. 1977;23(2):77-83.
7. Bhathena RK, Sheriar NK, Walvekar VR, Guillebaud J. Second trimester pregnancy termination using extra-amniotic ethacridine lactate. Br J Obstet Gynecol. 1990;97(11): 1026-9.
8. Lewis BV, Pybus A, Stilwell JH. The oxytocic effect of acridine dyes and their use in terminating mid-trimester pregnancies. J Obstet Gynecol Br Common. 1971;78(9):838-42.
9. Slaughter L, Ballard CA. Midtrimester abortion with intramuscular injection of 15-methyl-prostaglandin F2 alpha. Contraception. 1975; 11(5):533-40.

CHAPTER 26

Newer Contraceptive Drugs

Chandan Dubey, Reena Rani

INTRODUCTION

Contraceptive drugs are among the most frequently prescribed agents in clinical practice. With the changing needs of society, these drugs have witnessed tremendous advances. In this chapter we would be discussing the newer contraceptive drugs **(Table 26.1)**.

Table 26.1: Newer contraceptive drugs

Class	*Drug(s)*
New oral contraceptive pills	Low-dose combined oral contraceptives
	Drospirenone containing COCs*
	Continuous or extended COCs*
	Newer progestogen-only pills
Contraceptive patch	Ortho Evra
	Newer low-dose patch (Twirla)
Injections	Combined: Lunelle and Mesigyna
	Progesterone-only-Depot medroxy progesterone acetate (DMPA)-Norethisterone enanthate
Implants	Nonbiodegradable • Norplant • Jadelle • Implanon • Sino-implant • Uniplant • ST-1435 Biodegradable • Capronor • Annuelle
Contraceptive vaginal ring	NuvaRing
	Nestorone/Ethinyl estradiol (NES/EE) (under trial)
	Levonorgestrel ring (Varlevo 20 /sialistic 382) (under trial)
Newer intrauterine contraceptive device	Skyla GyneFix

*COCs—combined oral contraceptives

New Oral Contraceptive Pills

Latest developments in combined oral contraception are use of low-dose of estradiol, use of newer progesterones, and development of continuous oral contraceptive pills (OCPs).

Low-dose Combined Oral Contraceptives

Low-dose combined oral contraceptives (COCs) consist of 20–35 micrograms of ethinylestradiol (EE). Because they have low estrogenic side effects with comparable contraceptive efficacy hence are preferred over conventional COCs.[1]

Preparations

- Novelon—30 mcg EE and 0.15 mg desogestrel
- Femilon, Elogen—20 mcg EE and 0.15 mg desogestrel
- Loette—20 mcg EE and 0.10 mg levonorgesterel.

Combined Oral Contraceptives Containing Newer Progestogens: Drospirenone Containing COCs

These COCs contain newer progestogens such as desogestrel, gestodene, norgestimate and most recent drospirenone.

Drospirenone is a derivative of spironolactone. Unlike most other progestogens, it has antiandrogenic properties and antimineralocorticoid activity **(Fig. 26.1)**.[2]

Pharmacology: Drospirenone is an analog of the aldosterone antagonist, spironolactone, and the dose of drospirenone in COCs currently marketed has properties similar to 25 mg of this diuretic. Oral absorption is rapid and almost complete. Peak serum concentration reached in around 1–2 hours of ingestion. Bioavailability is 76–85%. In blood it binds to serum albumin and not with sex hormone binding globulin. Its metabolites are excreted in biliary and urinary system in ratio of about 1.2–1.4. It acts mainly by inhibition of ovulation.

Indications: Drospirenone containing COCs have following advantages over conventional contraceptives:

- Good contraceptive efficacy
- Decreases seborrhea, acne and hirsutism
- Low fluid retention related side effects such as weight gain, bloating, increase in BP, breast tenderness, and mood changes
- Improvement in lipid profile.

Therefore it is a preferred contraceptive in women with acne, hirsutism and hypertension.

Contraindication: Pregnancy, renal or adrenal insufficiency and hepatic dysfunction.

Dosage: One pill is taken every day for 21 days followed by one week off.

Adverse effect: It causes potassium retention leading to hyperkalemia.

Monitoring: Serum potassium level is recommended in the first month for patients chronically treated concomitantly with any drug associated with potassium retention, e.g. nonsteroidal anti-inflammatory drugs (NSAIDs), angiotensin II antagonists, aldosterone antagonists, angiotensin-converting enzyme (ACE) inhibitors, heparin and potassium-sparing diuretics.

Preparations: Yasmin and Dronis 30-contain ethinylestradiol 30 mcg and drospirenone 3 mg.

Safety during pregnancy and lactation: Category X drug in pregnancy. Therefore it is contraindicated during pregnancy. Drospirenone-ethinyl estradiol should be avoided during lactation as it is secreted (0.02%) in breast milk. Infants exposed to steroid contraceptives have been reported to develop jaundice and breast enlargement.

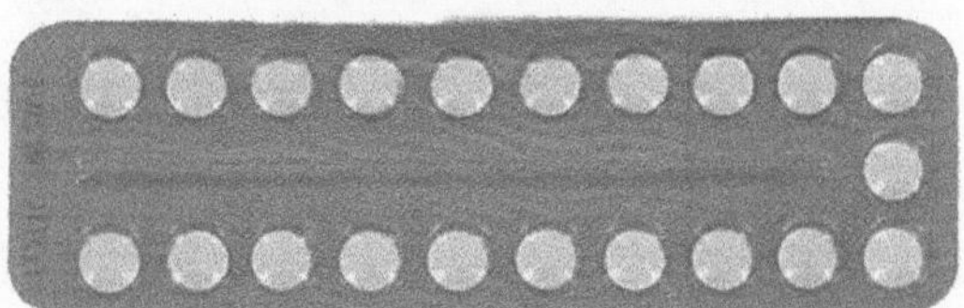

Fig. 26.1: Drospirenone containing combined oral contraceptives

Continuous or Extended COCs

Longer duration of active hormone is designed to minimize the number of withdrawal episodes.[3] A 13-week cycle is designed, that is 12 weeks of hormone use, followed by a week off for withdrawal menses. Mechanism of action is same as with other combined oral contraceptive pills **(Table 26.2)**.

Indications: Especially useful in conditions when minimal menstruations are required, e.g. in menorrhagia, dysmenorrhea and endometriosis.

Contraindication: Pregnancy, smoking and age over 35 years, breast or uterine cancer, uncontrolled hypertension, heart disease, a blood-clotting disorder, diabetes mellitus with nephropathy or retinopathy, abnormal uterine bleeding, acute or chronic liver disease, severe migraine headaches, jaundice, stroke and current embolism.

Side effects: Abnormal uterine bleeding and/or spotting, which generally resolves with persistent use. Nausea, vomiting, headaches, bloating or swelling, and breast tenderness.

Preparations and dosage

Interaction: They are less effective in preventing pregnancy when taken with drugs including antibiotics, hepatitis C medications, HIV/AIDS medications, seizure medications, or barbiturate sedatives.

Safety during pregnancy and lactation: Not to be used in pregnancy and should be avoided in lactation.

Newer Progestin-only Contraceptives: Desogestrel-only Mini-pill

The latest progestogen only pill contains new progestin desogestrel.

Pharmacology: It contains desogestrel 75 microgram (third generation progesterone). It acts via ovulation inhibition in 97% of users as compared to traditional POPs which inhibit ovulation only in 20–30% users.[4]

Indication: Lactating women, women over 40 years and those in whom estrogen is contraindicated.

Contraindication

- Absolute (Medical Eligibility Criteria 2009—Category 4)
  - Pregnancy
  - Breast cancer within 5 years
  - Unexplained vaginal bleeding
- Relative (Medical Eligibility Criteria 2009—Category 3)
  - Current deep vein thrombosis or pulmonary embolism
  - Acute liver disease/liver tumor
  - History of breast cancer with no evidence of disease in past 5 years
  - Breastfeeding and less than 4 week partum
  - Use of rifampicin or anticonvulsants such as phenytoin, carbamazepine, barbiturates.

Dosage and Regimen: It is taken continuously with no pill-free interval. Each pill contains 75 mcg of desogestrel. Following regimen should be followed:

Table 26.2: Composition of the available continuous COCs

Trade name	*Composition*		*Duration for which pill is taken*
	Ethinylestradiol (mcg)	*Levonorgesterel (mg)*	
Seasonale	30	0.15	12 weeks of active pill and 1 week of inert pill
Seasonique	30	0.15	12 weeks of active pill followed by 1 week of 10 mcg ethinylestradiol pill only instead of inert pills
Lybrel	20	0.09	One pill every day for 365 days

- Started on D1-D5 of cycle
- If started later then backup contraception is needed for 2 days and pregnancy should be ruled out.
- Can be started on D1-D7 after a first or second trimester abortion
- Has safety margin of 12 hours as compared to 3 hrs of traditional POPs
- If a pill is missed for more than 12 hours then user should take it as early as possible and continue taking pills as usual.

Side effects: Menstrual irregularity, acne, mastalgia, headache, nausea and mood changes.

Preparations: Cerazette-contains 75 mcg of desogestrel. It is the only mini-pill available in India.

Mini-pills Containing Other Progestine

These are described in **Table 26.3**. However none of these preparations are available in India.

Contraceptive Patch

Ortho Evra

Contraceptive patch consists of a 20 cm square three-layer system which is to be applied on the upper arm, buttocks, torso or on abdomen to release ethinylestradiol and a progestogen norelgestromin, (17-deacetyl-norgestimate) transdermally. Its contraceptive action comes via ovulation inhibition **(Fig. 26.2)**.[5]

Pharmacology: Transdermal application of a contraceptive patch provides a number of benefits compared to the oral route such as elimination of the variability in gastrointestinal absorption, avoidance of the hepatic first-pass metabolism, and loss of peaks and troughs in serum concentrations.

Indications: It is prescribed for contraception in those who are not willing to use daily oral COCs tablet.

Contraindications: These are same as COC's. (Medical Eligibility Criteria 2009).

Dosage: A new patch is started from the first day of the menstrual cycle. A new patch is applied every week for 3 weeks followed by one week off. Menstruation should happen in patch-free week. After abortion or miscarriage, if it happens before 20 weeks' gestation, the patch should be started immediately with no back-up contraceptive. If patch get detached for less than 24 hours, reapplication should be done and in cases of more than 24 hours patch detachment it should be reapplied and a back-up contraceptive is used for next 7 days.

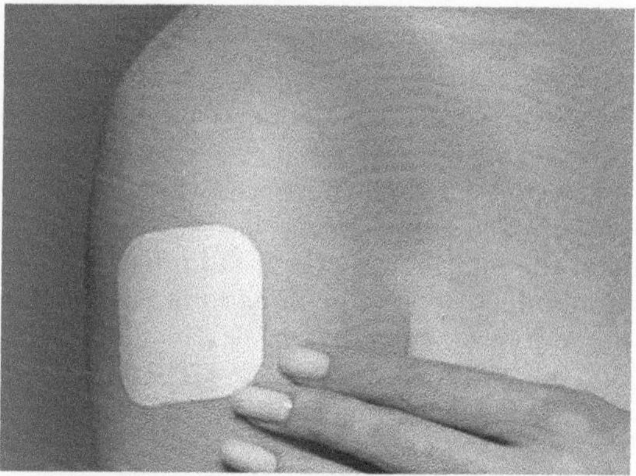

Fig. 26.2: Contraceptive patch

Table 26.3: Mini-pills containing progestines other than desogestrel

Progestin	*Concentration (mg)*	*Brand*
Norethindrone	0.350	Micronor, Noriday
Levonorgestrel	0.075	Neogest
Norgestrel	0.030	Microval, Norgeston
Ethynodiol diacetate	0.500	Femulen

Failure rates: 0.5% HWY (per hundred women years).

Adverse effects: Transient breast tenderness and skin site reactions may occur. There may be decrease in contraceptive effectiveness of the patch in women weighing 90 kg or more.

Preparations

- *Ortho Evra*: It consists of 6 mg of norelgestromin and 0.75 mg of ethinylestradiol and releases 150 mcg of norelgestromin and 20 mcg of ethinylestradiol into the blood per day.

Newer Low-dose Patch

Twirla: Newer low-dose patch and releases 100 mcg of levonorgestrel and 30 mcg of ethinyl estradiol daily. At present it is under phase III clinical trial.

Injections

Combined Injections

Pharmacology: Combined injectable contraceptives contain short-acting estradiol esters, e.g. cypionate or valerate which produce elevated estradiol serum levels within 15 days, followed by a rapid decrease which leads to an estrogen withdrawal bleeding 2–3 weeks after the injection. However the progestational component is found in blood in the detectable amount throughout the cycle. Ovulation inhibition remains for around 30 days. They are given as intramuscular injection of oily solution.[6] **(Table 26.4)**

Indications: Combined injectables are especially effective for couples who are willing to take monthly injections and who want:

- To avoid a method which requires daily use or use every time during act of intercourse
- An effective contraceptive method.

Contraindications

- Known or suspected pregnancy
- Abnormal genital tract bleeding
- Suspected malignancy of the breast
- Active thromboembolic disease
- Acute liver disease such as viral hepatitis.

Dosage and regimen: One injection is to be given every 4 weekly, not more than 33 days. Injection is given deep IM either on buttock, deltoid on anterior thigh. The injection can be given at the following times:

- D1- 5 days of menstrual cycle
- Postabortion immediately
- Breastfeeding woman—after 6 months postpartum.

Side effects: Irregular bleeding, amenorrhea, heavy or prolonged bleeding, body weight changes, headache and dizziness.

Preparations: The preparations available are described in **Table 26.4**.

Advantages over others

- Single injection is highly effective contraception for one month.
- *Failure rate*: 0.2–0.4% per hundred women year.

Progesterone-only Injections

Two types of progesterone only injections are available:

1. Depot medroxyprogesterone acetate (DMPA)
2. Norethisterone enanthate (NET-EN).

They are administered by intramuscular injection and are effective and safe long-acting reversible method of contraception.

Pharmacology: After a single intramuscular dose of DMPA, progesterone concentrations increase for first 3 weeks to reach to peak plasma concentrations of 1–7 ng/mL followed by an exponential decrease until they become undetectable (less than 100 pg/mL) between 6–7 months following injection. The half-life for medroxyprogesterone acetate following IM administration is approximately 50 days.[7]

It causes suppression of ovulation, endometrial atrophy and thickens the cervical mucus. Return of fertility takes 6–12 months of discontinuation.

Table 26.4: Combined injectable contraceptives

Trade	Estrogen	Progestogen
Lunelle	5 mg estradiol cypionate	25 mg medroxy progesterone acetate
Mesigyna	5 mg estradiol valerate	50 mg norethisterone enanthate
Cyclofem	5 mg estradiol cypionate	25 mg medroxyprogesterone acetate
Deladroxate	10 mg estradiol enanthate	150 mg dihydroxy-progesterone acetophenide

Indications: They are recommended in women who are breastfeeding and do not want to take daily pills.

Contraindications: According to WHO medical eligibility criteria, they are contraindicated in following conditions:

Catgeogories

Category 1: 18–45 years, heavy smokers, breastfeeding after six weeks postpartum, thyroid disorders, severe dysmenorrhea, uterine fibroids, STIs/PID, use of rifampicin or rifabutin, anticonvulsants, or any type of antiretroviral drugs.

Category 2: <18 or >45 years, adequately controlled hypertension, uncomplicated diabetes, gallbladder disease.

Category 3: Breastfeeding before 6 weeks postpartum, severe hypertension (≥160/≥100), vascular disease, acute deep vein thrombosis or pulmonary embolism, current or history of ischemic heart disease or stroke, complicated diabetes, severe liver disease and most liver tumors.

Category 4: Current breast cancer

Dosages and regimen

- DMPA-150 mg given by deep intramuscular injection in gluteal or deltoid region every 12 weekly. It can be given two weeks before or up to two weeks after three months.
- NET-EN—200 mg given as deep intramuscular injection every 8 weekly.

They can be given:

- On day 1–5 of menstrual cycle
- After 6 postpartum weeks if woman is breast feeding, additional contraceptive should be used for 7 days
- Immediately or within 7 days of abortion.

Reinjection should be done within 14 weeks in case of DMPA and if more than 14 weeks have passed back-up contraception should be used for 7 days.

Adverse effects: Irregular bleeding, amenorrhea on prolonged use (50% users experience it after one year and 80% after 2 years), osteoporosis, weight gain, headache, etc.

Preparation

- DMPA preparations are Depo-Provera, Depo Progestin, Khushi, Paree, etc.
- NET-EN preparations are Norigest, Norlutin enanthate, Nur-Isterate, etc.

Implants

There are nonbiodegradable and biodegradable implants. These are progesterone only implants.

Nonbiodegradable Implants: Implanon

The advantage associated with progesterone only nonbiodegradable implants is that they can be removed any time when required without difficulty. The pharmacological features of nonbiodegradable implants are summarized in **Table 26.5**.

Implanon is a long-acting reversible progesterone-only contraceptive consisting of a single-rod (length 40 mm and diameter 2 mm). It is made up of an ethylene vinyl acetate copolymer with a core containing 68 mg of etonogestrel (3-ketodesogestrel). The release

Table 26.5: Pharmacological features of different nonbiodegradable implants

Parameter/ brand	*Norplant*	*Jadelle*	*Implanon*	*ST-1435*	*Uniplant*
Progesterone	Levonorgestrel	Levonorgestrel	Etonogestrel	Nestorone	Nomegestrol acetate
No of rod (dose per rod)	6 (36 mg)	2 (70 mg)	1 (68 mg)	1	1 (55 mg)
Release of progesterone	50–80 mcg per day	70 mcg per day	30 mcg per day	100 mcg per day	150 mcg per day
Effective for	5 years	5 years	3 years	6 months	1 year
Polymer	Silicone	Silicone	Ethylene vinyl acetate	Silicone	Silicone
Pearl index	1.1	1.1	0.01	0	0.9

rate is 60–70 mcg per day initially and decreases to approximately 25–30 mcg per day at the end of the third year. Its contraceptive effectiveness lasts for 3 years.

Pharmacology: After subdermal injection etonogestrel (ENG) is approximately 100% bioavailable. ENG is around 32% bound to sex hormone binding globulin (SHBG) and 66% bound to albumin in blood. It is metabolized in liver microsomes by the cytochrome P450 3A4 isoenzyme. Its elimination half-life is approximately 25 hours. ENG and its metabolites are mainly excreted in urine and to a lesser extent in feces. Serum levels are maintained relatively stable through 36 months. Effect starts within 24 hours of insertion and back-up contraception is required for first day after insertion.

It acts by following mechanism:[8]
- Cervical mucus thickening
- Ovulation inhibition
- Endometrial changes unfavorable for implantation
- Endocrinal dysfunction preventing oocyte fertilization.

Timing of insertion
- *Regular menstruating woman*: Day 1-5 of the menstrual cycle without the need for additional contraceptive protection.
- *Amenorrheic woman*: At any time with 7 days of additional contraception after ruling out pregnancy.
- *Postpartum woman*: On or after day 21 with 7 days of additional contraception.

Insertion technique[9]: The average time for insertion is 0.5 to 1 minute. The cleaning and draping of upper arm is done and a local anesthetic is applied around the insertion area. A needle-like applicator is used to insert the rod under the skin into the subdermal tissue on the inner side of the arm between the biceps and triceps muscles in the nondominant arm 6–8 cm above elbow. This is followed by application of bandage on the insertion site for 24 hours. Bruising and mild discomfort are common after insertion.

Removal technique: By pop-out method. Implant is palpated and local anesthetic is injected under the implant. A 2 mm incision is given at caudal end and implant is pushed towards the incision.

Effectiveness: It is shown to be the most effective form of birth control available. The failure rate of Implanon is 0.01–0.05% per hundred women years.

Contraindications
- Pregnancy
- Allergy to etonogestrel
- History of breast cancer
- Unexplained vaginal bleeding
- Ffirst 6 weeks postpartum in breastfeeding women
- Severe liver disease.

Adverse effects: Menstrual irregularity, weight gain, mastalgia, headache and mood changes. Minor side effects such as bruising, skin irritation, or pain around the insertion site are common.

Preparation

Nexplanon and Implanon NXT.

Safety in pregnancy: It is not indicated for use during pregnancy. If a pregnancy does occur Implanon should be removed. However, there is no evidence to suggest that the implant has a negative effect on a developing fetus.

Advantages

- Works for up to 3 years
- Most effective form of birth control. Failure rate is 0.05% (1/2,000 women) for both perfect use and typical use.
- No estrogenic side effects
- Quick action after insertion
- No necessary actions prior to intercourse for contraception
- Quick return of fertility after removal.

Biodegradable Implants

Biodegradable implants need not to be removed. They are easier to insert.

Capronor (under trial)

- It consists of polycaprolactone capsule which contains levonorgestrel 21.6 mg
- 4 cm rod is promising development
- Advantage include no need for removal
- Quick return of fertility.

Hormonal microcapsules (under trial): They include norethindrone microcapsules and LNG-PLGA (Levonorgestrel in Poly lactic glycolic acid) microcapsules.

Contraceptive Vaginal Ring

NuvaRing

The vaginal contraceptive ring is made up of ethinyl vinyl acetate measuring 54 mm in diameter and 4 mm in cross-section. It contains 2.7 mg of ethinyl estradiol and 11.7 mg of etonogestrel. It releases on average 0.120 mg of etonogestrel and 15 mcg of ethinyl estradiol per day **(Fig. 26.3).**[10]

Pharmacology: After the insertion of NuvaRing, maximum serum concentrations of etonogestrel is achieved in approximately 1 week. The absorption bypasses first pass metabolism. Hence it is associated with low hormonal side effects with similar efficacy. Effect remains after 2 weeks of the recommended interval of 3 weeks.

Its contraceptive effect is achieved through ovulation inhibition.

Contraindication: Same as of COC's (Medical Eligibility Criteria 2009).

Dosage: It is inserted in vagina on first day of menstruation for 3 weeks and removed for 1 week. It can be removed during intercourse but not for more than 3 hours.

Adverse effect: Vaginitis, leucorrhea, unrecognized expulsion, etc.

Failure rates: After perfect use 0.03%.

Vaginal Rings Under Trial

- Nestorone/Ethinyl Estradiol (NES/EE) 1-year contraceptive vaginal ring (releases 150 mcg nestorone and 15 mcg ethinyl estradiol per day.) The ring is left in place for 3-week and removed for one week. Each ring is good for up to 13 cycles (one full year). It is under phase III clinical trial.
- Levonorgestrel ring (Varlevo-20/sialistic 382).

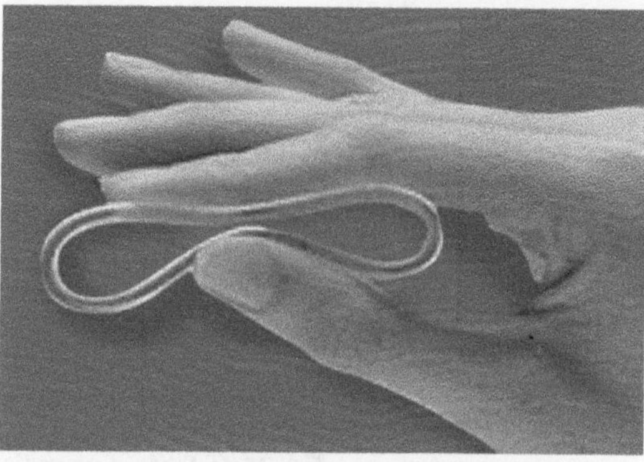

Fig. 26.3: NuvaRing

Newer Intrauterine Contraceptive Device

Skyla and GyneFix are two new intrauterine devices which have benefits over older IUCDs.

Skyla

It is a newer progestin-containing intrauterine device (IUD) which consists of a T-shaped polyethylene frame with a steroid reservoir having 13.5 mg levonorgestrel packaged within a sterile inserter. levonorgestrel (LNG) is released at rate of 14 mcg per day after 24 days and declines to 5 mcg per day after 3 years **(Fig. 26.4)**.

Insertion of skyla: Its insertion should be done by a trained healthcare provider under strict aseptic precautions. Patient should be re-examined and evaluated 4–6 weeks after insertion, then yearly or more often if required.

Removal of skyla: Skyla must be removed or replaced after 3 years.

Contraindications

- Suspected pregnancy. Not to be used for emergency contraception
- Distorted uterine cavity either due to congenital or acquired uterine anomaly
- Acute pelvic inflammatory disease (PID) or a history of PID
- Postpartum endometritis or septic abortion in the past 3 months
- Known or suspected uterine or cervical malignancy
- Known or suspected breast malignancy or other progestin-sensitive tumor
- Uterine bleeding of unknown etiology
- Untreated acute cervicitis, lower genital tract infections
- Acute liver disease or liver tumor (benign or malignant).

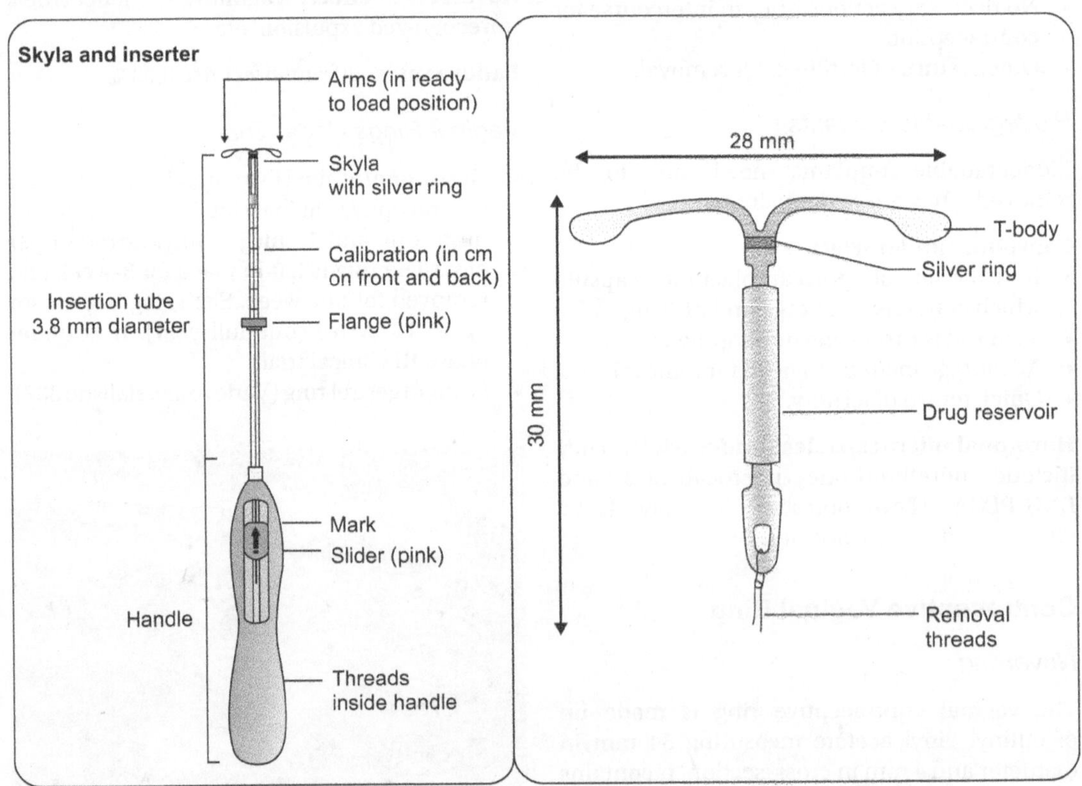

Fig. 26.4: Skyla, a newer intrauterine contraceptive device

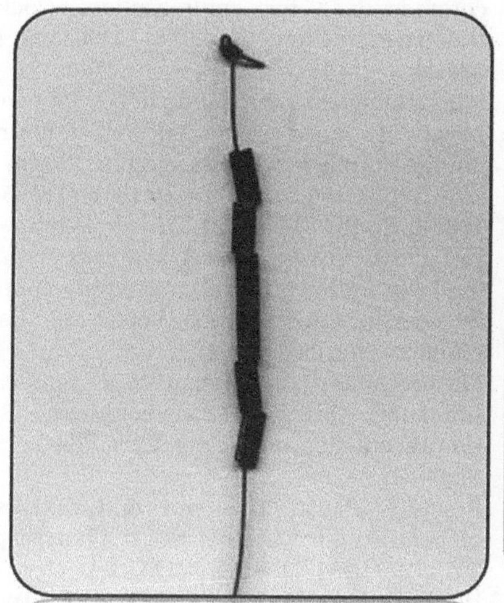

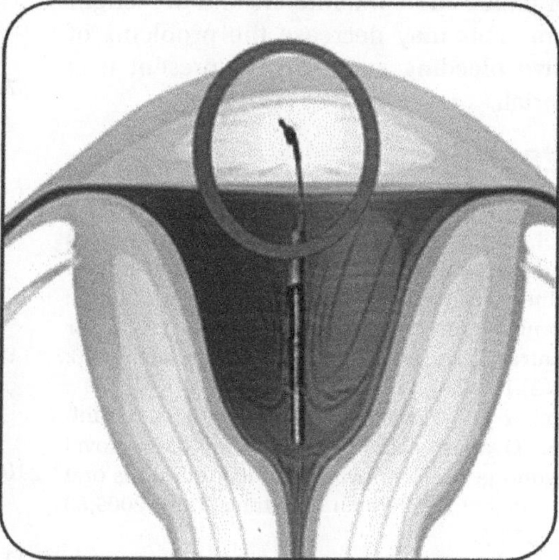

Fig. 26.5: GyneFix

Adverse effects: The most common adverse effects are bleeding pattern changes, vulvovaginitis, abdominal or pelvic pain, acne, seborrhea, ovarian cyst and headache, etc.

Drug interaction: Enzyme inducing drugs such as CYP3A4, may decrease the serum concentration of progestins.

GyneFix

GyneFix is a frameless intrauterine contraceptive device (IUCD). It consists of a monofilament polypropylene thread studded with six 5-mm-long copper sleeves. It contains copper with surface area of 330 cubic millimeter. The proximal end of the thread contains a knot which is anchored into the myometrium of the uterine fundus, thus ensuring the device in the uterine cavity. Insertion is done using a specially made inserter. It acts by inflammatory or foreign body reaction. It is effective for 5 years **(Fig. 26.5)**.[11]

Timing of insertion

It can be inserted at the same timings as has been for the conventional IUCDs:

- *Interval insertion*: First 7 days of menstrual cycle
- *Postabortal insertion*: Immediately following a first- or second-trimester abortion (spontaneous or induced)
- *Postpartum insertion*: Within 48 hours of delivery
- *Postplacental insertion*: Within 10 minutes of delivery of the placenta
- *Postcoital insertion*: Up to 5 days of unprotected intercourse.

Adverse effects

- Postinsertion bleeding and heavy menstruation in initial 2–3 cycles
- No protection from sexually transmitted diseases.

When properly inserted, GyneFix offers several important advantages over CuT380A:[12]

- Comparable efficacy
- Efficacy does not decrease with time
- Reduced expulsion rate
- Less bleeding
- Less pain
- Minimal chances of ectopic pregnancy.

A new frameless IUCD, GyneFix (Mini), has been developed with four instead of six copper cylinders with reduced total surface area of copper to 200 cubic millimeters and the length to 2 cm. This may decrease the problems of excessive bleeding and pain. At present it is under trial.

REFERENCES

1. Cianci A, De Leo V. Individualization of low-dose oral contraceptives. Pharmacological principles and practical indications for oral contraceptives. Minerva Ginecol. 2007;59(4):415-25.
2. Sitruk-Ware R. New progestogens for contraceptive use. Hum Reprod Update. 2006; 12(2):169-78.
3. Archer DF, Kovalevsky G, Ballagh SA, Grubb GS. Ovarian activity and safety of a novel levonorgestrel/ethinyl estradiol continuous oral contraceptive regimen. Contraception. 2009;80 (3):245-5.
4. Grimes DA, Lopez LM, O'Brien PA, Raymond EG. Progestin-only pills for contraception. Cochrane Database Syst Rev. 2013 Nov 13; 11:CD007541. Epub 2013;13.
5. Burkman RT. Transdermal hormonal contraception: benefits and risks. Am J Obstet Gynecol. 2007;197(2):134.e1-6.
6. Gallo MF, Grimes DA, Lopez LM, Schulz KF, d'Arcangues C. Combination injectable contraceptives for contraception. Cochrane Database Syst Rev. 2008:8;(4):CD004568. Epub 2008;8.
7. Wu L, Janagam DR, Mandrell TD, Johnson JR, Lowe TL. Long-acting injectable hormonal dosage forms for contraception. Pharm Res. 2015;32(7):2180-91. doi: 10.1007/s11095-015-1686-2. Epub 2015 Apr 22.
8. Horacio B Croxatto. Mechanisms that explain the contraceptive action of progestin implants for women. Contraception, Volume 65, Issue 1, January 2002, Pages 21-27.
9. Mascarenhas L. Insertion and removal of Implanon: practical considerations. Eur J Contracept Reprod Health Care. 2000;5(Suppl 2):29-34.
10. Brache V, Payán LJ, Faundes A. Current status of contraceptive vaginal rings. Contraception. 2013;87(3):264-72. Epub 2012 Oct 4.
11. Wildemeersch D, Batar I, Affandi B, Andrade A, Shangchun W, Jing H et al. The 'frameless' intrauterine system for long-term, reversible contraception: a review of 15 years of clinical experience. J Obstet Gynaecol Res. 2003;29:160-9.
12. O'Brien PA, Marfleet C.Frameless versus classical intrauterine device for contraception. Cochrane Database Syst Rev. 2005;25:(1):CD003282.

Section VII

GENERAL GYNECOLOGY

CHAPTERS

CHAPTER 27

Fibroid and Endometriosis

Bidisha Singha

INTRODUCTION

The goal of drug therapy in fibroid uterus is to relieve severe pain, correct anemia, reduce size of fibroid prior to myomectomy and to avoid hysterectomy. Indication of drug therapy in endometriosis is to suppress active symptomatic disease, as preoperative therapy in severe recurrent endometriosis to facilitate surgical excision, as postoperative therapy if excision is not complete or in the treatment of recurrent disease and for prevention of disease progression when conception must be delayed. Drugs used in medical management of fibroid are given in **Table 27.1**.[1-7]

Nonsteroidal Anti-inflammatory Drugs

Nonsteroidal anti-inflammatory drugs (NSAIDs) block the synthesis of the prostaglandins, which contribute to pain and inflammation in endometriosis.

Table 27.1 Drugs used in treatment of fibroid and endometriosis[8-14]

Class	*Drug(s)*
Non steroidal anti-inflammatory drugs	Mefenamic acid, ibuprofen, diclofenac sodium
Antifibrinolytics	Tranexamic acid
Combined contraceptives	Ethinyl estradiol plus levonorgestrel Contraceptive trans-dermal patch or vaginal ring
Progestins	Medroxyprogesterone acetate, Dienogest, dydrogesterone, depot medroxyprogesterone acetate
Intrauterine progesterone	LNG -IUS
Progesterone antagonist	Mifepristone
Anti-gonadotropic agents	Danazol, gestrinone
Gonadotrophin releasing hormone agonists	Leuprolide, goserelin, buserelin, nafarelin, triptarelin
GnRH antagonist	Cetrorelix, ganirelix
Aromatase inhibitors	Letrazole, anastrozole
Selective estrogen receptor modulators	Raloxifene
Selective progesterone receptor modulators	Asoprisnil, ulipristal
Newer drugs	Cabergoline, pirfenidone

NSAIDS are effective for relief of primary dysmenorrhea in endometriosis. However, the available evidences do not show whether any individual NSAID is more effective than another. Commonly used NSAIDs are mefenamic acid, ibuprofen and diclofenac sodium.

NSAIDS are reported not to be effective for treatment of menorrhagia in women with fibroids.

Antifibrinolytics

Tranexamic Acid

Pharmacology: It is a synthetic derivative of lysine. It causes reversible blockade of lysine binding sites on plasminogen molecules and inhibits the activation of plasminogen to plasmin, which in turn is responsible for fibrin degradation.

Indications of use: It is used as a first-line nonhormonal therapy for menorrhagia associated with uterine fibroids and dysfunctional uterine bleeding.

Contraindications: Disseminated intravascular coagulation, from upper, genitourinary bleeding tract, e.g. kidney and ureters.

Dosage

For menorrhagia: 10–15 mg/kg of body weight or 500 mg orally 2–3 times a day for up to 5 days during monthly menstruation for menorrhagia.

In severe bleeding: 500–1000 mg slow IV 2–3 times a day can be given.

Adverse drug reaction: Nausea, diarrhea, thromboembolic events, disturbed color vision, allergic reactions, etc.

Drug interaction: Antifibrinolytic agents, fibrinogen concentrates, hormonal contraceptives, tretinoin, etc.

Monitoring: No specific laboratory test is required. Watch for symptoms of severe allergic reactions and any changes in vision.

Preparation

- *Pause*: 500 mg and 1 g tablets, 500 mg injection per 5 mL vial
- *Texid*: 500 mg tablets, 500 mg injection
- *Tranarest*: 250, 500 mg tablets.

Safety during pregnancy: Pregnancy category B.

Combined Contraceptives

Combination contraceptives act by ovarian suppression. They acts by altering the estrogen and progesterone levels in the body and result in a low enough estrogen level and control the fibroid growth. It induces a thin pseudodecidualization of endometrium and therefore brings about atrophic changes in the endometriotic implants.

Initially a trial of continuous or cyclic COCs should be given for 3 months. If the patient's pain is relieved, this treatment is continued for 6–12 months. Subsequent pregnancy rates are 40–50% upon discontinuation of the contraceptive pill.

Dosage

- Ethinyl estradiol 0.03 mg plus levonorgestrel 0.15 mg daily taken either in cyclical or continuous manner.
- Contraceptive vaginal ring—releases on average 0.120 mg of etonogestrel and 15 mcg of ethinyl estradiol per day.
- Transdermal patch Ortho Evra—releases 150 mcg of norelgestromin and 20 mcg of ethinyl estradiol into the blood per day.

Progestins

Pharmacology: All progestational agents act by decidualization and atrophy of the endometrium. These effects are mediated directly by cellular hormonal receptors and are shown to include changes in estrogen metabolism in the endometrial tissue.

Use of this category of drugs relies on high-dose hormones which inhibits ovulatory function and induce amenorrhea. Progestins also have suppressive effect on the expression of endometrial matrix metalloproteinases which contributed to the pathogenesis of endometriosis.

Indications of use

- These are used to reduce uterine bleeding in cases of fibroid uterus. They reduce bleeding by 30–70%
- Endometriosis to reduce pelvic pain
- As progestin only contraceptives.

Progestin implants, injections or pills may be used.

Contraindications: Depot medroxyprogesterone acetate (DMPA) is contraindicated in infertile women as it causes profound amenorrhea and anovulation and the time required for ovulation to resume after discontinuation varies.

Dosage: The progestins used to reduce bleeding from fibroids and reduce pelvic pain in endometriosis are described in **Table 27.2**.

Adverse drug reaction: Nausea, weight gain, fluid retention, breakthrough bleeding, depression, mood disorders, etc.

Drug interaction: Ulipristal and progestins decrease efficacy of each other. Progestins decrease efficacy of anticoagulants.

Monitoring: Effect of treatment evaluated after 3–6 months of therapy.

Preparation

- Medroxyprogesterone acetate
  - *Meprate, Modus, Deviry*: 2.5 and 10 mg tablets
  - *Premella*: 2.5, 5 and 10 mg tablets
- Depot medroxyprogesterone acetate
  - *Depot provera*:150 mg per mL injection for IM use
- Dienogest
  - Dinofirst 2 mg capsule, dienofem 2 mg tablets, endoreg 2 mg tablets
- Lynestrenol
  - *Orgametril*: 5 mg tablets.

Table 27.2 Progestins dosages for use in fibroid and endometriosis

Progestin	Dosage
Medroxyprogesterone acetate	30 mg orally daily, max 100mg daily
Depot medroxyprogesterone acetate	150 mg IM every 3 months
Dienogest	2 mg once daily
Lynestrenol	10 mg daily orally

Dienogest

Pharmacology: It is a 19-nor-testoeterone derivative (C-19 progesterone). Its strong endometrial efficacy underlies its use to treat endometriosis, and gives it antiproliferative and anti-inflammatory effects in treatment of endometriotic lesions. It has no glucocorticoid or antimineralocorticoid activity. It has no antiestrogenic activity which suggest that it should not antagonize estradiol's beneficial effect.[15]

It has short plasma half-life of 10 hours and high oral bioavailability of more than 90%. After distribution 10% remains free and 90% binds to albumin but no binding to sex hormone binding globulin (SHBG) and corticosteroid binding globulin (CBG).

It metabolises by hydroxylation and conjugation. A steady state is reached after 2–3 days which is not influenced by SHBG levels. It has fewer hepatic side effects than other C-19 derivatives.

Indications of use: For long-term treatment of endometriosis.

Contraindications: Active venous thrombotic disorder, arterial and cardiovascular disease, diabetes mellitus with vascular involvement, liver tumors, known or suspected sex hormone dependent malignancies, undiagnosed vaginal bleeding, etc.

Dosage: 2 mg orally once daily.

Adverse drug reaction: Headache, breast discomfort, sleep disorder, abdominal pain, etc.

Drug interaction: It interact with phenytoin, barbiturates, carbamazepine, ketoconazole, itraconazole, erythromycin, ritonavir, etc.

Monitoring: Monitor for any sign of thromboembolic complications and vision change.

Safety during pregnancy: Contraindicated in pregnancy and lactation.

Intrauterine Progesterone

LNG-IUS

It induces endometrial glandular atrophy and decidual transformation of the stroma.[16]

Indications of use

- It is used for control of menorrhagia associated with fibroids when uterine size is not larger than 12 weeks with normal cavity. One study found that women with one fibroid smaller than 5 cm and less than 50% of fibroid in endometrial cavity (type 2) had 90% reduction in blood flow and increase in hemoglobin with 1 year of LNG-IUS insertion though expulsion rate was high (12%).
- In endometriosis significant improvement in severity, frequency of pain and menstrual symptoms is seen. It reduces endometriosis associated pain caused by peritoneal and rectovaginal endometriosis and risk of recurrence of dysmenorrhea after conservative surgery.

Contraindications: Pelvic inflammatory disease, liver disorders, suspected uterine or cervical cancer, etc.

Dosage: It releases 20 µg per day of levo-norgestrel.

Adverse drug reaction: Irregular bleeding, breast tenderness, acne, headache, etc.

Drug interaction: Insulin, warfarin, steroids.

Monitoring: Check for proper placement of intrauterine device (IUD).

Preparation: Mirena.

Safety during pregnancy: Mirena to be removed if woman becomes pregnant.

Progesterone Antagonists

Mifepristone

It is a 19-norsteroid derivative with potent antiprogestational and significant anti-glucocorticoid and anti-androgenic activity.[17-20]

Pharmacology: Mifepristone has a noncompetitive antiestrogen action. It blocks endometrial tissue to grow in response to estrogen, thereby used in treatment of endometriosis and fibroid.

It is orally active but only 25% is bioavailable. It is largely metabolized in liver and excreted in bile.

Indications of use: It is used for treatment of fibroid associated menorrhagia and to reduces size of fibroids. Around 48% decrease in mean uterine volume is noted after 6 months.

Contraindications

Long-term corticosteroid therapy, inherited porphyria, hemorrhagic disorders, adrenal failure, etc.

Dosage

- *In fibroid uterus*: 2.5–50 mg orally daily for 3 months
- *In endometriosis*: 25–50 mg orally daily for 3 months

Trials are still conducted for proper dose regimes. A study by Morales et al.[6] revealed that using mifepristone in dose of 25 mg daily for 3 months led to 50% decrease in the size of uterine myoma.

Adverse effects: Hot flushes, elevated liver enzymes, endometrial hyperplasia, etc.

Drug interactions: It interacts with *CYP3A4* inhibitors (erythromycin, ketoconazole) and the inducers (rifampin, anticonvulsants).

Preparations: *Mifegest, mifeprin, mifty, colestone*: 200 mg tablets.

Safety during pregnancy and lactation: Pregnancy category X. No data on excretion of mifepristone in breast milk.

Antigonadotropic Agents

They act by suppressing the hypothalamic-pituitary-ovarian axis, inhibiting the mid-cycle follicle-stimulating hormone (FSH) and luteinizing hormone (LH) surge and preventing steroidogenesis in the corpus luteum. They also suppress endometriosis at a local level.

Danazol

Pharmacology: It is a synthetic steroid analog with strong antigonadotropic activity. It inhibits luteinizing hormone (LH) and follicle-stimulating hormone (FSH) and has a weak androgenic action. Danazol displaces endogenous testosterone almost completely from its binding globulin, and this endogenous androgen contributes to the effect of drugs.

It suppresses pituitary-ovarian axis by inhibition of pituitary gonadotropin output and induces a state of hypoestrogenic, hyperandrogenic state that suppress ectopic endometrial growth.

It acts by interfering with autocrine and paracrine functions. It decrease the number of endometrial growth factor receptor, which has a potential role in maintenance of ectopic endometrial tissue. It also inhibits production of interlukin 1-β and tumor necrosis factor. It also interacts with intracellular androgen and progesterone receptors.

It causes direct inhibition of multiple enzymes of steroidogenesis and alteration of endogenous steroid metabolism.

It is well absorbed after oral administration. Peak levels are reached in 2 hours; it gets extensively metabolized in the liver to 2-hydroxymethyl ethisterone. Half-life is 15 hours. It is highly concentrated in liver, adrenals and kidney. Its complete clearance is done by liver in 8 hours and is excreted in feces and urine.

Indications of use
- Endometriosis
- *Fibroid*: It reduces fibroid size slightly and minimizes blood loss or even produce amenorrhea.

Contraindication: Pregnancy, breastfeeding, porphyria, undiagnosed abnormal genital bleeding, hypersensitivity, liver, renal and cardiac disease, etc.

Dosage
- Endometriosis
  - *Mild*: 200–400 mg/day orally twice daily
  - *Moderate-to-severe*: 800 mg/day orally twice daily.

  Dose should be titrated downward to a dose sufficient to maintain amenorrhea. Therapy is continued for 6 months or can be continued up to 9 months.
- *Fibroid*: 200–400 mg/day orally for 3 months.

Adverse drug reaction: Weight gain, acne, hirsutism, edema, hair loss, deepening of voice, flushing, etc.

Drug interaction: Warfarin, carbamazepine, statins, cyclosporine, etc.

Monitoring: LFT and KFT at 4 weeks interval, signs and symptoms of intracranial tension (papilledema, headache, nausea and vomiting), lipoproteins and androgenic changes.

Preparation
- *Gonablok, Gynazole*: 50, 100, 200 mg capsules
- *Endozol, gynadom*: 100 and 200 mg tablets.

Safety during pregnancy: Pregnancy category X, breastfeeding is contraindicated.

Gestrinone

It is a-19-nortestosterone derivative with androgenic, antiprogestogenic, antiestrogenic and antigonadotrophic activities.

Pharmacology: It acts centrally and peripherally to increase free testosterone and reduce sex hormone binding globulin (androgenic effect), reduces serum estradiol values to early follicular phase levels (antiestrogenic effect), reduce, mean LH levels and obliterate the FSH and LH surge (antigonadotrophic effect).

It causes cellular inactivation of endometriotic implants. Amenorrhea occurs in 50–100% of women and resumption of menses after 33 days of discontinuation. Half-life is 28 hours.

Indications of use: Fibroid uterus, endometriosis and benign breast disease.

Contraindications: It is contraindicated in pregnancy because it may lead to masculinization of female fetus. It is contraindicated in renal, hepatic, cardiac, metabolic and vascular disorders.

Dosage: 1.25–2.5 mg orally twice weekly, start on first day of cycle with second dose 3 days later, repeat on the same days of the week and preferably at the same time. It is taken for 6 months.

Adverse drug reaction: These are dose dependent and include nausea, muscle cramps, weight gain, acne, seborrhea, oily hair and skin, breast hypotrophy, etc.

Drug interaction: Antiepileptic drugs, rifampicin.

Preparation: Dimetrios, dimetros, florizel- 2.5 mg capsules.

Safety during pregnancy: Contraindicated in pregnancy. Pregnancy category X.

Gonadotropin-releasing Hormone Agonist

Gonadotropin-releasing hormone (GnRH) agonists produce a hypogonadotrophic-hypogonadism state by downregulation of the pituitary gland.

Indications of use: It used for 6 months in monthly dose to reduce fibroid volume by 30% and total uterine volume by 35%. Reduction of uterine size occurs in first 3 months. Following discontinuation of GnRH analog, menses return in 4–8 weeks' time and uterus returns to pretreatment levels in 4–6 months. It causes atrophy of the endometriotic implants in the same dose.

Contraindication: Pregnancy and breastfeeding.

Dosage: It is given in **Table 27.3**.

Adverse drug reaction: Osteoporosis, hot flushes, dry vagina, headache, depression, loss of libido, night sweats, breast atrophy, etc.

Interactions: Antidiabetic agents, mifepristone.

Monitoring: It is by bone densitometry prior to repeat course of treatment.

The dose of daily GnRH agonist can be regulated by monitoring estradiol levels. Their sides effects can be minimized by addition of low dose progestin or estrogen-progestin in add-back regimens.

Leuprolide

It is available as depot injections. It is used in management of endometriosis including relief in pain and reduction of the size. It is used for treatment of anemia caused due to fibroids.

Goserelin

It is available in form of implantable cylinder placed subcutaneously. It gets metabolized in liver and excreted in urine.

Table 27.3 Dosages of GnRH agonists in fibroid and endometriosis

GnRH	*Dosage*	*preparations*
Leuprolide	3.75 mg IM monthly 11.5 mg IM every 3 months	Lupron
Goserelin	3.6 mg SC monthly	Zoladex
Nafarelin	200 µg intranasal twice daily	Synarel

Implants containg goserelin 3.6 mg administered subcutaneously every 28 days. Add back therapy is given to prevent vasomotor symptoms and bone loss related to hypoestrogenic state.

Nafarelin

Pharmacology: It is a synthetic decapeptide and an agonist of luteinizing hormone releasing hormone (LHRH), desensitizes response to endogenous GnRH, which in turn reduces secretion of LH and FSH and subsequently causes decreased ovarian and testicular hormone production. Its peak serum time is 10–45 minutes, 78–84% is protein bound, degraded by peptidase and excreted in urine and feces.

Its initial effect occurs at 1 month and peak effect at 12 weeks on endometriotic implants.

Indications of use

- Endometriosis
- Fibroids–to shrink size of uterine fibroid, reduce meno-metrorrhagia, dysmenorrhea and pelvic discomfort.

Contraindications: Pregnancy, hypersensitivity, lactation, undiagnosed abnormal vaginal bleeding, etc.

Dosage

Endometriosis: Treatment begun on day 2–4 of menstrual cycle with initial dose of 1 spray twice daily maximum of mcg intranasally per day.

Adverse drug reaction: Withdrawal bleeding.

Add Back Therapy

One of the following can be given:

- *Progestin only*: Norethisterone 1.2 mg or norethindrone acetate 5 mg per day
- Combined estrogen and progestogen
  - Conjugated estrogen 0.625 mg plus medroxyprogestrone acetate—2.5 mg or norethindrone acetate—5 mg daily.
  - Estradiol 2 mg plus norethisterone acetate—1 mg daily.
- Raloxifne (SERM)—60 mg orally daily.

GnRH Antagonists

Cetrorelix and Ganirelix

Pharmacology: They cause immediate suppression of endogenous GnRH and are considered for medical treatment prior to surgery in cases of fibroid and endometriosis.

Rapidly absorbed subcutaneously, maximum plasma concentrations occur 1–2 hours after administration.

Indications of use: Ganirelix brings 29% reduction in fibroid volume in 3 weeks.

Contraindications: Hypersensitivity, GnRh analog, pregnancy and lactation, severe renal impairment.

Dosage

Fibroid: 3 mg SC, every 4 days for 2–4 weeks prior to surgery. Treatment is commenced on first day of periods.

Endometriosis: 3 mg SC, once a week for 8 weeks.

Adverse drug reaction: Hot flushes, vaginal dryness, mood swings, headaches, spotting.

Preparations

- *Cetorelix*: Cetrotide, cetace, Ovuralix—0.25 mg injection for subcutaneous use.
- *Ganirelix*: Orgalutran 250 mcg/0.5 mL for SC injection.

Safety during pregnancy: Contraindicated in pregnancy and lactation.

Aromatase Inhibitors

Letrazole and Anastrozole

There are the two aromatase inhibitors which are available.

Pharmacology: They blocks aromatase activity in extra-ovarian sites and suppress the conversion of androstenedione and testosterone to estrogen. It leads to suppression of endometriosis at a local level. Letrazole is rapidly absorbed with 100% bioavailability and causes decrease in E2 levels.

Indications of use: Fibroid and endometriois.

Contraindication: Pregnancy.

Dosage: Letrozole is given 5 mg orally daily for 3 months.

Anastrozole 1 mg daily orally for 3 months is effective in reducing the volume of fibroids by an average of 9.32% and control of symptoms without changes in levels of FSH and estradiol.

Adverse drug reaction: Hot flushes, nausea, diarrhea, dyspepsia, thinning of hair, bone loss, etc.

Due to the severe side effects, aromatase inhibitors should only be prescribed to women after all other options for medical or surgical treatment have failed.

Drug interaction: Tamoxifen.

Preparation
- Letrezole-Letroz, Letoval—2.5 mg tablets
- Anastrozole-Altraz, Armotraz—1 mg tablets.

Safety during pregnancy: Contraindicated in pregnancy.

Selective Estrogen Receptor Modulators

Raloxifene

Pharmacology: It acts as partial estrogen agonist in bone and CVS while acts as antagonist in endometrium and breast. It has long half-life so single dose is administered. It decreases size of fibroid but has no effect on uterine bleeding. Its role in endometriosis is unclear.

Contraindications: Active or past history of venous thromboembolism and coronary artery disease.

Dosage: 60 mg orally per day.

Adverse drug reaction: Hot flushes, leg cramps, vaginal bleeding, increased risk of DVT and pulmonary embolism, etc.

Drug interaction: Cholestyramine, diazepam, warfarin, lidocaine and hormone replacement therapy.

Monitoring: Lipid profile, endometrial sampling if indicated due to abnormal uterine bleeding, bone mineral density.

Preparation: Ralotab, Rolafen, Ralista, Gynista—60 mg tablets.

Safety during pregnancy: Not safe in pregnancy.

Selective Progesterone Receptor Modulators

Selective progesterone receptor modulator (SPRM) is a new class of progesterone receptor modulators.

They exert tissue selective progesterone agonist, antagonist or mixed agonist-antagonist effects on various tissues including the endometrium.

Preliminary study with SPRM has showed that it reduces the duration and amount of uterine bleeding in a dose-dependent manner.

Asoprisnil

Pharmacology: It is an orally active selective progesterone receptor modulator (SPRM).

It is used in management of symptomatic uterine leiomyomata, as it suppresses both the duration and intensity of menstrual bleeding in a dose-dependent manner. Its use causes statistically significant reduction in frequency and intensity of uterine bleeding and decreases fibroid size by 35–40%.

It acts by downregulation of collagen synthesis through upregulation of extracellular matrix metalloproteinase inducer.

Indications of use: Fibroids and endometriosis.

Dosage: 5–25 mg orally daily.

Adverse drug reaction: Bloating, flatulence, breast pain, hot flushes, night sweats, asymptomatic ovarian cysts, etc.

Ulipristal Acetate

Pharmacology: It is a selective progesterone-receptor modulator.[21,22]

Indications of use

Fibroid uterus: Two recent clinical trials (PEARL 1 and PEARL 2, 2012) revealed that ulipristal acetate brings about 42% reduction in the size of fibroid, and improvement in heavy menstrual bleeding (98% reduction in heavy periods and 89% achieved amenorrhea) at a daily dose of 10 mg. This is comparable to that achieved by GnRH analog (leuprolide acetate). A daily dose of 5 mg ulipristal appears to be marginally less effective than the 10 mg dose in achieving fibroid size reduction (36%) and amenorrhea (75%), but these differences were not statistically significant. Symptom improvement occurred by one week of treatment commencement and uterine volume reduction was maintained for at least 6 months after discontinuation of treatment.

Contraindications: Liver disorders (severe), genital bleeding of unknown etiology, uterine, cervical, ovary and breast cancers.

Dosage: 5 mg orally daily for only 3 months.

Adverse drug reaction: Headache, nausea, abdominal pain, etc.

Ulipristal was able to achieve effects comparable to three weeks for GnRH analog and had significantly less side effects than GnRHa. It had only 10% risk of hot flushes as compared to 40% risk of hot flushes with GnRHa.

Drug interaction: Antifungals, barbiturates, digoxin, hormonal contraceptives, etc.

Monitoring: Evaluate if persistent vaginal bleeding.

Preparation: Fibristal 5 mg tablet. It is a costly drug 16.70$ per tablet.

Safety during pregnancy: Pregnacy category X.

FDA approval: It has been licensed in Europe for use in medical treatment of fibroids since 2012.

The mechanim of action, effects on fibroid or endometriosis and adverse effects of all the drugs used in management of fibroid endometriosis is summarized in **Table 27.4**. Summary of therapeutic effects of these drugs on fibroid is given in **Table 27.5**.

Newer Drugs

Cabergoline

It is a lysergic acid derivative and a dopamine agonist.

Use it is in leiomyoma uteri.

It has inhibitory effect on the secretion of GnRH because of its dopaminergic action.

Only one study, from Iran, has compared the effects of GnRHa (diphereline 3.75 mg every 28 days, total of four injections) with cabergoline (0.5 mg once a week for 6 weeks) which found significant fibroid regression with both treatments. The extent of tumor regression correlated positively with the number of tumor nodules. Cabergoline was well tolerated and had fewer adverse effects compared with GnRHa.

More studies are required before any definitive conclusions are drawn.

Pirfenidone[23]

It is a new drug which that blocks the growth of existing fibroids and may stop formation of new fibroids.

Exact mechanism of action not known. It affect the production of collagen, a major component of fibroid and may have effect on cell growth factor. However, it not available and studies are under way to establish its safety and efficacy.

Table 27.4 Summary of drugs used in medical management of fibroid and endometriosis

Drug class	*Mechanism of action*	*Effect*	*Adverse effects/concerns*
Antifibrotics	Interfere with growth factors, leiomyoma cell proliferation and extracellular matrix/ collagen production	Interfere with fibroid growth	Long-term effects not known, further studies needed
Oral contraceptives	Endometrial stabilization, variable effects on leiomyomas	May improve uterine bleeding, but no significant decrease in fibroid size	Use judiciously—both estrogen and progesterone may promote fibroid growth (increased mitotic activity)
Progestin only	Endometrial stabilization/ atrophy, variable effects on leiomyomas	Mixed results—both fibroid shrinkage and enlargement have been shown; may induce amenorrhea	Use judiciously—progesterone may promote fibroid growth (increased mitotic activity)
Antiprogestins	Antiprogesterone effect—reduces action and number of progesterone receptors in fibroids and myometrium	Improved symptoms in 60–75%, may induce amenorrhea, reduction in fibroid volume 25–50% within 3 months	Side effects include hot flashes, elevated hepatic enzymes, and endometrial hyperplasia
Androgens	Combination hormonal and vascular effects (androgenic, progestogenic, antiprogestogenic, and antiestrogenic actions)	24% fibroid size reduction in 4 months, may improve bleeding symptoms	*Side effects*: Weight gain, edema, acne, oily skin, hirsutism, voice changes, headaches, hot flashes, altered libido, decreased breast size, and muscle cramps
GnRH agonists	Suppression of ovarian steroidogenesis production – delayed pituitary downregulation	Fibroid size and symptom reduction up to 50% within 3–6 months	*Hypoestrogenic side effects*: Hot flashes, vaginal dryness, headaches. Prolonged use associated with reduced bone mineral density
GnRH antagonists	Suppression of ovarian steroidogenesis production–immediate pituitary downregulation	Reduction in fibroid size 25–40% and symptom improvement within 3 weeks	*Hypoestrogenic side effects*: Hot flashes, vaginal dryness, headaches. Prolonged use associated with reduced bone mineral density
Aromatase inhibitors	Reduces estrogen synthesis and effects	Fibroid size reduced 60–70% within 1–2 months in a case report	Hypoestrogenic side effects; further studies needed
Mixed estrogen receptor antagonist/ agonists	Estrogen antagonist effects on fibroid and endometrium	Inconsistent results— trend to decreased fibroid size in small heterogeneous studies	*Side effects*: Leg cramps, hot flashes. Increased risk of thromboembolic events
Mixed progesterone receptor antagonist/ agonists	Local progesterone-mediated effects on leiomyomas and endometrium	Decreased menstrual bleeding (up to 80%) and fibroid size reduction up to 36% within 12 weeks, may induce amenorrhea	Maintains follicular phase estrogen levels, no adverse endometrial effects—causes nonphysiologic secretory changes (clinical relevance unknown)

Table 27.5 Summary of outcomes of medical therapy in fibroid

Type of drug	*Product*	*Outcome on fibroid size*	*Outcome on abnormal uterine bleeding*	*Outcome on fertility*
Nonhormonal	NSAIDs and Tranexamic Acid	No effect on fibroid size	Decrease by 30%	No effect
Hormonal	Combined oral Contraceptive	No data	Decrease 20–30%	Contraceptive
	GnRH analog (3–6 months duration of therapy)	Decrease 30%	Decrease > 80%	Contraceptive
	Oral progestins	Decrease 30%	Decrease > 60%	Contraceptive
	Long acting reversible contraceptive (e.g. Depo-provera, Implanon	Decrease uterine volume by 35%	Breakthrough bleeding	Contraceptive
	Levonorgestrel intrauterine device (Mirena)	Decrease 20–30%	Decrease 40% No systemic side effects	Contraceptive

REFERENCES

1. Owen C, Armstrong AY. Clinical management of leiomyoma. Obstet Gynecol Clin North Am. 2015;42:67-85.
2. Diamond, et al. Medical treatment of endometriosis. In: wallach and Zacur (Eds). Reproductive Medicine and Surgery. Ist edition. Mosby Publishers, 1995.
3. Endometriosis. In clinical gynaecologic endocrinology and infertility. Fritz, Speroff. Lippincott Publisher, 8th edition; 2011.pp.1221-48.
4. Lindsay SF, Luciano DE, Luciano AA. Emerging therapy for endometriosis. Expert Opin Emerg Drugs. 2015;20:449-61.
5. Hormones and related drugs. In: KD Tripathi (Ed). Essentials of Medical Pharmacology. Jaypee Publishers, 7th edition, 2013
6. Peitsidis P, Koukoulomati A. Tranexamic acid for the management of uterine fibroid tumors: a systematic review of the current evidence. World J Clin Cases. 2014;2:893-8.
7. William H. Parker. Uterine myoma management. 2007;88:255-71.
8. Edyta J Frackeiwicz. Endometriosis: an overview of the disease and its treatment. J Am Pharm Assoc. 2000;40(5):1-10.
9. Srividya Sankaran. Medical management of fibroid. Best practice and research clinical obstetrics and gynecology. 2000;22:655-76.
10. Nirma l Duhan. Current and emerging treatments for uterine myoma: an update. Int J Women's Health. 2011;3:231-41.
11. British fibroid trust.www. British Fibroid Trust. org.uk.
12. Management of uterine fibroid: an update of the evidence. Evidence/Report/Technology/ Assesment No. 2007;154.
13. Dsouza J, Kumar S, Hande PC, Singh SN. Uterine artery embolisation for uterine fibroids: our experience at a tertiary care service hospital. Med J Armed Forces India. 2015;71(3):233-8.
14. Dunselman, et al. ESHRE guidelines: Management of women with endometriosis. Human Reproduction. 2014;29:400-12.
15. XiangyanRuan et al. The pharmacology of dinogest. Maturitas. 2012;71:337-44.
16. Kumar Sushil, et al. Therapeutic use of LNG intrauterine system (Mirena) for menorrhagia due to benign lesion: an alternative to hysterectomy? J Obstet Gynecol India. 2005; 55:541-3.
17. Esteve, Acosta, Perez, et al. Mifepristone versus placebo to treat uterine myoma: a double blind, randomized clinical trial. International Journal of Women's Health. 2013;5:361-9.
18. M Engmam, et al. Mifepristone for treatment of uterine leiomyoma: a prospective randomized placebo controlled trial. Human Reprod. 2009; 24:1870-9.

19. Kettel LM, et al. Treatment of endometriosis with antiprogesterone mifepristone. Fertil Steril. 1996;65(1):23-8.
20. Low dose mifepristone in medical management of uterine leiomyoma: an experience from a tertiary care hospital from North India. Indian J Medical Res. 2013;137:1154-62.
21. Darlene K Taylor and Phyllis C Luppert. Treatment for uterine fibroids: searching for effective drug therapy. Drug discovery today. Ther Strategy. 2001;29(1):e41-e49.
22. ACOG committee opinion. Aromatase inhibitors in gynecologic practice. Obstet Gynecol. 2008; 112:405-7.
23. Lee BS, Margolin SB, Nowak RA. Pirfenidone: a novel pharmacological agent that inhibits leiomyoma cell proliferation and collagen production. J Clin Endocrinol Metab. 1998;83 (1):219-23.

CHAPTER **28**

Menstrual Disorders

Madhavi M Gupta, Purnima Gupta

INTRODUCTION

Menarche occurs between 11 and 13 years of age during pubertal development while average age of menopause is 51 years. From onset of menstruation until it stops, is the time period when a woman can have deviation from normal menstrual pattern, called as menstrual disorders. Normal menstruation has following characterstics:[1]

- Frequency = 24–38 days
- Regularity = ± 2–20 days
- Duration = 4–8 days
- Volume of monthly blood loss = 5–80 mL.

Flow chart 28.1 depicts the signal pathway that leads to menstruation.

Management of these disorders can be medical or surgical. Various drugs are used for either diagnostic evaluation or therapeutic purposes. The medical management of various menstrual disorders in adolescent and reproductive age group women is discussed separately **(Table 28.1)**.

ADOLESCENT

Amenorrhea

Absent or cessation of menstruation is called as amenorrhea. It can further be classified as primary and secondary amenorrhea. Primary amenorrhea describes patients who have never menstruated and secondary amenorrhea describes those who have menstruated previously but now do not.

Primary amenorrhea can be caused due to defect anywhere in the hypothalamo-pituitary-ovarian axis, gonads or the genital tract. Uterine and vaginal structural defects need surgical correction. Gonadal dysgenesis, Müllerian agenesis and androgen insensitivity syndrome constitute the common causes of primary amenorrhea. Ovaries are mainly involved in conditions causing chronic anovulation (polycystic ovarian syndrome, obesity, thyroid disorder, hyperprolactinemia) and conditions causing complete ovarian failure like chromosomal abnormalities (gonadal dysgenesis), genetic disorders (Turner syndrome), and autoimmune disorders (Addison's disease). Besides, cause specific treatment, these girls need supplementation of sex steroids for normal pubertal development in case of primary amenorrhea due to premature ovarian insufficiency or premature ovarian failure (POF). Pitutary and hypothalamic causes will be discussed later.

Turner Syndrome

Patients with Turner syndrome need growth hormone for optimum height before starting estrogen therapy.

Flow chart 28.1: Signal pathway that leads to menstruation

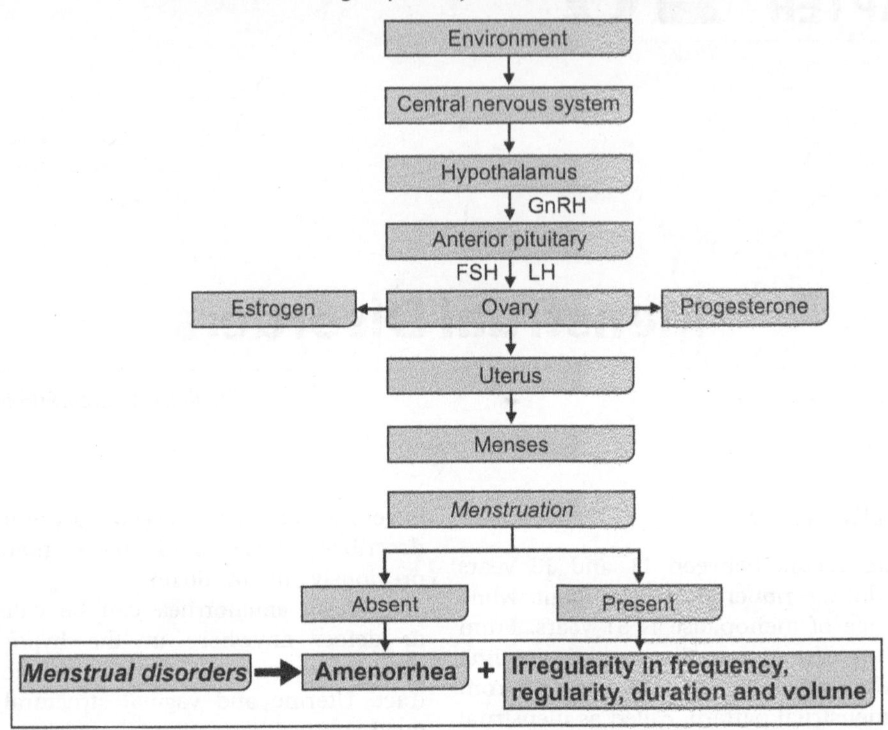

Growth Hormone

Pharmacology

- Growth hormone acts on its receptor belonging to the cytokine 1 receptor superfamily, ultimately leading to tyrosine phosphorylation of cytoplasmic proteins that mediate downstream signaling events.[2]
- It causes stimulation of long bone growth and increase in bone density by differentiation of prechondrocytes to chondrocytes and stimulation of osteoclast and osteoblast proliferation.[3]
- The circulating half-life of growth hormone is 20 minutes, the biological half-life is in the range of 9–17 hours.[3]
- In patients of Turner syndrome, this should be started as soon as the height falls below the fifth percentile for normal woman growth.
- Final height depends on the dose and duration of GH treatment before estrogen therapy begins and with early diagnosis and treatment final height of around 150 cm can be achieved in these patients.

Dosage

- *Genotropin*: 0.33 mg/kg given subcutaneously every week—divided into equal daily doses or on 3 alternate days.
- *Norditropin*: 0.067 mg/kg/day.
- *Nutropin and Nutropin AQ*: 0.375 mg/kg given subcutaneously every week—divided into equal doses 3–7 times per week
- Side effects.

Generally includes increased intracranial hypertension, visual changes with papilledema, headache, vomiting, high blood sugars, carpal tunnel syndrome or worsening of scoliosis.[3]

Estrogen Supplementation

In 1930s, ovarian hormone, estrogen was first isolated by Edgar Allen and Edward Doisy.

Table 28.1: Medical management of various menstrual disorders

Adolescent	Primary Amenorrhea	*Turner syndrome* Growth hormone Estrogen supplementation Progesterone supplementation
Reproductive age group	Anovulatory cycles	Progestin therapy Estrogen progesterone therapy Estrogen only
	Hirsutism	Combined oral contraceptives (COCs) Progesterone only Anitandrogens—spironolactone, cyproterone acetate, flutamide, eflornithine hydrochloride Insulin sensitizers—metformin, thiazolidonediones
	Heavy menstrual bleeding	**Nonhormonal treatment** *NSAIDs:* Cyclooxygenase-1 inhibitors Salicylates—aspirin Indoleacetic acid analogs—indomethacin Aryl propionic acid derivative—naproxen, ibuprofen Fenamates—mefenamic acid, meclofenamic acid Cyclooxygenase 2 inhibitors Coxibs—celecoxib, refecoxib **Antifibrinolytic**—Trenaxamic acid Others—Ethamsylate **Hormonal treatment** Oral progesterone—Norethisterone Medroxyprogesterone acetate Dihydrogesterone Intrauterine progestogens—Levonorgestrel IUCD Progestasert IUCD Combined estrogen/progestogens—OCPs HRT *Others*: Danazol Gestrinone GnRH analog Mifepristone
	Menstrual migraine	Triptans COCs Estrogen only Nonhormonal therapy
	Premenstrual syndrome and premenstrual dysphoric disorder	Serotonin reuptake inhibitors Benzodiazepine group Gonadotropin-releasing hormone agonists Oral contraception or progesterone
	Secondary amenorrhea	Premature ovarian failure Micronized estradiol Conjugated equine estrogen Progesterone—Micronized progesterone MDPA **Prolactinoma** Cabergoline Bromocriptine

In 1939, urine of pregnant horses was used for extracting estrogen for clinical use in humans producing sodium salt from sulfate esters of various estrogen.

This conjugated estrogen (premarin) was used for clinical use in 1942 in USA.[4-7]

Pharmacology: 17β-estradiol is the most potent naturally occurring estrogen in humans, is followed by estrone and estriol. All of them contain phenolic A ring with a hydroxyl group at carbon 3, and a β-OH or ketone in position 17 of ring D.[8] Estrogen receptors are nuclear receptors and cause ligand activated decrease or increase in transcription of target genes. The estrogen and progesterone production by the ovaries regulate events in fallopian tubes, uterus, cervix, and vagina. Many nonreproductive tissues, including bone, vascular endothelium, liver, CNS, immune system, gastrointestinal tract, and heart also express both type of estrogen receptors.[8] It gets readily absorbed because of its lipophilic nature. It undergoes rapid hepatic biotransformation and is converted to estriol in the end. Estrogens also undergo enterohepatic recirculation via sulfate and glucuronide conjugation in the liver. Then it gets secreted in bile, hydrolysis in the gut (largely by bacterial enzymes) takes place, followed by reabsorption.[8]

Estrogen preparations are as follows:
- Conjugated estrogen
- Micronized estradiol
- Estropipate
- Ethinyl estradiol
- Esterified estrogen
- Transdermal estradiol.
- Ideally, in patients with turner syndrome, estrogen therapy should begin between 12 and 15 years of age.
- Low dose (0.25–0.5 mg micronized estradiol or its equivalent) should be started initially, increasing gradually at intervals of 3–6 months according to response (Tanner stage, bone age).
- Sexual maturation usually achieved over 2–3 years.

Contraindications include—estrogen should not be used in women with any of the following conditions:
- Undiagnosed abnormal genital bleeding
- Known, suspected, or history of breast cancer
- Known or suspected estrogen-dependent neoplasia
- Known anaphylactic reaction or angioedema to estradiol
- Known liver impairment
- Known protein C, protein S, or antithrombin deficiency, or other known thrombophilic disorders
- Known or suspected pregnancy
- Active deep vein thrombosis (DVT), pulmonary embolism (PE), or history of these conditions
- Active arterial thromboembolic disease (for example, stroke and myocardial infarction), or a history of these conditions.

Side effects: Include premature closure of epiphysis, if given before growth hormone therapy.
- Estrogen supplementation may have various side effects as follows:
  - *Gastrointestinal:* Nausea, vomiting, abdominal cramps and bloating, cholestatic jaundice, pancreatitis and derangement of liver function tests are seen with estrogen use.
  - *Cardiovascular:* It has been seen that estrogen supplementation decreases the risk of coronary heart disease.
  - *Metabolic:* Increased HDL and decreased cholesterol and LDL levels are favorable alterations in lipid profile with the estrogen use.
  - *Hematological:* With increased coagulability, increased risk of deep vein thrombosis, thrombophlebitis and pulmonary embolism is there with its use.
  - *Oncological:* Increased risk of endometrial carcinoma with intact uterus if taken without progesterone supplementation. The increased risk of breast cancer due to estrogen is controversial.
  - *Nervous:* Nervous side effects include irritability, mood swings, dementia,

dizziness, depression, headache, nervousness and exacerbation of migraine headache.
- *Dermatological:* Chloasma, melasma, pruritus, erythema multiforme, scalp hair loss and purpura have been seen with estrogen use.
- *Musculoskeletal:* Its use may lead to arthralgia and leg cramps.
- *Others:* Estrogen use has been associated with fibrocystic disease, mastodynia, nipple discharge, fluid retention, edema and alterations in libido.

Progesterone Supplementation

Pharmacology

The progestins include:

- Progesterone (naturally occurring hormone)
- 17a-acetoxyprogesterone derivatives of the pregnane series
- 19-nortestosterone derivatives (estranes)
- Norgestrel and similar compounds of the gonane series. Medroxyprogesterone acetate and megestrol acetate are C21 steroids having activity similar to that of progesterone itself.[9] The progesterone receptor (PR) favors a D4-3-one A-ring structure in an inverted 1b, 2a-conformation.[10] There are two types of progesterone receptors—PR-A and PR-B. stimulatory activities of progesterone are carried out via PR-B receptor.
- PR-A inhibits stimulatory action of PR-B and is also a transcriptional inhibitor of other steroid receptors.[11] Progesterone is metabolized primarily in the liver to hydroxylated metabolites and their sulfate and glucuronide conjugates.[9]
- Acts as antiestrogen by following mechanisms:
  - They have stimulatory activity on 17-β-hydroxysteroid dehydrogenase and sulfotransferase enzymes that convert estradiol to estrone sulfate (which is rapidly cleared from the body)
  - They inhibit estrogen action on induction of its own receptor (estrogen receptor replenishment)
  - They also suppress estrogen-mediated transcription of oncogenes.
- When a girl with Turner has first vaginal bleeding or has taken estrogen therapy for 12–24 months, a progestin (medroxyprogesterone acetate) should be added.

Indications: It helps in preventing dysfunctional uterine bleeding and protects the endometrium from the effect of unopposed estrogen.

Contraindications

- Current or past history of thrombophlebitis, thromboembolic disorders, or cerebral apoplexy.
- Liver dysfunction or disease.
- Known or suspected malignancy of breast or genital organs.
- Undiagnosed vaginal bleeding.
- Known sensitivity to progesterone injection.

Dosage

10 mg once a day from day 16 to day 25.

Adverse drug reaction

Side effects include:

- *Gastrointestinal:* Abdominal pain, bloating, diarrhea, nausea, dry mouth, dyspepsia, constipation and vomiting are reported side effects. Increase in liver transaminases levels may be seen during its use.
- *Cardiovascular:* Associated with hypertension, angina pectoris and syncope.
- *Musculoskeletal:* Joint pain, back pain, arthritis, leg cramps, hypertonia, muscle disorder, and myalgia.
- *Nervous:* Depression, anxiety, insomnia and forgetfulness.
- *Dermatological:* Acne, pruritus, verruca, rash and skin discoloration.
- *Respiratory:* May lead to bronchitis, nasal congestion, pharyngitis and sinusitis.
- *Other:* May cause breast pain, breast enlargement, cystitis, fatigue, irritability, night sweats, anorexia and edema.

Secondary amenorrhea in adolescent group can be seen in girls suffering from eating disorders and primary premature ovarian failure. Treatment used for eating disorders comprises of cognitive behavioral therapy and adequate nutrition. Medical management includes antidepressants (primarily selective serotonin reuptake inhibitors).

REPRODUCTIVE AGE GROUP

Abnormal uterine bleeding is the major menstrual complaints in this age group. Important causes are anovulation, hormonal contraception, complications of pregnancy, infections, endocrine disorders, and polyps and myomas.

Anovulatory Cycles

Progestin Therapy

- Mainstay of treatment of anovulatory bleeding
- In acute anovulatory bleeding high dose progestin alone are beneficial[12-14]
  - Medroxyprogesterone acetate = 10–20 mg two times a day
  - Megestrol acetate = 20–40 mg two times a day
  - Norethindrone (Norethisterone) = 5 mg two times a day

  ↓

  After 7–10 days, dose can be decreased to once daily and continued up to 3 weeks. For long-term management patient can be offered cyclic progestin treatment or estrogen-progesterone combination treatment.
- In chronic anovulatory irregular bleeding, cyclic progesterone therapy is a good option **(Table 28.2).**

Estrogen-Progesterone Therapy

- As already discussed, women with anovulatory bleeding and sexually active are best managed by combination therapy.
- It reduces menstrual blood loss by 60%.[15]
- In acute anovulatory prolonged bleeding, high-dose estrogen-progesterone therapy may be used (endometrium should be normal or increased in thickness):
  - Initially one pill twice daily is started, bleeding usually slows down within 24–48 hours. Dose can be changed to one pill a day and given up to 2 weeks.
- Estrogen-progesterone combination induces structural changes that organize and stabilize the endometrium.

Estrogen Only

- This has an important role when endometrium is too thin to be acted upon by progesterone as incase of estrogen

Table 28.2 Management of chronic anovulatiory irregular bleeding

Bleeding pattern	*Regimen*	*Disadvantages*
1. Chronic anovulatory irregular bleeding (in patients who are compeletely anovulatory and sexually not active)	Cyclic progesterone (Medroxy-progesterone acetate 5–10 mg daily) for 12–14 days each month is given	Will not prevent random ovulation
2. Chronic anovulatory irregular bleeding (in patients who still ovulate and want contraception)	Estrogen-progesterone combination	Gastrointestinal intolerance
3. Chronic anovulatory irregular bleeding (in patients who cannot take combination therapy but need contraception)	Depot medroxyprogesterone acetate (150 mg intramuscularly every 3 months)	• Episodic breakthrough bleeding • Once given, it cannot be withdrawn

breakthrough bleeding and acute heavy bleeding leading to thin, denuded endometrium.

- Estrogen stimulates endometrial re-epithelialization, proliferation and stabilizes lysosomal enzymes.
- In hemodynamically, unstable patients:
  - Intravenous estrogen therapy (25 mg conjugated equine estrogen 4 hourly) given until bleeding stops (usually avoided because of increased risk of thrombosis)

    ↓

    Oral high-dose estrogen therapy (2.5 mg conjugated estrogen or 2 mg micronized estradiol) every 4 hour, tapering to a once daily dose after bleeding is controlled is given[16]

    ↓

    After 14–21 days either progesterone (medroxyprogesterone acetate 5–10 mg daily for 7–10 days) or estrogen-progesterone combination can be started.

    Chronic anovulation may be associated with polycystic ovaries, androgen excess and insulin resistance. For regulation of menstrual cycle above described regimens can be used but associated other symptoms and their management is as follows:

Hirsutism

- **Combined estrogen-progesterone contraception (COC)**

  Pharmacology:

  They reduce androgen by following mechanism:
  - Inhibition of LH relase and thus decrease ovarian androgen production
  - Increase SHBG
  - Reduce DHEAS production
  - Reduction in 5 alpha-reductase activity
  - Low dose oral contraception (containing 20–35 μg ethinyl estradiol) are used
  - Estrogen induces a dose dependent increase in serum SHBG.[17,18]
  - Contraceptive progestins have variable effect on SHBG.
  - Drospirenone, a derivative of spironolactone, has some intrinsic antiandrogenic properties, used with estrogen in COC.
  - Around 60–100% of women report improvement in their hirsutism during treatment with oral contraceptives.[17]
  - Transdermal patch (delivering 20 μg ethinyl estradiol and 150 μg norelgestromin daily) and vaginal ring (releasing 15 μg ethinyl estradiol and 120 μg etonogestrel daily) can be used.
- **Progesterone only:**
  - For those who cannot tolerate combined preparation
  - MDPA 150 mg intramuscularly every 3 months or oral 10–20 mg daily is given
  - Progesterone also increases testosterone clearance due to induction of hepatic enzyme activity.
- **Antiandrogens (Table 28.3)**

Insulin Sensitizers

Biguanides

Metformin

Pharmacology

- Biguanide oral insulin-sensitizing agent
- Metformin is absorbed primarily in the small intestine. The drug does not bind to plasma proteins, and is excreted unchanged in the urine. It has a short half-life of about 2 hours.
- It reduces hepatic glucose production, glucose uptake in the small intestine, increases peripheral insulin sensitivity and also inhibits lipolysis.
- Its mode of action consists of the adenosine monophosphate-activated protein kinase pathway in liver and skeletal muscles.

Dosage

250 or 500 mg bd or tds.

Table 28.3 Antiandrogens

Name	*Mechanism of action*	*Absorption and elimination*	*Dose*	*Side effect*
Spironolactone	• Aldosterone antagonist having structural similarity to progestins • Androgen receptor antagonist competing with dihydrotestosterone (DHT) for binding to androgen receptor[19]	It gets absorbed partially (65%), metabolized extensively in liver and also undergoes enterohepatic circulation[20]	50–100 mg BD	Diuresis, diarrhea, gastritis, peptic ulcer, hyperkalemia, skin rashes fatigue[20]
Cyproterone acetate	• Derivative of 17-alpha hydroxyprogesterone • Potent progestational activity, inhibits gonadotropin secretion • Antiandrogenic	Similar to progestins	2 mg combined with estrogen[21]	Fatigue, loss of libido, edema, weight gain, and mastalgia
Flutamide	• Androgen receptor antagonist	• After absorption, flutamide is quickly α-hydroxylated to its primary active form, hydroxyflutamide. • It is excreted in urine as being 2-amino-5-nitro-4-(trifluoromethyl) phenol	250–750 mg daily[22]	Hepatotoxicity
Eflornithine hydrochloride	• Inhibitor of ornithine decarboxylase, an enzyme active in dermal papilla that is essential for hair growth	• Low degree of percutaneous absorption and excreted in urine unchanged[23]	Twice daily	Relatively safe

Side effects

- Nausea, vomiting, constipation, diarrhea, bloating, flatulence, heartburn, metallic taste.
- Lactic acidosis is a rare complication and therefore the drug should be avoided in patients with renal insufficiency, liver disease or alcohol abuse.[24]
- Interferes with the absorption of vitamin B_{12}. Hence, high doses can cause B_{12} deficiency

Thiazolidinediones

Pharmacology

- Synthetic agonists for the peroxisome proliferator-activated receptor gamma, which serves as a nuclear transcription factor in the regulation of genes involved in carbohydrate, lipid and protein metabolism.
- Well absorbed from the GI tract.
- Metabolized by the liver
- Can be administered to patients with renal dysfunction but should be avoided if there is active hepatic disease or significant elevations of serum liver transaminases and also in CHF.
- They include rosiglitazone and pioglitazone.
- Metabolization of rosiglitazone occurs by hepatic cytochrome P450 (CYP) 2C8, whereas pioglitazone is metabolized by CYP3A4 and CYP2C8.

- Failure of oral contraception may occur during pioglitazone therapy.

Side effects: Have been associated with cardiac complications, however limited studies are available.

Heavy Menstrual Bleeding

Treatment of abnormal uterine bleeding (AUB) is mainly medical management. **Table 28.4** lists the drugs used in heavy menstrual bleeding.[25] The pharmacology of different drugs used for heavy menstrual bleeding is given in **Table 28.5**.

Dysmenorrhea

Many associated pathologies like endometriosis, adenomyosis, fibroid uterus and pelvic inflammatory diseases can lead to pain during menstruation.

Prostaglandins and leukotrienes have been identified in increased concentrations in women with dysmenorrhea. Despite medical management of pain only, many cases need etiology directed therapy also to reduce pain during cycles.

NSAIDs

- If woman wishes to avoid contraception, NSAIDs are effective treatment. No particular NSAIDs recommended. Paracetamol and codeine may be used in addition.
- NSAIDs provide relief in pain in 70–90% of patients.
- Patients exhibit variations in response to different NSAIDs.
- Side effects are gastrointestinal irritation.

Oral Contraceptives

- Best suited for sexually active women who need contraception also
- They inhibit ovulation, thereby decrease the endometrial prostaglandin production.
- Two regimens can be used:
  - *Standard cyclic regimen*: 21–24 active pills followed by 4–7 inactive pills.
  - *Extended cyclic regimen*: Active pills for 12 weeks continuously followed by 7 pills that are inactive or contain low dose estrogen only.

Table 28.4 Drugs used in the management of heavy menstrual bleeding

Nonhormonal treatment	*Hormonal treatment*
Nonsteroidal anti-inflammatory drugs (NSAIDs) • Cyclooxygenase-1 inhibitors – Salicylates- aspirin – Indoleacetic acid analogs—indomethacin – Aryl propionic acid derivative—naproxen, ibuprofen – Fenamates—mefenamic acid, meclofenamic acid • Cyclooxygenase 2 inhibitors – Coxibs—celecoxib, refecoxib *Antifibrinolytic* • Tranexamic acid *Others* • Ethamsylate	*Oral progesterone* • Norethisterone • Medroxyprogesterone acetate • Dihydrogesterone *Intrauterine progestogens* • Levonorgestrel IUCD • Progestasert IUCD *Combined estrogen/progestogens* • Oral contraceptives • Hormone replacement therapy *Other* • Danazol • Gestrinone • GnRH analog • Mifepristone

Table 28.5 Pharmacology of drugs used for menstruation bleeding

Drugs	*Mechanism of action*	*Absorption and elimination*	*Doses*	*Efficacy*	*Side effects*
NSAIDs	• Inhibit prostaglandin synthesis • Fenmates bind to prostaglandin receptors also	• Rapidly absorbed from the GI tract • Peak concentrations occurring within 1–4 hours • Food tends to delay its absorption • Most NSAIDs are 95–99% protein-bound and undergo hepatic metabolism and renal excretion	Fenmates—500 mg tds from day 1 to day 5 of cycle	• Reduction of blood loss by 20–49% • COX 1 inhibitors also improve menstrual pain	Gastrointestinal irritation
Antifibrinolytics	Plasminogen activator inhibitors	• Absorbed from GI tract • Oral bioavailability is 34% • Food does not affect absorption	2–4.5 g/day for 4 – 7 days	• Reduction of blood loss by 29-58% • Effect superior to mefenamic acid and luteal phase norethisterone	Gastrointestinal complaints
Ethamsylate	Reduces capillary fragility	• Absorbed from GI tract • Eliminated in urine (unchanged) • Also excreted in breast milk	50 mg 8 hourly for 5 days	Blood loss reduction –not significant	Headache, skin rash, nausea
Oral progestogens Norethisterone	19-nortestosterone derivative. Has intrinsic weak estrogenic, weak androgenic, anabolic and strong anti-ovulatory action	Discussed above	5 mg tds from day 5 to day 26	• Blood loss reduction by 83% • Less effective than LNG-IUS	• Weight gain, headache, bloatedness

Contd...

Contd...

Drugs	*Mechanism of action*	*Absorption and elimination*	*Doses*	*Efficacy*	*Side effects*
Intrauterine progesterone LNG-IUS (Mirena) Progestasert (withdrawn)	Local effect on endometrium	—	Delivers 20 µg of levonorgestrel over 24 hours for 5 years	• Blood loss reduction by 71–90% after 12 months of use • NICE guidelines recommends as the first line treatment provided long-term use is anticipated • Patient satisfaction comparable to endometrial ablation	• Progestasert—risk of ectopic therefore has been withdrawn from the market • Frequently occurring variable bleeding and spotting
Danazol	• It is an isoxazol derivative of 17 alpha-ethinyl-testosterone • Has weak androgenic and weak progestational effect • Acts on hypothalamic-pituitary axis and on endometrium to produce atrophy	• After oral administration, peak concentration reaches within 2–4 hours • Metabolized and excreted in urine in form of 2-hydroxymethyl Danazol and ethisterone	200–800 mg daily in two to four divided doses	• Reduces blood loss by 50% • More effective than placebo, progestogen, NSAIDs	• Androgenic side effects (weight gain, muscle cramps, acne, hirsutism) • Hepatotoxicity • Additional contraception needed as it causes virilization of fetus
Gestrinone	• 19-nortestosterone derivative • Antiprogestogenic activity. Anti-estrogenic and androgenic activity	Similar to progesterone	—	Reduces blood loss by 79%	• Androgenic side effects • Contraception needed
GnRH agonists	Downregulation of expression of GnRH receptors	—	Leuprolide acetate 6.6 mg intradermal implant	Mainly used in fibroid-associated bleeding	Osteoporosis
Antiprogestogens Progesterone receptor modulators- • Mifepristone (RU- 486) • Asoprisnil (selective)	• Inhibit ovulation • Disrupts endometrial integrity		5 mg per day	• Reduces blood loss by 83% • Have major role in fibroid associated bleeding	Endometrial hyperplasia

Intrauterine Devices

If contraception is also needed, LNG-IUS is excellent choice but the woman should be made aware about irregular bleeding especially during initial months.

Menstrual Migraine

Headaches that occur exclusively in association with menses.

Triptans

Pharmacology

They are 5-HT1-Receptor Agonists:

- When given subcutaneously, peak plasma concentration of sumatriptan is achieved in approximately 12 minutes. Bioavailability is approximately 97%.
- Peak plasma concentrations occur within 1–2 hours after oral administration with bioavailability of only 14–17%.
- The half-life of triptan is approximately 1 to 2 hours. After being metabolized by MAO-A, metabolites are excreted in the urine.
- Well absorbed orally.
- Triptans inhibit the release of vasoactive peptides, promote vasoconstriction and inhibit neurotransmission in trigeminal nucleus.

Dosage

- Treatment of acute menstrual migraine is serotonin agonists (triptans)
  - Sumatriptan = 50–100 mg
  - Rizatriptan =10 mg
  - Frovatriptan = 2.5 mg
- For prevention of migraine episode both hormonal and nonhormonal methods can be used.

a. Combined Oral Contraceptive Formulations

- Hormonal methods aim either to eliminate or minimize premenstrual decline in serum estrogen level:
  - Extended cyclic oral contraception or standard formulations may help these women, but estrogen supplementation is needed during placebo period.
- Oral contraceptive use is discouraged in women over 35 years whose migraine is associated with focal neurological signs or symptoms because of increased risk of stroke.

Estrogen Only

- In women with contraindications to oral contraceptives, estrogen supplement can be done at the end of the cycle.
- It is started just before the onset of menstruation and continued for a total 7 days.
- Transdermal patch (0.1 mg/day) or gel (1.5 mg/day) are effective.

b. Nonhormonal Therapy

- Treatment with NSAIDs, beginning 7 days before onset and continuing through the end of the menses is helpful in prevention.
- Sumatriptan 25 mg 3 times a day beginning 2–3 days before menses and continuing up to 5–6 days is effective regimen for prevention.

Premenstrual Syndrome and Premenstrual Dysphoric Disorder

Drugs used are as follows:

Serotonin Reuptake Inhibitors

- They inhibit reuptake of serotonin at the nerve terminals.
- Well absorbed orally.
- CNS and plasma elimination half-life may differ for different SSRIs

  Dosage:
  - Fluoxetine = 20 mg OD
  - Sertraline = 50–150 mg OD
  - Paroxetine = 20–30 mg OD
  - Citalopram = 20–30 mg OD
  - Venlafaxine = 50–200 mg OD (inhibits reuptake of both serotonin and Nor-epinephrine (NE)).
- These drugs can be administered either on a continuous daily basis or as intermittent regimen at the time of onset of symptoms.

- Side effects are nausea, nervousness, agitation or restlessness, dizziness, reduced libido, drowsiness, insomnia, weight gain or loss, headache. They can cause major malformations, particularly cardiac defects when used during pregnancy.

Alprazolam

- It is a drug belonging to benzodiazepine group.
- Rapidly absorbed from GI tract.
- Undergoes hepatic metabolism-oxidation followed by conjugation and metabolites are primarily excreted in urine.
- It reaches peak blood level within 1–2 hours.
- It enhances the effect of neurotransmitter Gamma-aminobutyric acid (GABA) at GABA receptors.
- It mainly relieves depressive symptoms.
- Used intermittently.
- Side effects include addictive potentials, cognitive dysfunction.

Gonadotropin-releasing Hormone Agonists

- It induces medical menopause and more effective for relieving irritability and physical symptoms.
- Treatment with GnRH agonist may induce hypoestrogenic state and bone mineral depletion on prolonged use.

Oral Contraception or Progesterone

- Newer oral contraceptives containing drosperinone are effect in eliminating variety of symptoms of PMS including behavioral and mood symptoms.
- Progesterone is not considered as an effective treatment of PMS.

Secondary Amenorrhea

- There can be problem at any level in hypothalamo-pitutary-ovarian axis or in the uterus itself leading to amenorrhea.
- In case of premature deficiency of sex steroid hormones in the body, a woman will need it from exogenous source.
- Various important causes of secondary amenorrhea and their management are as follows:

Premature Ovarian Failure

The mainstay of treatment consists of estrogen replacement therapy and is recommended till the time of natural menopause. Combined estrogen-progesterone pills or HRT may be used.

Dosage

- Micronized estradiol = 1–2 mg daily
- Conjugated equine estrogen = 0.625–1.25 mg daily

  or

  Transdermal patch = 0.1 mg/24 hours

  +

  Progesterone

  (micronized progesterone—200 mg daily or MDPA 10 mg daily for 12–14 days).
- Estrogen supplementation decreases the risk of osteoporosis, dementia, cardiovascular disease and Parkinsonism. Women with POF who are receiving HRT may require higher doses of estrogen in order to relieve vasomotor symptoms. Persistent complaints of decreased libido or sexual dysfunction can be managed by testosterone supplementation.
- Non-estrogen based regimen, such as strontium ranelate, bisphosphonates or raloxifene are not recommended in women with POF.
- No added risk of breast cancer by estrogen replacement in women with POF is seen, therefore screening mammography is not needed in early phase.

Prolactinoma

- Dopamine agonists are the mainstay of treatment for functional prolactinoma of all sizes.
- They effectively lower prolactin levels and decreases the size of more than 90% of such tumors.

a. Cabergoline

Pharmacology

- It is an ergot derivative, selective dopamine receptor type 2 (D2) agonist, which is longer acting (t1/2 >60 days)
- It is orally administered without regard to meals
- It has greater efficacy, more potency in restoring normal prolactin levels in women with lactotroph adenoma and fewer side effects than bromocriptine.

Dosage: 0.25 mg twice weekly to be started with and can be increased guided by serum prolactin levels at monthly intervals.

Contraindication

- It is associated with hypertrophic valvular heart disease after long-term use. It is contraindicated in patients with known sensitivity to ergot derivatives and in uncontrolled hypertension.
- It is category B drug for use in pregnancy.
- It decreases milk production in lactating mothers.
- Vaginal preparation is also available for those who cannot tolerate oral preparation.

Side effects

- Nausea, constipation, headache, abdominal pain, dizziness, asthenia, fatigue, somnolence are common side effects.

b. Bromocriptine

Pharmacology

- It has agonist action at dopamine receptor D2 and various serotonin receptors. By reversing glutamate GLUT 1 transporter, it also inhibits the release of glutamate.[26]
- Activates dopaminergic receptors on lactotrophs (anti-galactopoietic) which in turn decreases prolactin release from the pituitary
- Absorbed from GI tract and peak plasma level reaches within 1 hour after oral administration.[27]
- Usually well tolerated. Some side effects like nausea, vomiting and postural hypotension may be present initially but usually weans off with time.
- It is excreted in bile and feces.
- Less efficacious than cabergolin.

Dosage

- 1.25 mg at bedtime to start with and then the dose is gradually increased.

Contraindications

- It can lead to increase in size of tumor during pregnancy, therefore should be stopped once pregnancy is diagnosed.[28]
- As it is also a ergot derivative, therefore should not be used in patients with uncontrolled hypertension.

REFERENCES

1. Fraser IS, Critchley HO, Munro MG, Broder M. A process designed to lead to international agreement on terminologies and definitions used to describe abnormalities of menstrual bleeding. Fertil Steril. 2007;87(3):466-76.
2. Herrington J, Carter-Su C. Signaling pathway activated by the growth hormone receptor. Trends Endocrinol Metab. 2001;12: 252-7.
3. Parker KL, Schimmer BP. Pituitary hormones and their hypothalamic releasing hormones. In: Brunton LL, Lazo JS, Parker KL. Goodman and Gilman's: The Pharmacological Basis of Therapeutics, 11th edn. 2006.
4. Medvei VC. The History of Clinical Endocrinology. The Parthenon Publishing Group, New York, 1993.
5. O'Dowd MJ, Philipp EE. The History of Obstetrics and Gynaecology. The Parthenon Publishing Group, New York, 1994.
6. Speert H. Obstetric & Gynecologic Milestones Illustrated. The Parthenon Publishing Group, New York, 1996.
7. Sneader W. The discovery of oestrogenic hormones. J Br Menopause Soc. 2000;129.
8. Loose DS, Stancel GM. Estrogens and progestins-estrogens and progestins: introduction. In: Brunton LL, Lazo JS, Parker KL (Eds). Goodman and Gilman's: The Pharmacological Basis of Therapeutics, 11th edn. 2006.
9. Sung JH, An HS, Jeong JH, Shin S, Song SY. Megestrol acetate increases the proliferation, migration and adipogenic differentiation of adipose-derived stem cells via glucocorticoid receptor. Stem Cells Transl Med. 2015;4(7): 789-99.

10. Duax WL, Griffin JF, Weeks CM, Wawrzak Z. The mechanism of action of steroid antagonists: insights from crystallographic studies. J Steroid Biochem. 1988;31:481-92.
11. McDonnell DP, Goldman ME. RU486 exerts antiestrogenic activities through a novel progesterone receptor A form-mediated mechanism. J Biol Chem. 1994;269:11945-9.
12. Bayer SR, DeCherney AH. Clinical manifestations and treatment of dysfunctional uterine bleeding. JAMA. 1993;269(14):1823-28.
13. Aksu F, Madazli R, Budak E, Cepni I, Benian A. High-dose medroxyprogesterone acetate for the treatment of dysfunctional uterine bleeding in 24 adolescents. Aust NZJ Obstet Gynaecol. 1997;37:228.
14. Munro MG, Mainor N, Basu R, Brisinger M, Barreda L. Oral medroxyprogesterone acetate and combination oral contraceptives for acute uterine bleeding: A randomized controlled trial. Obstet Gynecol. 2006;108:924-9.
15. Nelson L, Rybo G. Treatment of menorrhagia. Am J Obstet Gynecol. 1971;110:713.
16. DeVore GR, Owens O, Kase N. Use of intravenous premarin in the treatment of dysfunctional uterine bleeding: A double-blind randomized control study. Obstet Gynecol. 1982;59:285.
17. Zupi E, Zullo F, Marconi D, Sbracia M, Pellicano M, Solima E, Sorrenti G, Hysteroscopic endometrial resection versus laparoscopic supracervical hysterectomy for menorrhagia: A prospective randomized trial. Am J Obstet Gynecol. 2003;188:7.
18. Lo JS, Pickersgill A. Pregnancy after endometrial ablation: English literature review and case report. J Minim Invasive Gynecol. 2006;13:88.
19. Young RL, Goldzieher JW, Elkind-Hirsch K. The endocrine effects of spironolactone used as an antiandrogen. Fertil Steril. 1987;48:223.
20. Jackson EK. Diuretics: introduction. In: Brunton LL, Lazo JS, Parker KL. Drugs affecting renal and cardiovascular function. Goodman and Gilman's: The Pharmacological Basis of Therapeutics, 11th edn. 2006.
21. Belisle S, Love EJ. Clinical efficacy and safety of cyproterone acetate in severe hirsutism: Results of a multicentered Canadian study. Fertil Steril. 1986;46:1015.
22. Venturoli S, Marescalchi O, Colombo FM, Macrelli S, Ravaioli B, Bagnoli A, et al. A prospective randomized trial comparing low dose flutamide, finasteride, ketoconazole, and cyproterone acetate-estrogen regimens in the treatment of hirsutism. J Clin Endocrinol Metab. 1999;84:1304.
23. Malhotra B, Noveck R, Behr D, Palmisano M. Percutaneous absorption and pharmacokinetics of eflornithine HCl 13.9% cream in women with unwanted facial hair. J Clin Pharmacol. 2001;41(9):972-8.
24. Mosconi G, Gambaretto C, Zambianchi L, Lifrieri F, De Fabritiis M, Cristino S, et al. Metformin-associated lactic acidosis. G Ital Nefrol. 2015;32(4).
25. Quinn S, Higham J. Available management options for heavy menstrual bleeding [online]. Available from-http://onlinelibrary.wiley.com/doi/10.1002/psb.1245/pdf
26. Elaine Sanders-Bush, Steven E Mayer. 5-hydroxytryptamine (serotonin): receptor agonists and antagonists-5-hydroxytryptamine (serotonin): receptor. In: Brunton LL, Lazo JS, Parker KL. Drugs acting at synaptic and neuroeffector junction sites. Goodman and Gilman's: The Pharmacological Basis of Therapeutics, 11th edn. 2006.
27. Ralph A. DeFronzo. Bromocriptine: A sympatholytic, D2-dopamine agonist for the treatment of type 2 diabetes. Diabetes Care. 2011;34(4):789-94.
28. Ciccarelli E1, Camanni F. Diagnosis and drug therapy of prolactinoma. Drugs. 1996;51(6): 954-65.

Section VIII

REPRODUCTIVE ENDOCRINOLOGY

CHAPTERS

CHAPTER 29

Polycystic Ovary Syndrome, Hirsutism and Hyperprolactinemia

Anjali Tempe, Komal Rastogi

Polycystic ovary syndrome (PCOS) is one of the most common endocrine disorders in women of reproductive age group. It affects 5–10% of women worldwide. It is characterized by a combination of chronic anovulation, hyperandrogenism, and polycystic ovaries. Management of women with PCOS depends on the symptoms and includes (A) treatment of menstrual dysfunction, (B) treatment of ovulatory dysfunction-related infertility, (C) treatment of metabolic dysfunction and (D) treatment of androgen-related symptoms (**Table 29.1**).

Table 29.1: Drugs used in PCOS

Menstrual dysfunction	Estrogen-progestin contraceptives
Infertility	Clomiphene citrate
	Aromatase inhibitors
	Exogenous gonadotropins
Prevention of metabolic syndrome	Metformin
	Thiazolidinediones
	Myo-inositol and D-chiro-inositol
	Statins
Androgen related symptoms (hirsutism and acne)	Estrogen-progestin contraceptives
	Anti-androgens

WEIGHT REDUCTION

Weight loss improves endocrine profile and ovulatory function, thereby increasing pregnancy rates and also possibly decreases the risk for miscarriage. Even small reduction in weight (2–5%) can result in normalization of the menstrual cycles and improvement in ovulatory function.[1] Weight loss also increases sex hormone-binding globulin (SHBG) concentrations and reduces free androgen levels. Hence, weight reduction is the first treatment for obese women with PCOS.

TREATMENT OF MENSTRUAL DYSFUNCTION

Due to chronic anovulation, obesity, and hyperinsulinemia, PCOS patients are at increased risk of developing endometrial hyperplasia and carcinoma.[2] Overall, the risk for developing endometrial cancer may be increased by as much as 3-fold. Hence, endometrial biopsy should be considered in patients with PCOS who have not had menstrual bleeding for a year or longer. Estrogen-progestin contraceptives are most commonly used for the treatment of menstrual abnormalities associated with chronic anovulation because they induce regular cyclic menses and attenuate endometrial growth. In those who have a contraindication to the use of estrogen-progestin contraceptives, cyclic or continuous progestins can be used. Estrogen-progestin contraceptives also reduce ovarian androgen production and may be particularly beneficial. Metformin is another alternative that can restore ovulatory menses in many women with PCOS. However, results vary widely and may require up to 6 months of treatment before they are known.[3,4]

Infertility

Chronic anovulation is one of the most common causes of infertility. In women with PCOS, other factors relating to oocyte quality or endometrial and implantation abnormalities, also might contribute.[5] Infertile anovulatory women who want to conceive are candidates for ovulation induction.

Clomiphene Citrate

Clomiphene citrate is the first drug of choice for ovulation induction in these patients. It is economical, requires little monitoring and has few adverse effects.

Pharmacology: Clomiphene citrate is an estrogen receptor antagonist. It interferes with negative feedback effect of estrogen, resulting in increased availability of FSH. Increased FSH levels lead to follicular growth, followed by an LH surge and ovulation.

Dosage: It is administered in dosage of 50–150 mg for 5 days, starting on days 3 or 5 of menstrual cycle. Clomiphene induces ovulation successfully in 70–80% of women.[6,7] The cumulative pregnancy rate with clomiphene treatment is approximately 50% after three induced ovulatory cycles, and approaches 75% within 6–9 cycles of treatment.[8] The risk for multiple gestation is approximately 5–8%. Approximately, 20% of the patients prove refractory to clompihene treatment, most of those having severe hyperandrogenism or obesity.

Tamoxifen is another ovulatory agent that has the same mechanism of action as clomiphene citrate, but it does not have any antiestrogenic effect on the cervix and endometrium. Tamoxifen can be used as an alternative to clomiphene citrate in case of clomiphene citrate resistance or failure. Treatment with insulin sensitizing agents can increase ovulation rates in some women with PCOS. Metformin has been used widely for that purpose.

Aromatase Inhibitors

Pharmacology: Anastrozole and letrozole are triazole derivatives that act as potent, competitive, nonsteroidal inhibitors of aromatase. Aromatase is an enzyme which catalyzes the rate-limiting step in estrogen production. Letrozole inhibits estrogen production in the hypothalamus-pituitary axis, which results in compensatory increase in gonadotropin-releasing hormone (GnRH) and FSH and stimulates ovarian follicular development. Letrozole does not have peripheral anti-estrogenic effects on the endometrium and stimulates monofollicular growth.[9]

Dosage: Letrozole (2.5–5 mg daily) or anastrozole (1 mg daily) is given for 5 days and may be accompanied by exogenous gonadotropins and human chorionic gonadotropin trigger (hCG; 10,000 IU) in order to program the ovulation.

Aromatase inhibitors have similar efficacy as that of clomiphene for ovulation induction, they can also be used in clomiphene-resistant anovulatorywomen.Theymayalsobeconsidered for women who respond to clomiphene but exhibit grossly poor endometrial proliferation. Though early preliminary data suggested that they might have significant fetal toxicity, studies have found no evidence to indicate that birth defects are more common in children conceived after treatment with aromatase inhibitors than in those conceived naturally or after treatment with clomiphene citrate.[10,11] However, letrozole is at present not approved by drug controller of India for ovulation induction.

Exogenous Gonadotropins

Exogenous gonadotropins are the second line of therapy after resistance to clomiphene citrate in women with PCOS. Gonadotropins act by inducing ovulation, maintaining optimum follicle growth via their controlled administration, in order to achieve a follicle capable of being fertilized. Gonadotropins do not have a peripheral antiestrogenic effect which is a problem with clomiphene citrate. Ovulation induction with exogenous gonadotropins is highly effective, but is expensive, time consuming and requires careful monitoring to avoid the risks of multiple pregnancy and ovarian hyperstimulation syndrome (OHSS). OHSS is an iatrogenic complication of ovulation induction with exogenous gonadotropins, characterized by increased capillary permeability mediated by increased production of vasoactive substances including vascular endothelial growth factor (VEGF), elements of rennin-angiotensin system and other cytokines.[12]

Several treatment protocols have been advocated, such as step-up, low-dose step-up, and step-down regimens. Ovarian hyperstimulation, higher risks of multiple pregnancy, and the expense and frustration associated with canceled cycles usually can be avoided by using a "low-slow" treatment regimen involving low doses (37.5–75 IU daily), small increments, and a longer duration of stimulation. hCG is administered to trigger ovum release, it leads to maturation of the oocyte, rupture of the follicle, and formation of the corpus luteum. The step-down regimen starts with the maximum recommended dose (150–225 IU daily), which is reduced gradually in order to promote continued development of only the more sensitive dominant follicle. Insulin resistant women may be less sensitive to gonadotropin stimulation. In such women, metformin treatment before and during gonadotropin stimulation can help to improve response, limit the number of smaller developing follicles[13] and reduce the likelihood of cycle cancelation for excessive stimulation.[14]

No response with six cycles of gonadotropins signifies resistance. Hence, a maximum of six cycles with gonadotropins are recommended.

In Vitro Fertilization

Infertility is a problem in PCOS patients in general, because of anovulation that conceptually is not an indication for *in vitro* fertilization techniques. IVF techniques are used when treatments with clomiphene citrate, exogenous gonadotropins, and letrozole have failed as a last resort. IVF techniques are the first choice in PCOS patients having other additional factors like severe endometriosis, tubal factor infertility, mild male factor infertility that reduce the effectiveness of other techniques. Ovulation induction by exogenous gonadotropins in anovulatory women with PCOS has increased risk of multiple gestations (up to 10%). IVF is a reasonable alternative for women seeking pregnancy as IVF with a single embryo transfer significantly reduces the risk of multiple gestations. IVF also allows for cryopreservation of embryos, with transfer of a single embryo in a subsequent cycle with endometrial but not ovarian stimulation.

Several stimulation protocols can be used for the treatment of patients with PCOS undergoing IVF, including combinations or isolated use of clomiphene, human menopausal gonadotropins, recombinant FSH, GnRH agonists, and GnRH antagonists. Women with PCOS are at increased risk for developing OHSS. The smaller follicular cohorts observed in antagonist cycles may help to reduce the risk of OHSS. The use of antagonist also provides the opportunity to use an agonist instead of hCG to induce final oocyte maturation, thereby further decreasing the risk of OHSS.[15] Patients with PCOS have similar IVF outcomes as that of patients without PCOS, which implies that PCOS does not intervene in embryo implantation.

PREVENTION OF METABOLIC SYNDROME

Insulin Sensitizers

Metformin

Pharmacology: Metformin is a biguanide and an oral insulin-sensitizing agent. It is approved by the US Food and Drug Administration (FDA) for management of type 2 diabetes mellitus. Metformin treatment increases insulin sensitivity and decreases weight, BMI, blood pressure and LDL-cholesterol. Metformin improves menstrual cyclicity, ovulatory function, and reduces circulating androgen levels.[16] Metabolic benefits are enhanced in the presence of weight loss, and weight loss itself may be enhanced in the presence of metformin.[17]

Mechanism of action: Metformin primarily inhibits hepatic gluconeogenesis. It decreases intestinal glucose uptake and increases insulin sensitivity in peripheral tissues. Metformin also decreases circulating concentrations of free fatty acids by inhibiting lipolysis, which further helps to reduce hepatic gluconeogenesis. Metformin helps in improving ovulation induction in women with PCOS through a variety of actions. It acts by reducing insulin levels and altering the effect of insulin on ovarian androgen production, theca cell proliferation, and endometrial growth. In addition, it directly inhibits ovarian gluconeogenesis and thus reduces ovarian androgen production.

Pharmacokinetics: Plasma half-life of metformin is one and half hour to three hours. It is excreted unchanged by kidney. The clearance of metformin approximates glomerular filtration rate. In renal failure, it may accumulate and increase the risk of lactic acidosis.

Indications: Metformin should be used in women with impaired glucose tolerance or diabetes, those with obvious evidence of severe insulin resistance (acanthosis nigricans),[18] and women having other features of the metabolic syndrome, such as central obesity, dyslipidemia, and hypertension. In these patients, metformin helps in preventing or slowing progression to type 2 diabetes and reduces long-term risks for cardiovascular disease.

To define the exact role of metformin in ovulation induction, it is crucial to distinguish two different indications. In PCOS patients, metformin has been shown to improve ovulation rates as compared with placebo, but no significant advantage of metformin was observed over clomiphene citrate with respect to ovulation, pregnancy, or livebirth rates.[19] Therefore, metformin is not used as a first choice for ovulation induction. The combination of metformin and clomiphene citrate is not better than clomiphene citrate or metformin monotherapy in PCOS patients.[20] In PCOS patients with resistance to clomiphene citrate, no benefit of metformin monotherapy was observed over placebo with respect to ovulation, pregnancy, and livebirth rates, but the combination of metformin and clomiphene citrate significantly improved ovulation and pregnancy rates when compared with clomiphene citrate alone. However, no significant improvement was observed in terms of livebirth rates.[21] Hence, pretreatment with metformin improves the efficacy of clomiphene citrate in PCOS patients with clomiphene citrate resistance.

Contraindications: Metformin is contraindicated in presence of renal diseases, acute or chronic metabolic acidosis and in case of hypersensitivity to metformin hydrochloride.

Dosage: Several dose regimens have been proposed.[17] To improve patient tolerance and decrease side effects, metformin is started with a low dose (500 mg daily) with food. The dose is increased to 1000 mg after one week for another week and then to 1500 mg daily. The target dose is 500 or 850 mg three times daily (1500–2550 mg/day). Clinical response is usually seen at the dose of 1000 mg daily.

Adverse effects: Nausea and diarrhea are the most common adverse effects of metformin. Lactic acidosis may occur and has been described mainly in patients with congestive heart failure, renal impairment, and sepsis.

Abdominal pain, anorexia are other side effects. Metformin may also cause vitamin B_{12} deficiency as it interferes with its absorption.

Drug interactions: Cimetidine may cause increase in plasma concentration of metformin as it reduces metformin clearance by the kidneys. Cephalexin may also increase plasma concentration of metformin by same mechanism.

Preparations: Tablets Glyciphage and Glycomet 500 mg and 850 mg.

Safety during pregnancy and lactation: Metformin is FDA approved pregnancy category B drug and is safe during pregnancy. Metformin is secreted in breast milk and should be used with caution while nursing premature infants and infants with renal impairment.

Thiazolidinediones

Pharmacology: Thiazolidinediones are another type of insulin-sensitizing agents which have been used to improve insulin resistance in women with PCOS. They include rosiglitazone, pioglitazone and formerly troglitazone (withdrawn from the market due to concerns about liver toxicity).

Mechanism of action: Thiazolidinediones are nuclear peroxisome proliferator-activated receptor gamma agonists which enhance the transcription of several insulin responsive genes. They stimulate *GLUT4* expression and translocation which improves entry of glucose into muscle and fat and help in reversing insulin resistance. They also activate genes regulating fatty acid metabolism and lipogenesis in adipose tissue which further contributes to the insulin sensitizing action.

Pharmacokinetics: Plasma half-life of rosiglitazone is 4 hours and of pioglitazone is 3–5 hours. Both drugs are metabolized in liver. Rosiglitazone is metabolized by *CYP2C8* and pioglitazone is metabolized by both *CYP3A4* and *CYP2C8*. Failure of oral contraception may occur during pioglitazone therapy.

Indications: Thiazolidinediones are used for the treatment of type 2 diabetes mellitus. Rosiglitazone in a dose of 8 mg/day, improves insulin sensitivity and enhances both spontaneous and clomiphene-induced ovulation in women with PCOS. Pioglitazone also appears to be effective; however, the studies with pioglitazone are limited.

Contraindications: Thiazolidinediones are contraindicated in liver diseases and congestive heart failure.

Dosage: Rosiglitazone is given in a dose of 8 mg/day. Recommended dose of pioglitazone is 15–45 mg/day.

Adverse effects: Thiazolidinediones may cause plasma volume expansion, edema and weight gain. Headache and myalgia may occur. Cases of hepatic dysfunction have been reported and congestive heart failure (CHF) may be precipitated or worsened.

Drug interactions: As pioglitazone is metabolized by both *CYP3A4* and *CYP2C8*, failure of oral contraception may occur. Metabolism of pioglitazone is inhibited by ketoconazole. Drug interactions are less marked with rosiglitazone.

Preparations: Tablet Reglit 2, 4, 8 mg and tablet Pionorm 15 mg and 30 mg.

Safety during pregnancy: Both rosiglitazone and pioglitazone have little short-term risk but fetal safety with these drugs has not been established. These drugs belong to pregnancy category C of the US FDA guidelines. Hence, if used, these drugs should be discontinued as soon as pregnancy is established.

Though thiazolidinediones improves insulin sensitivity, overall experience with them is quite limited and they have been associated with cardiac complications. Metformin is better than thiazolidinediones in improving insulin sensitivity and currently is the preffered insulin-sensitizing agent for women with PCOS.[22,23]

Myo-inositol/Myoinositol and D-chiro-inositol Combination

Pharmacology: Inositol is a physiological compound belonging to the sugar family.

Myo-inositol and D-chiroinositol are the two main inositol stereoisomers present in our body. Myo-inositol is the precursor of inositol triphosphate which is a second messenger and regulates many hormones such as insulin, FSH and TSH. D-chiroinositol is synthetized by conversion of myo-inositol into D-chiroinositol by an insulin-dependent epimerase.

Mechanism of action: In PCOS patients, administration of myo and/or D-chiroinositol has been shown to improve insulin sensitivity. Myo-inositol produces second messengers for glucose uptake and D-chiroinositol provides second messengers which promote glucose uptake and glycogen synthesis.

Indications: Combination of Myo-inositol and D-chiro-inositol can be used for the treatment of PCOS. Myo-inositol and D-chiroinositol have been shown to improve insulin resistance, restore regular menstrual cycles, induce ovulation and improve hyperandrogenism in PCOS women.[24,25] In IVF cycles, treatment of PCOS women with myoinositol before hormonal stimulation increases the quality of oocytes and embryos.[26] In IVF cycles for myo-inositol to be effective, it should be given preferably 3 months prior to ovarian stimulation. The combination of myo-inositol plus D-chiroinositol has also been seen to reduce the cardiovascular risk in PCOS women.

Dosage: Combination of myo-inositol and D-chiro-inositol is used in a ratio of 40:1. Currently available formulations contain 13.8 mg of D-chiroinositol and 550 mg of myo-inositol.

Adverse effects: Side effects are nausea, headache and dizziness.

Preparation: Tablet Normoz.

Statins

Dyslipidemia is common in women with PCOS, with many having decreased HDL-cholesterol or increased total and LDL-cholesterol or triglycerides. Statins may offer a promising approach to the treatment of women with PCOS who are at risk for developing diabetes and cardiovascular disease.

Pharmacology and mechanism of action: Statins acts by competitively inhibiting the conversion of 3-Hydroxy-3-methyl glutaryl coenzyme A (HMG CoA) to mevalonate which is the rate limiting step in cholesterol synthesis catalyzed by the enzyme HMG CoA reductase. Therapeutic doses of statins reduce cholesterol synthesis by 25–50%. As a result of which there is compensatory increase in LDL receptor expression on liver cells leading to increased receptor mediated uptake and catabolism of LDL.

Pharmacokinetics: Simvastatin has a half-life of 2–3 hours. It is lipophilic and given in the lactone precursor form. Except rosuvastatin, all statins are metabolized primarily by CYP3A4. Inducers and inhibitors of this isoenzyme respectively decrease and increase statin blood levels.

Indications: Statins are used for the treatment of high cholesterol levels and to lower the risk of heart attack, stroke or other cardiovascular conditions in patients with type 2 diabetes.

Contraindications: Statins are contraindicated in liver diseases, during pregnancy and lactation.

Dosage: 5–20 mg/day (maximum 40 mg).

Adverse effects: All statins are well tolerated. Notable side effects are: Headache, nausea, bowel upset, rashes, sleep disturbances, rise in serum transaminase, muscle tenderness and rise in creatine phosphokinase (CPK) levels. Myopathy is the only serious adverse effect of statins, but is rare.

Drug interactions: Risk of muscle problems may increase when statins are used with nicotinic acid, gemfibrozil or CYP3A4 inhibitor like erythromycin, HIV protease inhibitor and ketoconazole.

Preparations: Tablet Atorva 10 mg and 20 mg, and tablet Simcard.

Safety during pregnancy and lactation: Atorvastatin is FDA pregnancy category X and its use is contraindicated in pregnancy. Use of statins in pregnancy has been associated with increased risk of skeletal malformations in the fetus. Statins are contraindicated in lactation.

TREATMENT OF ANDROGEN-RELATED SYMPTOMS

Hirsutism (Table 29.2)

Table 29.2: Drugs used in hirsutism

Estrogen-progestin contraceptives	
Antiandrogens	Spironolactone
	Cyproterone acetate
	Flutamide
	Finasteride
Insulin sensitizers	Biguanides (Metformin)
	Thiazolidinediones
GnRh agonists	
Glucocorticoids	
Eflornithine hydrochloride	

Hirsutism is defined as excessive male-pattern facial and body hair and affects 5–10% of women in reproductive age group. It is a clinical sign and is not a disease by itself, and the presence of hirsutism does not always require treatment. However, perception of having male-type pattern body hair, irrespective of its objective severity, may have profound adverse effects on the psychological wellbeing of women with even mild hirsutism. Therefore, treatment of hirsutism should consider the extent to which the patient views it as a problem, and her therapeutic and reproductive goals.

Mild hirsutism can be managed using cosmetic measures such as shaving, plucking, waxing, and depilatory agents. However, a pharmacological approach is usually required when hirsutism is moderate to severe and/or is widespread in androgen-sensitive areas. Pharmacological therapy is only partially effective on terminal hairs. Therefore, for management of clinically important hirsutism dual approach is used which includes pharmacological therapy to reduce androgen secretion and/or androgen action, and removal of terminal hair already present.

Before treatment begins, it is important to foster reasonable expectations regarding its likely impact. Finer, lighter and slower hair growth, and the prevention of new terminal hair growth, all can be expected; a complete cessation or elimination of hair growth cannot. No significant reduction in hair growth may occur for up to 6 months, which approximates the half-life of a hair follicle growth cycle. After 6 months, a change in dose, drug, or the addition of a second drug should be considered if patient judges her response inadequate. In general, treatment should be continued indefinitely because the problem rarely goes away and almost always recurs when treatment is discontinued. Patients planning to attempt pregnancy are the obvious exception, because most treatments prevent pregnancy or are contraindicated during pregnancy due to the risk of adverse impact on sexual development in a male fetus.

Estrogen-Progestin Contraceptives

Pharmacology: Estrogen-progestin contraceptives have a number of complementary non-contraceptive actions that make them a logical and effective treatment for hirsutism and have been the mainstay for hirsutism therapy for decades.

Mechanism of action: Androgen production in hirsute women is an LH-dependent process. Estrogen-progestin contraceptives suppress pituitary LH secretion and thus also suppress ovarian androgen production.

- The high level of estrogen in combination contraceptives stimulates hepatic SHBG production; thereby increasing binding capacity for circulating androgens and decreasing the amount of free/active androgen.
- Directly or indirectly, estrogen-progestin contraceptives can decrease adrenal DHEA-S secretion.[27]

- Contraceptive progestins inhibit 5 alpha reductase activity in skin,[28] which decreases the production of dihydrotestosterone (DHT), the major nuclear androgen in hair follicles and sebaceous glands.

Pharmacokinetics: Ethinyl estradiol has a half-life of 12-24 hours. Most of the synthetic progestins have half-life of 8-24 hours. These drugs undergo enterohepatic circulation.

Indications: Estrogen-progesterone contraceptives are used for the prevention of unwanted pregnancy, treatment of menstrual dysfunction, hirsutism and acne.

Contraindications

- Presence of or a history of thromboembolic, coronary and cerebrovascular disease.
- Moderate to severe hypertension.
- Presence of hepatoma, active liver disease or history of jaundice during past pregnancy.
- Suspected or overt malignancy of genitals and breast.
- Porphyria.
- Impending major surgery—to avoid postoperative thromboembolism.

Mild hypertension, migraine, and smoking are relative contraindications.

Dosage: Low-dose oral contraceptive pills containing 20–35 μg ethinyl estradiol and a progestin with low androgenicity (neutral progestin), such as desogestrel or gestodene, or the spironolactone-derivative drospirenone, or an antiandrogen, such as cyproterone acetate, chlormadinone acetate, are the choice of treatment for hirsutism because all of these drugs provide adequate normalization of testosterone levels.[29,30] If the clinical response obtained with OCPs containing a neutral progestin is unsatisfactory, the OCP formulation should be changed to include an antiandrogenic progestin. Subjectively, 60–100% of women report improvement in their hirsutism during treatment with OCPs.[31,32]

The transdermal contraceptive patch (delivering 20 μg ethinyl estradiol and 150 μg norelgestromin daily) and the vaginal contraceptive ring (releasing 15 μg ethinyl estradiol and 120 μg etonogestrel daily) also can be used for the treatment of hirsutism, although data relating to their effects on androgens are limited.

Adverse effects: Third generation low dose OCP formulations are not associated with unfavorable metabolic profile which was a problem with older formulations. These formulations may even have beneficial effects on the lipid profile[33] even in obese PCOS patients who are insulin-resistant.[34] However, these newer OCP formulations may lead to a mild increase in blood pressure.[35] Third-generation OCPs may have deleterious effects on coagulation, especially among smokers [36] and may also increase the risk of non-fatal venous thromboembolism.

Drug interactions: Contraceptive failure may occur with enzyme inducers such as phenytoin, phenobarbitone, rifampin. Contraceptive failure may also occur by drugs like tetracycline which cause suppression of intestinal microflora due to interruption of enterohepatic circulation.

Preparations: Yasmin (3 mg drospirenone and 0.03 mg ethinyl estradiol), Yaz (3 mg drospirenone and 0.02 mg ethinyl estradiol).

Safety during pregnancy and lactation: Oral contraceptive pills belong to pregnancy category X and use of these drugs is contraindicated during pregnancy. Oral contraceptive pills are not associated with any deleterious effects on breast-fed infants but these drugs may decrease milk production.

Oral contraceptive pills besides improving hirsutism also provide the effective contraception recommended for the concomitant use of antiandrogens. These formulations regularize menstrual cycle in women with PCOS, hence reducing the risk of endometrial hyperplasia.

Antiandrogens

Antiandrogens are an effective treatment for hirsutism, but are best used in combination with oral contraceptives or another means of highly effective contraception, because they have potential to adversely affect sexual development in a male fetus, if the patient conceives during treatment.

Spironolactone

Pharmacology and mechanism of action: Spironolactone is an aldosterone antagonist having structural similarity to progestins. The drug also acts as an androgen receptor antagonist and to varying extent, also inhibits ovarian and adrenal androgen synthesis.[37]

Pharmacokinetics: Spironolactone is highly bound to plasma proteins and completely metabolized in liver and gets converted to its active metabolites. Spironolactone has a plasma half-life of 1-2 hours while half-life of its active metabolite is 18 hours.

Indications: Spironolactone is used in moderate to severe hirsutism, hypertension and treatment of fluid retention (edema) due to congestive heart failure.

Contraindications: Spironolactone is contraindicated in presence of kidney disease, Addison's disease and hyperkalemia.

Dosage: The effects of spironolactone are dose-dependent and best results are achieved with doses of 50–100 mg twice daily. Maximal effects are observed only after approximately 6 months of therapy.

Adverse effects: Side effects are relatively few, including diuresis in the early days of treatment and occasional complaints of fatigue and dysfunctional uterine bleeding. Although the drug can cause hyperkalemia, the effect is rare and monitoring of potassium levels is not necessary in women with normal renal function.

Drug interactions: Dangerous hyperkalemia may occur if spironolactone is given with potassium supplements. Hyperkalemia may also occur if drug is used with ACE inhibitors and angiotensin receptor blockers (ARBs). Aspirin blocks the action of spironolactone by inhibiting tubular secretion of canrenone, which is an active metabolite of spironolactone.

Preparations: Tablet Aldactone 25 mg and 100 mg.

Safety during pregnancy and lactation: Spironolactone is pregnancy category C drug according to FDA and is used in pregnancy only when benefit outweighs risk. There is a risk of feminization of male fetus when spironolactone is used in pregnancy. Spironolactone may cause serious adverse effects in nursing infants and is not used in lactation.

Cyproterone Acetate

Pharmacology and mechanism of action: Cyproterone is a derivative of 17 alpha hydroxyprogesterone (17OHP) having potent progestational activity that inhibits gonadotropin secretion, but also acts as a competitive androgen receptor antagonist and inhibits enzymes involved in androgen synthesis, like spironolactone.

Pharmacokinetics: Bioavailability of cyproterone is almost 88%. It is metabolized by CYP3A4 and 15 beta-hydroxy cyproterone acetate is the main metabolite of cyproterone. Its plasma half-life is 1.9 days. Most of the drug is excreted in urine and bile.

Indications: Cyproterone acetate is used for the treatment of excessive hair growth, acne, and androgenic alopecia. It is also used for the treatment of prostate cancer in males.

Contraindications: Contraindications to the use of cyproterone containing contraceptives are: pregnancy, lactation, presence or history of hepatic tumors, hepatic disease, Dubin-Johnson syndrome, Rotor syndrome, presence or a history of breast cancer or cancer of genital organs, history of thromboembolism, heart attack and stroke, presence of hypertension, migraine and liver disease.

Dosage: Cyproterone acetate is the progestin in the combined estrogen-progestin oral contraceptive called "Diane" which contains 2 mg of cyproterone acetate. The drug also has been used in higher doses (12.5–100 mg), alone or in combination with estrogen. Combined treatment with cyproterone acetate and ethinyl estradiol yields comparable results to those achieved with oral contraceptives and other treatments.

Adverse effects: The most common side effects associated with cyproterone treatment are fatigue, edema, loss of libido, weight gain, and mastalgia.

Drug interactions: Medicines used for the treatment of epilepsy, HIV and barbiturates may decrease the efficacy of cyproterone containing pills.

Preparations: Tablet Diane (2 mg cyproterone acetate and 50 µg ethinyl estradiol), tablet Diane 35 (2 mg cyproterone acetate and 35 µg ethinyl estradiol), tablet Dianette.

Safety during pregnancy and lactation: Cyproterone has been assigned as pregnancy category X and is contraindicated during pregnancy and lactation.

Flutamide

Pharmacology and mechanism of action: Flutamide is a nonsteroidal androgen receptor antagonist.

Pharmacokinetics: Flutamide has a plasma half-life of 5–6 hours. After absorption, it gets converted to its active form 2-hydroxyflutamide which is responsible for its actions. It is excreted in urine.

Indications: Flutamide is primarily used in the treatment of prostate cancer. It can also be used for treatment of moderate to severe hirsutism.

Contraindications: Flutamide is contraindicated in presence of liver diseases.

Dosage: The drug (250–750 mg daily) inhibits hair growth directly.

Adverse effects: Side effects of flutamide include breast tenderness and hepatotoxicity.

Drug interactions: Flutamide may increase the side effects of warfarin.

Preparations: Tablet Cytomid 250 mg, and tablet Flutide 250 mg.

Safety during pregnancy: Flutamide is FDA category D for pregnancy.

Though it is as effective as spironolactone, its higher cost and potential for causing severe hepatotoxicity make it an unattractive therapeutic choice, by comparison.[38] Flutamide is currently not approved by FDA for the treatment of hirsutism.

Finasteride

Pharmacology and mechanism of action: Finasteride is a competitive inhibitor of the enzyme 5 alpha reductase which blocks the conversion of testosterone into more active dihydrotestosterone which is responsible for androgen action. The enzyme exists in two forms, with type 1 most prevalent in skin and type 2 predominating in reproductive tissues.[39] Although finasteride inhibits the type 1 enzyme only to a limited extent, evidence from clinical trials indicates its efficacy is comparable to those of spironolactone and flutamide.[40,41]

Pharmacokinetics: Finasteride is metabolized in liver, metabolites are excreted in urine and feces. Its plasma half-life is 4–8 hours.

Indications: Finasteride is used for the treatment of hirsutism. It is also used for the treatment of benign prostatic hyperplasia and male pattern baldness in males.

Contraindications: Finasteride is contraindicated during pregnancy and lactation.

Dosage: Finasteride is given in a dose of 5 mg/day.

Adverse effects: Finasteride is well tolerated by most patients. Skin rashes and swelling of lips may occur.

Drug interactions: No clinically significant drug interaction of finasteride has been reported till now.

Preparations: Tablet Proscar 5 mg.

Safety during pregnancy and lactation: Finasteride is FDA category X for pregnancy. It is contraindicated during pregnancy and lactation. It may cause feminization of male fetus if used during pregnancy.

Antiandrogens have the potential to adversely affect sexual development in a male fetus if the patient conceives during treatment and should be used in combination with highly effective contraception. These drugs can be used in combination with oral or transdermal contraceptives. In patients with contraindication to oral contraceptives; for instance in heavy smokers older than 35 years or in women at risk for thrombophilia, an alternative means of reliable contraception (e.g. an intrauterine device or surgical sterilization) must be used. These medications when given alone may cause menstrual disturbances or even amenorrhea because of their strong progestin effects.

In summary, antiandrogens are used:

- In women presenting with moderate or severe hirsutism in combination with OCPs, or in those with a milder hirsutism when satisfactory control of hirsutism is not obtained after using oral contraceptive pills for 1 year.
- As single drugs in cases where OCPs are contraindicated along with a reliable method of contraception.

Insulin-Sensitizing Drugs

Insulin sensitizers are widely used in patients with PCOS because insulin resistance is a common feature of this disorder. Treatment with insulin sensitizers decrease circulating insulin levels, improve insulin resistance, menstrual dysfunction and decrease serum androgen concentrations but do not have any significant effect on hirsutism. A recent systematic review and meta-analysis including 9 placebo-controlled trials concluded that insulin-sensitizing drugs have no important benefits for the treatment of hirsutism.[42] According to the guidelines issued by the Endocrine Society, these drugs should not be used for the treatment of hirsutism.[43]

OTHER DRUGS

Gonadotropin-Releasing Hormone Agonists

GnRH agonists can be used in women with severe hyperandrogenism who fail to respond to or cannot tolerate treatment with estrogen-progestin contraceptives and antiandrogens. GnRH analogs are potent inhibitors of ovarian steroid production, they suppress LH-dependent ovarian androgen production. These drugs induce a reversible menopause and may be combined with OCPs (to eliminate estrogen deficiency symptoms and prevent bone loss). Considering their side effects due to estrogen deficiency and high economic cost, these drugs are not recommended for routine use and use should be restricted to the selected patients with severe hyperandrogenism of ovarian origin not responding to other drugs.

Glucocorticoids

Glucocorticoids are used to suppress endogenous ACTH secretion in the long-term management of women with classical congenital adrenal hyperplasia (CAH). They also have been used for the treatment of hirsutism in women with nonclassical, late-onset, form of the disorder, but with limited benefit. Although glucocorticoids suppress serum adrenal androgen levels effectively in women with nonclassical CAH, they are less effective than oral contraceptives or antiandrogens for the treatment of hirsutism.[44,45]

Eflornithine Hydrochloride

Pharmacology and mechanism of action: Eflornithine was initially developed for the treatment of trypanosomal sleeping sickness. It is an irreversible inhibitor of L-ornithine decarboxylase, an enzyme that converts ornithine to putrescine, a polyamine that is essential for the regulation of cell growth and differentiation within the hair follicle.

Pharmacokinetics: Plasma half-life of eflornithine is 3.4 hours. Its oral absorption is 27.5%. Most of the drug is excreted through kidneys.

Indications: Eflornithine hydrochloride (13.9% cream) is used in the topical treatment mild facial hirsutism. It can also be used as an adjuvant to permanent or long-term depilation and along with medical treatment for hirsutism. It is also used for the treatment of sleeping sickness.

Contraindications: Eflornithine is contraindicated in patients those are hypersensitive to eflornithine.

Dosage: Twice daily topical application of eflornithine (13.9% cream) produced noticeable improvement in facial hair growth in up to 70% of patients treated.[46,47] Eflornithine is not approved for the treatment of hirsutism in areas other than the face, and has a relatively high cost. The drug must be used continuously, because hair growth reverts to pretreatment characteristics within approximately 8 weeks after the treatment is discontinued.[47]

Adverse effects: Acne is the most frequently reported side effect of eflornithine. Other side effects are skin problems such as dry skin, burning, tingling sensation, itching, redness or rash.

Drug interactions: No significant drug interaction has been reported with topical application of eflornithine.

Preparation: Vaniqa (13.9% cream).

Safety during pregnancy and lactation: Eflornithine is an FDA pregnancy category C drug and its excretion in breast milk is not known.

ACNE

Acne is a skin condition that is often exacerbated in women with PCOS as a result of androgen overproduction. Oral contraceptive pills reduce androgen production; limit androgen bioactivity and effectively reduce acne. OCPs are recommended as the first line of treatment for PCOS women with acne. Antiandrogens may also be added to improve outcome.

HYPERPROLACTINEMIA

Drugs used in hyperprolactinemia	
Dopamine agonists	1. Cabergoline
	2. Bromocriptine

Plasma levels of immunoreactive prolactin are 5–27 ng/mL throughout the normal menstrual cycle. An elevated level should always be rechecked because of the variability prolactin secretion and inherent limitations of radioimmunoassay. In a case of elevated prolactin levels medications and hypothyroidism should first be ruled out as a cause. Pituitary gland imaging must be considered when otherwise unexplained and persistent prolactin elevation is present. Imaging is not necessary in patients with clearly identifiable drug induced or physiologic hyperprolactinemia, unless hyperprolactinemia is associated with symptoms such as headache and visual field defects which suggest a mass lesion. MRI of the sella and pituitary gland with gadolinium enhancement provides the best anatomic detail.

HYPOTHALAMIC DISORDERS

Prolactin release in the anterior pituitary is inhibited by dopamine. Lesions arising from the suprasellar area, pituitary gland, infundibular stalk, and lesions from adjacent bone, brain, cranial nerves, dura, leptomeninges and vessels may disrupt dopamine release resulting in hyperprolactinemia.

PITUITARY DISORDERS

Lactotroph Adenomas (Prolactinomas)

Functional lactotroph adenomas are common, accounting for approximately 40% of all clinically recognized pituitary adenomas. Most arise from clonal expansion of a single cell, presumably due to somatic mutation. They may also occur as a part of MEN 1 syndrome. Prolactin levels in serum mostly correlate with the size of adenoma. Microadenomas (<1 cm) usually are associated with serum prolactin levels less than 200 ng/mL and macroadenomas with higher levels. Elevations in prolactin may cause amenorrhea, galactorrhea, both, or neither.

Expectant Management

Expectant management can be used in women having microadenomas and those having hyperprolactinemia without any evidence of adenoma, if infertility is not a concern. Hormonal contraceptives or estrogen replacement with typical hormone replacement regimens can be used in patients with amenorrhea or irregular menses. If there are no symptoms of pituitary enlargement, repeat imaging may be done in 12 months and less frequently thereafter, to assess further growth of the microadenoma, if prolactin levels remain stable.

Medical Treatment

Dopamine agonists are the first treatment of choice for women with functional prolactin secreting lactotroph adenomas of all sizes because they effectively lower prolactin levels and decrease the size of more than 90% of such tumors.[48]

Cabergoline

Pharmacology and mechanism of action: It is a selective dopamine receptor type 2 agonist and has fewer side effects, greater potency, and is more effective than bromocriptine in restoring normal prolactin levels.

Pharmacokinetics: It is longer acting and has a plasma half-life of more than 60 days.

Indications: Hyperprolactinemia either idiopathic or due to prolactinomas causing infertility, amenorrhea and galactorrhea.

Contraindications: Cabergoline is contraindicated in presence of valvular heart disease, uncontrolled high blood pressure and allergy to ergot derivatives.

Dosage: To minimize side effects, treatment should begin with a low dose, i.e. 0.25 mg twice weekly and increased gradually, guided by serial prolactin levels obtained at approximately monthly intervals. In women with large macroadenomas and very high prolactin levels, doses of cabergoline up to 1.5 mg twice weekly may be required.

Adverse effects: Cabergoline may cause dizziness, nausea and vomiting which may be avoided by intravaginal administration of cabergoline. An increased risk of cardiac valve regurgitation was observed in recent studies in patients of Parkinson disease who were treated with high doses of cabergoline. It is postulated that 5HT2b-receptor stimulation leading to fibromyoblast proliferation[49] was responsible for this adverse outcome.

Drug interactions: The risk of side effects of cabergoline may be increased by macrolides. Butyrophenones (haloperidol), phenothiazines and metoclopramide may decrease the effectiveness of cabergoline.

Preparations: Tablet Caberlin 0.5 mg, and tablet Camforte 0.5 mg and 1 mg.

Safety during pregnancy and lactation: Cabergoline belongs to pregnancy Category B of FDA guidelines and drug should be used in pregnancy only when need has been clearly established. As cabergoline interferes with lactation, it is not given to women who are breastfeeding.

Bromocriptine

Pharmacology and mechanism of action: Bromocriptine is an ergot alkaloid, it is a potent dopamine agonist. It has greater action on D2 receptors and decreases prolactin synthesis and reduces overall size of prolactinomas by decreasing DNA synthesis and cell multiplication.

Pharmacokinetics: Absorption of bromocriptine is only 1/3 of an oral dose. It has high first pass metabolism in liver which further lowers its bioavailability. Metabolites are mainly excreted in bile. Plasma half-life of bromocriptine is 3–6 hours.

Indications: Hyperprolactinemia either idiopathic or due to prolactinomas causing infertility, amenorrhea and galactorrhea.

Contraindications: Bromocriptine is contraindicated in presence of uncontrolled high blood pressure, allergy to ergot alkaloids and during pregnancy and lactation.

Dosage: Bromocriptine is given in a dose of 1.25 mg once a day for one week followed by 1.25 mg twice a day during the second week. The dose is then increased to 1.25 mg in the morning and 2.5 mg in the evening during the third week followed by 2.5 mg twice a day during the fourth week and thereafter. The lowest dose that maintains the prolactin level in the normal range is continued.

Adverse effects: Nausea, vomiting, constipation, nasal blockage, postural hypotension may occur. In women who cannot tolerate oral treatment, bromocriptine may be administered vaginally. Psychotic reaction is a rare adverse effect of bromocriptine. Symptoms include changes in mood, delusional ideas, and auditory hallucinations. These symptoms quickly resolve after discontinuation of the drug.

Drug interactions: Excessive increase in blood pressure may occur if bromocriptine is used with triptans such as sumatriptan (used for migraine), azole antifungals, beta-blockers and macrolide antibiotics may increase the risk of side effects with bromocriptine.

Preparations: Tablet Proctinal 1.25 mg and 2.5 mg, and tablet B-crip 2.5 mg.

Safety during pregnancy and lactation: Bromocriptine belongs to pregnancy category B according to FDA guidelines. Although no teratogenic effect of bromocriptine has been reported, it should be stopped when pregnancy occurs. As bromocriptine suppresses lactation, it is contraindicated during lactation.

Medications such as metergoline or pergolide may be used when cabergoline or bromocriptine cannot be used.

Prolactin levels typically decrease within 2–3 weeks after treatment begins and can be normalized in virtually patients with microadenomas and in nearly all of those with macroadenomas.[50] In women with macroadenomas causing visual impairment, significant improvement can be observed within days after treatment begins and increases gradually over a period of months. Shrinkage of adenomas may begin as early as 6 weeks and can be assessed more confidently by repeating MRI after 3–6 months of treatment.

In women with both microadenomas and macroadenomas trial discontinuation can be attempted if prolactin levels have been normal for 2 years or more and MRI reveals no evidence of the adenoma.

Surgical treatment: In those patients who are resistant to or cannot tolerate dopamine agonist treatment, trans-sphenoidal surgery is an appropriate alternative. Surgery might also be considered for women with very large macroadenoma (e.g. >3 cm) who want to attempt pregnancy, even when their tumor responds to medical treatment.

Management during pregnancy: There is a risk of tumor growth during pregnancy, which is 1–2% in women with microadenomas and 15–20% in those with macroadenomas.[51,52] Regardless of the size of the adenoma, there is no indication for treatment with dopamine agonists during pregnancy in the absence of symptoms. In few women with macroadenomas who experience significant tumor growth during pregnancy, headache and visual disturbances may occur in any trimester. The symptoms regress promptly with resumption of dopamine agonist treatment without any risk to the fetus. Breastfeeding poses no significant risk for tumor growth in women with microadenomas or macroadenomas that remain asymptomatic during pregnancy, but is contraindicated for those with neurologic symptoms at the time of delivery.[53] Dopamine agonist treatment should not resume until after cessation of nursing.

REFERENCES

1. Patel SM, Nestler JE. Fertility in polycystic ovary syndrome. Endocrinol Metab Clin North Am. 2006;35(1):137-55.
2. Balen A. Polycystic ovary syndrome and cancer. Hum Reprod Update. 2001;7(6):522-5.
3. Glueck CJ, Wang P, Fontaine R, et al. Metformin-induced resumption of normal menses in 39 of 43 (91%) previously amenorrheic women with the polycystic ovary syndrome. Metabolism. 1999;48:511.
4. Essah PA, Apridonidze T, Iuorno MJ, et al. Effects of shortterm and long-term metformin treatment on menstrual cyclicity in women with polycystic ovary syndrome. Fertil Steril. 2006;86:230
5. Legro RS. Pregnancy considerations in women with polycystic ovary syndrome. Clin Obstet Gynecol. 2007;50:295.
6. Imani B, Eijkemans MJC, Habbema JDF, et al. Predictors of patients remaining anovulatory during clomiphene citrate induction of ovulation in normogonadotropic oligoamenorrheic infertility. J Clin Endocrinol Metab. 1998;83:2361.
7. Homburg R. Clomiphene citrate—end of an era? A mini-review. Hum Reprod. 2005;20:2043.
8. Imani B, Eijkemans MJ, Habbema JD, et al. Predictors of chances to conceive in ovulatory patients during clomiphene citrate induction of ovulation in normogonadotropic oligoamenorrheic infertility. J Clin Endocrinol Metab. 1999;84:1617.
9. Carroll N, Palmer JR. A comparison of intrauterine versus intracervical insemination in fertile single women. Fertil Steril. 2001;75(4):656-60.
10. Tulandi T, Martin J, Al-Fadhli R, Kabli N, Forman R, Hitkari J, et al. Congenital malformations among 911 newborns conceived after infertility treatment with letrozole or clomiphene citrate. Fertil Steril. 2006;85:1761.
11. Forman R, Gill S, Moretti M, Tulandi T, Koren G, Casper R. Fetal safety of letrozole and clomiphene citrate for ovulation induction. J Obstet Gynaecol Can. 2007;29:668.
12. Delbaere A, Bergmann PJM, Gervy-Decoster C, et al. Increased angiotensin II in ascites during severe ovarian hyperstimulation syndrome: role of early pregnancy and ovarian gonadotropin stimulation. Fertil Steril. 1997;67:1038.
13. De Leo V, la Marca A, Ditto A, Morgante, et al. Effects of metformin on gonadotropin-induced ovulation in women with polycystic ovary syndrome. Fertil Steril. 1999;72:282.
14. Yarali H, Yildiz B. Metformin and FSH for induction of ovulation in women with polycystic ovary syndrome. Hum Reprod. 2002;17:3007.
15. Itskovitz-Eldor J, Kol S, Mannaerts B. Use of a single bolus of GnRH agonist triptorelin to trigger ovulation after GnRH antagonist ganirelix treatment in women undergoing ovarian stimulation for assisted reproduction, with special reference to the prevention of ovarian hyperstimulation syndrome: preliminary report: short communication. Hum Reprod. 2000;15:1965.
16. Sam S, Dunaif A. Polycystic ovary syndrome: syndrome XX? Trends Endocrinol Metab. 2003;14(8):365-70.
17. Harborne LR, Sattar N, Norman JE, et al. Metformin and weight loss in obese women with polycystic ovary syndrome: comparison of doses. J Clin Endocrinol Metab. 2005;90(8):4593-8.
18. Dunaif A, Green G, Phelps RG, Lebwohl M, Futterweit W, Lewy L. Acanthosis nigricans, insulin action, and hyperandrogenism: clinical, histological, and biochemical findings. J Clin Endocrinol Metab. 1991;73:590.
19. Palomba S, Orio F Jr, Zullo F. What is the best first-step therapeutic approach in treating anovulatory infertility in patients with polycystic ovary syndrome? Questions that are still unanswered. Gynecol Endocrinol. 2007;23(5):245-7.
20. Moll E, Bossuyt PM, Korevaar JC, et al. Effect of clomifene citrate plus metformin and clomifene citrate plus placebo on induction of ovulation in women with newly diagnosed polycystic ovary syndrome: randomised double blind clinical trial. BMJ. 2006;332(7556):1485.
21. Creanga AA, Bradley HM, McCormick C, et al. Use of metformin in polycystic ovary syndrome: a meta-analysis. Obstet Gynecol. 2008;111(4):959-68.
22. Yilmaz M, Biri A, Karakoc A, Toruner F, Bingol B, Cakir N, et al. The effects of rosiglitazone and metformin on insulin resistance and serum androgen levels in obese and lean patients with polycystic ovary syndrome. J Endocrinol Invest. 2005;28:1003.
23. Ortega-Gonzalez C, Luna S, Hernandez L, Crespo G, Aguayo P, Arteaga-Troncoso G, et al. Responses of serum androgen and insulin resistance to metformin and pioglitazone in obese, insulin resistant women with polycystic ovary syndrome. J Clin Endocrinol Metab. 2005;90:1360.

24. Nestler JE, Jakubowicz DJ, Reamer P, et al. Ovulatory and metabolic effects of D-chiroinositol in the polycystic ovary syndrome. N Engl J Med. 1999;340:1314-20.
25. Iuorno MJ, Jakubowicz DJ, Baillargeon JP, Dillon P, Gunn RD, Allan G, et al. Effects of d-chiroinositol in lean women with the polycystic ovary syndrome. Endocr Pract. 2002;8:417-23.
26. Ciotta L, Stracquadanio M, Pagano I, Carbonaro A, Palumbo M, Gulino F. Effects of Myo-Inositol supplementation on oocyte's quality in PCOS patients: a double blind trial. Eur Rev Med Pharmacol Sci. 2011;15(5):509-14.
27. Madden JD, Milewich L, Parker CR Jr, Carr BR, Boyar RM, MacDonald PC. The effect of oral contraceptive treatment on the serum concentration of dehydroisoandrosterone sulphate. Am J Obstet Gynecol. 1978;132:380.
28. Cassidenti DL, Paulson RJ, Serafini P, et al. Effects of sex steroids on skin 5a-reductase activity in vitro. Obstet Gynecol. 1991;78:103.
29. Sobbrio GA, Granata A, D'Arrigo F, et al. Treatment of hirsutism related to micropolycystic ovary syndrome (MPCO) with two low-dose oestrogen oral contraceptives: a comparative randomized evaluation. Acta Eur Fertil. 1990;21:139-41.
30. Porcile A, Gallardo E. Long-term treatment of hirsutism: desogestrel compared with cyproterone acetate in oral contraceptives. Fertil Steril. 1991;55:877-81.
31. Guido M, Romualdi D, Giuliani M, et al. Drospirenone for the treatment of hirsute women with polycystic ovary syndrome: a clinical, endocrinological, metabolic pilot study. J Clin Endocrinol Metab. 2004;89:2817-23.
32. Dewis P, Petsos P, Newman M, et al. The treatment of hirsutism with a combination of desogestrel and ethinyl oestradiol. Clin Endocrinol (Oxf). 1985;22:29-36.
33. Vermeulen A, Rubens R. Effects of cyproterone acetate plus ethinylestradiol low dose on plasma androgens and lipids in mildly hirsute or acneic young women. Contraception. 1988;38:419-28.
34. Lemay A, Dodin S, Turcot L, et al. Rosiglitazone and ethinyl estradiol/cyproterone acetate as single and combined treatment of overweight women with polycystic ovary syndrome and insulin resistance. Hum Reprod. 2006;21:121-8.
35. Luque-Ramirez M, Alvarez-Blasco F, Botella-Carretero JI, et al. Comparison of ethinyl-estradiol plus cyproterone acetate versus metformin effects on classic metabolic cardiovascular risk factors in women with the polycystic ovary syndrome. J Clin Endocrinol Metab. 2007;92:2453-61.
36. Luque-Ramirez M, Mendieta-Azcona C, Maties M, et al. Effects of an antiandrogenic oral contraceptive pill compared with metformin on blood coagulation tests and endothelial function in women with the polycystic ovary syndrome: influence of obesity and smoking. Eur J Endocrinol. 2009;160:469-80.
37. Young RL, Goldzieher JW, Elkind-Hirsch K. The endocrine effects of spironolactone used as an antiandrogen. Fertil Steril. 1987;48:223.
38. Wysowski DK, Freiman JP, Tourtelot JB, et al. Fatal and nonfatal hepatotoxicity associated with flutamide. Ann Intern Med. 1993;118:860.
39. Russell DW, Wilson JD. Steroid 5a-reductase: two genes/two enzymes. Ann Rev Biochem. 1994;63:25.
40. Moghetti P, Tosi F, Tosti A, Negri C, Misciali C, Perrone F, et al. Comparison of spironolactone, flutamide, and finasteride efficacy in the treatment of hirsutism: a randomized, double blind, placebo-controlled trial. J Clin Endocrinol Metab. 2000;85:89.
41. Swiglo BA, Cosma M, Flynn DN, Kurtz DM, Labella ML, Mullan RJ, et al. Clinical review: Antiandrogens for the treatment of hirsutism: a systematic review and metaanalyses of randomized controlled trials. J Clin Endocrinol Metab. 2008;93:1153.
42. Cosma M, Swiglo BA, Flynn DN, Kurtz DM, Labella ML, Mullan RJ, et al. Clinical review: Insulin sensitizers for the treatment of hirsutism: a systematic review and metaanalyses of randomized controlled trials. J Clin Endocrinol Metab. 2008;93:1135.
43. Martin KA, Chang RJ, Ehrmann DA, Ibanez L, Lobo RA, Rosenfi eld RL, et al. Evaluation and treatment of hirsutism in premenopausal women: an Endocrine Society clinical practice guideline. J Clin Endocrinol Metab. 2008;93:1105.
44. Spritzer P, Billaud L, Thalabard JC, Birman P, Mowszowicz I, Raux-Demay MC, et al. Cyproterone acetate versus hydrocortisone treatment in late-onset adrenal hyperplasia. J Clin Endocrinol Metab. 1990;70:642.
45. Frank-Raue K, Junga G, Raue F, et al. Therapy of hirsutism in females with adrenal enzyme defects of steroid hormone biosynthesis: comparison of dexamethasone with cyproterone acetate. Klin Wochenschr. 1990;68:597.
46. Lapidoth M, Dierickx C, Lanigan S, et al. Best practice options for hair removal in patients with

unwanted facial hair using combination therapy with laser: guidelines drawn up by an expert working group. Dermatology. 2010;221:34-42.

47. Wolf JE Jr, Shander D, Huber F, Jackson J, Lin CS, Mathes BM, et al. Randomized, double-blind clinical evaluation of the efficacy and safety of topical eflornithine HCl 13.9% cream in the treatment of women with facial hair. Int J Dermatol. 2007;46:94.
48. Vance ML, Evans WS, Thorner MO. Drugs five years later. Bromocriptine, Ann Intern Med. 1984;100:78.
49. Roth BL. Drugs and valvular heart disease. N Engl J Med. 2007;356:6-9.
50. Di Sarno A, Landi ML, Marzullo P, Di Somma C, Pivonello R, Cerbone G, et al. The effect of quinagolide and cabergoline, two selective dopamine receptor type 2 agonists, in the treatment of prolactinomas. Clin Endocrinol (Oxf). 2000;53:53.
51. Kupersmith MJ, Rosenberg C, Kleinberg D. Visual loss in pregnant women with pituitary adenomas. Ann Intern Med. 1994;121:473.
52. Molitch ME. Management of prolactinomas during pregnancy. J Reprod Med. 1999;44:1121.
53. Bronstein MD, Salgado LR, de Castro Musolino NR. Medical management of pituitary adenomas: the special case of management of the pregnant woman. Pituitary. 2002;5:99.

CHAPTER 30

Ovulation Induction Drugs

Sudha Prasad, Aswathy Kumaran, Supriya Hajela

INTRODUCTION

Ovulation Disorders

Ovulatory dysfunction accounts for subfertility in 18–25% of couples who are anxious to conceive.

The World Health Organization (WHO) classified different categories of anovulation into three categories:[1]

1. *WHO group I*: Hypothalamopituitary failure (10%)
   Hypogonadotropic hypogonadal anovulation
2. *WHO group II*: Hypothalamopituitary dysfunction (85%)
   Normogonadotropic anovulation—polycystic ovarian syndrome (PCOS)
3. *WHO group III*: Ovarian failure (5%)
   Hypergonadotropic hypogonadal anovulation.

Other endocrine pathology mainly hyperprolactinemia and thyroid dysfunction contribute to ovulatory dysfunction and infertility. Treating the respective pathology restores ovulation and hence fertility.

Treatment of Ovulatory Dysfunction

Ovulation induction (OI) is stimulating the ovaries to achieve monofollicular development in women with anovulatory cycles.

Ovarian stimulation, in contrast, is stimulating otherwise ovulatory ovaries for multifollicular development. In IUI cycles, ovaries are stimulated so that 2–3 dominant follicles develop and ovulate; where as in assisted reproduction cycles (ART cycles) multifollicular development and multiple oocyte retrieval is the target.

Ovulation induction drugs are thus those aimed at stimulating and inducing ovulation in women with functional/responsive ovaries and are used in:

- Subfertile women falling in WHO categories 1 and 2 **(Table 30.1)**

Table 30.1 WHO classification of ovulatory dysfunction and management[1]

Cause of anovulation	*Treatment*
WHO 1 Hypogonadotropic hypogonadal anovulation	
Hypothalamic dysfunction	GnRH analogs
Pituitary dysfunction	Gonadotropins
WHO 2 Normogonadotropic normoestrogenic anovulation	
Polycystic ovarian syndrome	Clomephene citrate (CC) Aromatase inhibitors Tamoxifen Gonadotropins
WHO 3 Hypergonadotropic hypogonadal anovulation	
Ovarian failure	Donor oocyte IVF

- Controlled ovarian stimulation and hyperstimulation for IUI and ART cycles
- Hyperprolactinemia
- Thyroid dysfunction.

Thyroid dysfunction is managed based on the causative etiology with either thyroid suppressing or hormone replacement therapy and adjuncts as required. The treatment for hyperprolactinemia is with dopaminergic drugs like bromocriptine after evaluating the causative pathology and ruling out pituitary macro adenomas, which might require surgical correction. The adequate correction of thyroid dysfunction and hyperprolactinemia **(Table 30.2)** removes the ovulatory dysfunction caused by it. If both co-exist, thyroid dysfunction is managed first and correction of prolactinemia is done if required. However, these therapeutic interventions are generally not used per se to stimulate ovaries hence are not being covered extensively in this chapter.

Table 30.2 Other common causes of anovulation with treatment

Cause	*Treatment*
Hyperprolactinemia	Bromocriptine Cabergoline
Thyroid dysfunction	
Hypothyroidism	Thyroxine
Hyperthyroidism	Antithyroid drugs

OVULATION INDUCTION DRUGS

Ovulation induction (OI) drugs may be divided broadly into three groups:

1. Drugs for stimulating follicular development and dominant follicle recruitment.
2. Drugs to prevent premature endogenous gonadotropin surge and oocyte maturation.
3. Those used for final oocyte maturation and triggering ovulation.

Drugs for follicular stimulation		*Drugs to prevent gonadotropin surge and premature ovulation*	*Triggers of final oocyte maturation*
Oral tablets • Nonsteroidal SERMs Clomiphene citrate (CC)—1st line for non-ART OI tamoxifen • Aromatase inhibitors (3rd generation) Letrozole Anastrozole	Parenteral • Gonadotropins • Gonadotropin-releasing hormone (GnRH)—portable pump pulsatile infusion	• GnRH releasing Hormone agonist (GnRHa) • GnRH antagonist (GnRH antagonist)	• Urinary/recombinant human chorionic gonadotropin (hCG) • GnRH releasing hormone agonist (GnRHa) • Dual/double trigger • Recombinant LH—not used now

1. Drugs for Follicular Stimulation[2-5]

A. Clomiphene Citrate (Siphene, Clomid)

Clomiphene citrate is a nonsteroidal compound related to diethylstilbestrol. It is a racemic mixture constituted by 38% of cis isomer zuclomiphene and 63% transisomer enclomiphene of which enclomiphene is metabolically more active. It has been FDA approved for ovulation induction from 1967. It is the first line treatment for OI in type II anovulation and stimulated IUI cycles.

Pharmacology: It is available as oral tablets, metabolized in liver and excreted in bile and feces.

Dose: t ½ for 5 days.

Although the average t½ is only 5 days, antiestrogenic action of zuclomiphene.

Persists into midcycle and luteal phase.

Mechanism of action: It is a selective estrogen receptor modulator with potent antiestrogenic action.

Competitive attachment of CC to hypothalamic estrogen receptors
↓
Blocks negative feedback of hypothalamus by the circulating endogenous
↓
GnRH release
↓
Gonadotropin release
↓
Follicular stimulation.

Indications of use	*Contraindications*
WHO group II ovulatory dysfunction—PCOD Mild IVF	Pregnancy Ovarian cysts Chronic liver disease Scotoma

Advantages	*Draw backs*
• Inexpensive orally effective medication • Ovulation occurs in 60–85% of anovulatory patients treated with CC, resulting in a 10–20% pregnancy rate per cycle • May be combined with gonadotropins and adjuvants to improve OI outcomes. • No teratogenic risk.	• Multifollicular development→ multiple pregnancies in 7–10% pregnancies • Ovarian hyper-stimulation syndrome (OHSS)—rare with only CC stimulation • Due to long half-life, antiestrogenic effect persisting into luteal phase causes – Unfavorable cervical mucus – Decreased endometrial receptivity • Risk of ovarian cancer increased by 11% if more than 12 cycles of CC OI given

Dosage

Treatment protocols: For intrauterine insemination (IUI)/Timed intercourse (TI) cycles.

Clomiphene citrate only	For 5 days from D2–5
CC+ HMG/CC + FSH	hCG as ovulation trigger/ovulation confirmation by LH kit
CC+ metformin	Timed intercourse (TI)/Intrauterine insemination (IUI)

CC+ HMG/CC + FSH

CC 100 mg from day 2/3 for 5 days and hMG/FSH (75–150 units 3–5 doses from day 3 of CC or after the last dose of CC.

hCG trigger for ovulation→ TI/IUI

CC+ metformin

CC 100 mg from day 2/3 for 5 days

Metformin 500 mg BD or TDS or 850 mg BD daily throughout the cycle. Metformin acts as an insulin sensitizer and improves OI rates in obese PCOS women.

In mini/micro/mild ART cycles

Stimulation and monitoring with combination of clomiphene with or without low dose injectable medications
↓
One or two quality oocytes are retrieved after trigger
↓
All matured eggs are injected with sperm (ICSI)
↓
Embryos are cryopreserved
↓
Frozen embryo transfer (FET) done in next cycle.

Monitoring

- Ultrasound—follicular imaging to ensure recruitment and follicular growth and to decide trigger.
- LH kits/hCG trigger—to confirm final oocyte maturation.

Clomiphene Resistance

Clomiphene resistance is when CC stimulation fails to induce ovulation in six consecutive cycles inspite of stepping up the dose to 150 mg. This occurs in 15–20% patients.

Management
- Adding adjutants like metformin, myo-inositol and D-chiro-inositol in obese PCO patients
- Combination with gonadotropins.
- Extending the days of administration from 5 days to 10 days
- CC stimulation after laparoscopy and ovarian drilling
- Changing to other oral OI agents like letrozole or tamoxifen.

Clomiphene Failure

Failure to conceive even after three ovulatory cycles following CC stimulation.

Here other causes of infertility other than anovulation need to be reconsidered.

Dosage: Clomiphene 50 or 100 mg is prescribed orally daily for 5 days, is usually prescribed from between day 2 to day 5 of periods. The dose may be stepped up to 150 mg/day in the next cycle if ovulation was not achieved. Stepping up the dose by 50 mg/cycle have been described to a maximum of 200 mg daily but doses more than 150 mg daily are not recommended due to increased antiestrogenic effect and OHSS risk.

Maximum 4–6 consecutive cycles
Maximum dose 750 mg/cycle.

Adverse Effects
- Bloating
- Stomach or pelvic pain
- Hot flashes
- Visual symptoms—blurred vision, decreased or double vision or other vision problems, seeing flashes of light (reversible).

B. Tamoxifen: "Off Label Use"4

Tamoxifen is a SERM with agonistic action on endometrial receptors and antagonistic action on estrogen receptors of hypothalamus and pituitary. Unlike clomiphene citrate, tamoxifen only contains only one isomer. Tamoxifen was FDA approved from 1977 for cancer breast treatment. It is less commonly used for OI compared to CC or letrozole and is used "off label".

Advantages	*Disadvantages*
• Beneficial effects on cervical mucus • Agonistic effect at the endometrium • Ovulation occurs in 50–90% and pregnancy in 30–50% over 6 months cumulatively • No increased risk of multiple pregnancies or OHSS • Inexpensive	• Stigma of tamoxifen being a cancer-treating drug • Potential risk for endometrial cancer from more cycles of tamoxifen OI.

Indications: "Off Label Use"

- Clomiphene citrate resistant PCOS
- Ovulation induction in women who have had breast cancer.

Contraindications: Pregnancy and breast-feeding, stroke, deep vein thrombosis.

Dosage: 20 mg orally BD from day 2–5 of cycle for 5 days.

C. Aromatase Inhibitors[1,6]

Letrozole (Letsi, Letroz)

Letrozole is an aromatase inhibitor that was approved for use in 1997 for the treatment of breast cancer. It has been found to induce ovulation and this has led to its "off label" use for ovulation induction. It is not yet FDA approved. In India, letrozole was being used "off label" until 2011 since when its use for ovarian stimulation was banned. It is still legal for off label use in UK and USA.

Mechanism of action: Temporary inhibitor of aromatase enzyme that converts androgens to estrogens → reduces the production of estrogen temporarily → inhibition of negative feedback of hypothalamus and pituitary → FSH and LH release → ovarian stimulation.

Letrozole is orally effective and is cleared rapidly from the body. Half-life—45 hours.

Indications

- Clomiphene failure/resistance
- Poor ET build up in CC cycles
- Type II ovulatory disorders
- Mild IVF.

Advantages	*Disadvantages*
• Shorter half-life, hence no antiestrogenic effect on luteal phase endometrium and cervical mucus. • Induces mono ovulation • Lower multiple pregnancy 2–4% • Pregnancy rates similar to CC OI • Better in unexplained infertility • Less expensive than CC + gonadotropin stimulation	• Lack of FDA approval • Theoretical risk of birth defects—heart and bone defects in the newborns

Dosage and prescribing regimens: Tablet letrozole 2.5 mg is to be started orally from between day 2 to day 5 of periods for 5 days. Ovulation is confirmed by ultrasound follicular imaging and LH surge kits or is triggered by hCG after follicular imaging.

Higher dose regimens of 5-7.5 mg per day have also been described in anovulatory cycles.

Extended regimen: Letrozole 2.5 mg daily orally for 10 days to be started from day 2/3 of cycle. The extended letrozole regimen is considered to have superior efficacy compared to CC in patients with unexplained infertility undergoing super ovulation and IUI.

Side effects: Nausea and hot flushes.

Anastrazole (Adova)

Newer aromatase inhibitor

Dose: 1 mg tablet to be started from second or third day of periods for five days.

Indications: Clomiphene resistant PCOS Pregnancy or miscarriage rates with anastrozole and letrozole when used for clomiphene resistant Type 2 anovulation are similar.

D. Gonadotropins

Exogenous gonadotropins induced ovulation and pregnancies have been reported from as early as 1963. These mimic the action of the endogenous gonadotropins released from pituitary. FDA has approved them for OI from 1997 **(Table 30.3)**.

Preparations Available

- Purified urinary follicle stimulating hormone (Urofollitropin, <1 IU LH) IM injection
- Highly purified urinary follicle stimulating hormone (<0.001 IU LH) SC injection
- Recombinant FSH (rFSH)
- Human menopausal gonadotropins combination of urinary FSH and LH
- Recombinant LH (rLH)
- Human chorionic gonadotropin (hCG)

Indications

- Ovulation induction in type I ovarian dysfunction
- More commonly in controlled ovarian hyperstimulation (COH) in ART protocols
- Along with oral OI agents in IUI cycles that are less responsive to oral agents
- For only gonadotropin stimulation, IUI cycles in resistant PCOS with patients with normal tubes.

Principles of Gonadotropin Stimulation

- Daily treatment frequently adjusted according to clinical response—most effective
- Direct relationship between body weight and dose requirement, however, response threshold cannot be predicted
- FSH only stimulation better in PCOS and young patients
- hMG or rFSH + hCG/LH regimens in older patients (>35 years) and women with Type 1 ovulatory dysfunction

- Urinary FSH used more in IUI cycles while more potent and expensive recombinant gonadotropins are used in assisted reproduction (ART cycles).

Advantages	Disadvantages
Potent stimulator of follicular development	Higher risk of OHSS-15-30%
COH may be done under GnRHa/antagonist coverage	Premature LH surge/ ovulation if cycles not properly planned
Integral part of ART protocols	Expensive-constitute bulk of the ART expenses
Higher ovulation and pregnancy rates	Luteal phase support required
	Painful daily injections

Dosage

- Dose and duration varies among women and among cycles within women
- Doses from 75–150 IU to 300–450 IU.

FSH Treatment Principles

Step down

- Higher dose (150–225 IU) started and gradually dose is reduced according to follicular progression. The follicles must grow at 1–1.7 mm per day in early follicular phase and 2–3 mm/day once they are dominant.
- The dose reduction allow selective continued development of FSH sensitive dominant follicles.

Step up: Ovulation induction started at low daily dose of 75 IU and under follicular monitoring guidance and dose maintained/ gradually increased until effective threshold of response is achieved.

Low slow

- In PCOS patients, gonadotropins-FSH/hMG 37.5–75 IU started at low doses and gradually stepped up over 2–3 weeks until desired follicular maturation is achieved.
- Small increments and longer duration.

Table 30.3 Various follitropins and routes of administration

Preparation	Source	Constituents per amp/vial	Half-life	Mode of administration
Human menopausal gonadotropins (HMG) (Menotas HP)	Urine of menopausal women	75 IU FSH and LH	55 hours	IM injection
Purified urinary follicle stimulating hormone (uFSH)—Urofollitropin	Urine of menopausal women	75 IU FSH <0.1–1 IU LH	15–20 hours	IM injection
Highly purified urinary follicle stimulating hormone	Urine of menopausal women	75 IU FSH <0.001 IU LH	15–20 hours	SC injection
Recombinant FSH (rFSH)—Follitropins (Folisurge)	*In vitro* production by genetic engineering	Follitropin alpha or beta	2 hours	SC injection
Recombinant corifollitropin alpha (FSH-CTP)	Genetic engineering	Co-expression of the α subunit and chimeric FSH β-subunit	Extended half-life—1 inj = 7 daily injections of rFSH	SC injection

Monitoring: In ART cycles, COH with gonadotropins are done for 9–11 days under the cover of either GnRH agonists or antagonist to prevent premature LH surge/ ovulation. Follicular imaging is done to tailor the doses on daily injections and final oocyte maturation trigger when more than 3 follicles are greater than 18 mm in diameter. Serum estradiol (E2) monitoring—150 pg/mL for each follicle more than 15 mm tells us regarding the quality of follicles and risk of ovarian hyper stimulation syndrome (OHSS). COH should be stopped/reduced if more than 20 follicles are developing and serum E2 > 3500 pg/mL as the patient will develop life threatening OHSS.

"Coasting"—is when FSH stimulation withdrawn altogether—larger follicles continue to function as low concentrations of endogenous LH act on their LH receptors; smaller FSH dependant follicles regress and hence risk of OHSS decreases as evidenced by the decreasing serum E2 levels.

This prevents—OHSS.

Recombinant Corifollitropin Alpha (FSH-CTP)—injection

Long-acting recombinant follicle stimulating hormone—the most recently developed gonadotropin that has promising potential.

Pharmacology

- FSH-CTP appeared to be a potent inducer of multiple follicular growth
- Compared with a single SC injection of corifollitropin alfa achieves equivalent efficacy seven once-daily injections of rFSH
- 120 µg FSH-CTP induced multifollicular growth similar to that induced by 150 IU rFSH given daily for 7 days
- The half-life is 60–75 hours.
- Provides a well tolerated and more convenient treatment option COH in ART cycles
- No increased risk of OHSS
- Disadvantage—no control over doses once administered.

Recombinant Human Luteinizing Hormone

- Comparable to human pituitary LH
- Each vial delivers 75 IU
- Used along with FSH in women requiring additional LH for follicular growth → an alternative to HMG (FSH + LH combination).

Role of LH

- The final stages of ovulation dependant on LH
- Low doses of LH selectively promote larger follicle growth and hasten regression of smaller follicles.

Human Chorionic Gonadotropin (hCG)

- Structurally similar to LH
- Similar action as LH on its receptors
- Less expensive
- May used in place of LH in late follicular phase

Ashrafi et al[7] found that use of low-dose hCG in the mid to late follicular phase of COH can

- Provide adequate ovarian estradiol secretion, oocyte maturation, and acceptable fertilization rates.
- Significant reduction of FSH dosage and reduced cost of treatment
- Has no adverse effects on the number of oocyte retrieved/pregnancy rate but can prevent the occurrence of OHSS.

E. Pulsatile Gonadotropin-Releasing Hormone

Synthetic Gonadotropin Releasing Hormone (GnRH)

Ideal for OI in type I anovulation that is hypogonadotropic hypogonadism.

Endogenous gonadotropin releasing hormone is released from the hypothalamus in small amounts about once every 90 minutes. The pulsatile release of GnRH from the hypothalamus into the blood-stream stimulates the pituitary gland to secrete LH and FSH.

If GnRH is not being released properly, i.e. in Type I ovulatory dysfunction, it can be given in a pulsatile manner by a special drug delivery system that includes a belt holding a lightweight pump. The pump delivers a small volume of fluid every 60-90 minutes through a needle placed beneath the skin (usually in the abdomen) or into a blood vessel.

Mode of Administration: Parenteral→ IV/SC: Most commonly intravenous administration by portable, programmable mini-pump—for continuous pulsatile administration→ which mimic the endogenous GnRH secretion.

Indications of use

- Type I ovulation dysfunction
  - Functional hypothalamic amenorrhea
  - Kallmann syndrome

Dosage—until ovulation

- 75 ng/kg GnRH IV via portable mini infusion pump for GnRH
- Low dose (2.5 mcg) every 60-90 minutes; if LH remains low, increase to 5 mcg/pulse
- Continue till ovulation.

Post ovulation

- GnRH at slower pulse frequency (every 120/240 min) or
- Discontinue pump and small doses of hCG 2000 IU every 3 days/progesterone can be given for luteal phase support.

Advantages	Disadvantages
Metabolized rapidly—GnRH secretion—half-life 10–40 minutes	However, requires maintenance of in dwelling catheter over a period of 2–3 weeks
Mimics the normal pattern of pulsatile hypothalamic pituitary vs continuous low level of stimulation (SC)	Expensive, not available in India
Less multiple births and OHSS risks with synthetic GnRH	Not ideal for type II ovulation dysfunction
Simple to use No extensive/costly monitoring	

2. Drugs to Prevent Gonadotropin Surge and Premature Ovulation in Assisted Reproductive Technology Cycles

Controlled ovarian hyperstimulation (COH) is the initial important component of ART protocols. The main goal of COH is multi-follicular development of good quality oocytes. COH is achieved by hyperstimulation of the ovaries with gonadotropins that is controlled by GnRH releasing hormone agonist or GnRH antagonists. Understandably, the ART protocols are labeled agonist or antagonist based on which regulating hormone was used to prevent the premature gonadotropin surge.

A. GnRH Releasing Hormone Agonist (GnRHa) Protocols

Isolation of first GnRH decapeptide was in 1971 by Nobel Laureates Guilleman and Schally et al. marked a new era in the history of ART.

Mechanism of action

- Down regulation of the pituitary gonadotropin production
- Allows COH by gonadotropins along with preventing premature LH surge, until the oocytes are fully mature.

Commonly used Synthetic GnRH Analogs

- *Leuprolide acetate:* FDA has approved (subcutaneous injection) for use from 1985.
- Pharmacology:
  - Subcutaneous or intramuscular injection
  - 0.2–1 mg daily injections used
  - 50%—protein bound
  - Hepatic metabolism and urinary excretion
  - Elimination t ½—3 hours
  - Caution in hepatic and renal impairment
- *Nafarelin acetate* (intranasal spray)
- *Buserelin acetate* (subcutaneous injection or intranasal spray)
- *Triptorelin* (subcutaneously)

Disadvantages

- Flare up effect
- Increased cost and duration of treatment

- Prolonged hormonal exposure causes menopausal symptoms
- Pituitary responsiveness not readily restored following discontinuation
- More chance of ovarian hyperstimulation syndrome (OHSS).

B. GnRH Releasing Hormone Antagonist (GnRH Antagonist)

Pharmacology

- Binds to membrane receptors in pituitary
- Prevents the action of endogenous GnRH pulses
- Blocks imminent LH surge within 6–8 hours of administration
- Metabolized by cytochrome P 450
- Cautious use in renal and hepatic impairment
- *Elimination t ½:* Cetrorelix—5 hours, Ganirelix—13 hours
- Excreted in feces and urine.

Drugs

- Cetrorelix 0.25 mg (Ovucet)
- Ganirelix 0.25 mg (Orgalutran)
- *Smallest effective dose:* 0.25 mg.

Administration: Subcutaneous Injections

Multiple Dose Regimen

Fixed regimen

- Minimal dose to prevent LH surge is 0.25 mg
- Cetrorelix/ganirelix 0.25 mg SC started after 5 days of gonadotropin stimulation with gonadotropins, i.e. on sixth day of stimulation.
- The antagonist continued till the day of hCG trigger

Flexible regimen based on follicular growth noted by ultrasound monitoring:

- Gonadotropin stimulation started from day 2/3 of cycle
- Cetrorelix/ganirelix 0.25 mg SC given when the largest growing follicle on is more than 14 mm in size irrespective of day of stimulation.

Single Dose

Three mg antagonist given SC on day 7 of cycle, which suppresses the premature LH surge for 96 hours.

GnRH Agonist Protocols

Long protocol	*Short (flare up protocol)*	*Ultra-short protocol*
• GnRH-a is given for two to three weeks till pituitary gland is down regulated • Confirmed by low E2 levels • The GnRH is usually started on day 21 of previous cycle • FSH/hMG therapy is started after down regulation	• GnRH-a is started on day one or two of the cycle • r FSH administration is started on cycle day 3 for follicular stimulation, while complete pituitary down regulation is maintained by GnRHa	• GnRHa is given for only three days with the flare up technique • LH is suppressed till middle of the cycle
Advantages: • Better pregnancy rates • Long agonist has been proven to have the highest pregnancy rate of all the agonist protocols	*Advantages:* • Shortens the time of stimulation • Reduces the amount of agonist used • Reducing the amount of gonadotropin used • Less expensive	*Advantages:* • More oocytes are retrieved with very small risk of premature LH surge
Disadvantages: • It is more expensive takes longer time • Larger dose of GnRH analog • More doses of gonadotropins	*Disadvantages:* • Unphysiological • Increased LH levels in early follicular phase is detrimental to the follicular growth	

Advantages	*Disadvantages*
• No flare up effect and hence no cyst formation • Flexibility, simplicity and reversibility of action • Shorter duration of gonadotropin usage, hence chance of OHSS decreases • Less cost to patient	• Cycle scheduling difficult • Suppresses LH to very low levels

Agonist versus Antagonist Protocols

Various published literature[8] show that clinical and ongoing pregnancy rates between the two protocols were comparable. The antagonist protocol is becoming more favored as its more patient friendly and less expensive.

3. Triggers of Final Oocyte Maturation

Induction of final maturation of oocytes is a procedure that is usually performed as part of controlled ovarian hyperstimulation to render the oocytes fully developed and ready for ovulation. It is also used in non ART OI to ensure ovulation and to time IUI.

When to Trigger?

These triggers are administered when leading follicles more than 17-18 mm, the endometrium is triple line and more than 7 mm and when the serum E2 is more than 150 pg/mL per follicles larger than 15 mm. Oocyte pick up is done 34-36 hours later when the oocyte maturation is complete. Ovulation occurs 37-40 hours following the trigger.

A. Urinary/Recombinant Human Chorionic Gonadotropin (Fertigyn/Ovitrelle)

- Urinary hCG (5000-10000 IU IM) is the standard trigger used in most IUI cycles
- FDA approval for use from 2000
- It can be used to trigger ovulation in agonist and antagonist ART cycles.

Pharmacology and mechanism of action: Creates a surrogate to LH surges and trigger final oocyte maturation induction.

Pharmacokinetics

- Excreted in urine
- Eliminated in biphasic manner
- *Elimination t ½:* 23 hours (rhCG-29 hours)
- Caution in hepatic and renal disease.

Route of administration and dosage

- Recombinant hCG—250 mcg equivalent to 5000-10000 IU urinary hCG
- Recombinant hCG—250-500 mcg SC injection
- Urinary hCG—5000-10000 urinary hCG IM injection
- Low dose trigger 2500-5000 IU uhCG to be given in patients high risk for OHSS.
- Cochrane review 2011 found that urinary and recombinant gonadotropins equally effective as ovulation trigger.

Disadvantages

- Long half-life
- Increased luteotrophic effect
  - Luteal phase defect (more E2, Prog→ LH suppression)
  - Increased risk of OHSS (more VEGF, E2)
- No FSH surge (less physiologic)
  - May affect oocyte quality.

Caution: In case a patient is prone for OHSS as evidenced by more than 20 growing follicles and serum E2 more than 3500 pg/mL, always avoid a high dose hCG trigger. Instead, go for a low dose hCG trigger or an agonist trigger and opt for segmented IVF. This involved cryopreserving all embryos of the current cycle and then transferring them in another cycle after adequate endometrial preparation.

Serum E2 more than 700 pg/mL leads to high risk of multiple pregnancy in IUI cycles.

B. GnRH Releasing Hormone Agonist (GnRHa) Trigger

Itskovitz et al. first introduced this possibility in 1988.

GnRH agonist triggers can only be given in antagonist ART cycles. They are preferred in:

- Triggers in donor oocyte cycle
- High risk of OHSS.

Short-acting GnRHa are used as triggers.

- Triptorelin 0.2 mg
- Buserelin 0.5 mg
- Leuprolide acetate 1 mg
- Leuprolide acetate 1.5 mg

Single subcutaneous injection When >3 follicles more than 18 mm dm.

Advantages	*Disadvantages*
• Induces biphasic endogenous LH surge (~24–36 hours)—more physiologic • Induces an FSH surge also • Oocyte quality better • Low OHSS risk	• Profound luteal phase defect—needs modified luteal phase support if fresh ET planned • Poor fresh ET pregnancy rates • More early pregnancy losses

hCG versus Agonist Trigger[9]

Cochrane review by Youssef et al. in 2014 comparing the ovulation triggers concluded that human chorionic gonadotropin (hCG) is being routinely used effectively for final oocyte maturation in IVF/ICSI. But use of hCG may have drawbacks as it does not cause an FSH surge along with LH and because it is associated with higher risk for OHSS. GnRH agonists present an alternative to hCG in antagonist cycles especially for segmented IVF and oocyte donation programs.

C. Dual/Double Trigger[10]

GnRH agonist + single dose hCG.

Dosage

- Triptorelin acetate, decapeptyl 0.2 mg + recombinant hCG—250 mcg has all benefits of GnRHa trigger
  - Very low OHSS risk
  - Endogenous surge LH and FSH
  - Improved oocyte quality
  - Patient comfort due to short luteal phase

But

Without the severe luteolysis that is opposed by the luteotrophic effect of hCG. Research published by Lin et al. in 2013 found that dual trigger improves:

- Implantation and pregnancy rates
- Live birth rates.

D. Recombinant LH (rLH)

Very high doses are required for triggering ovulation that was found to adversely affect the ART outcomes significantly. Therefore, rLH triggers no longer advocated.

THE FUTURE

Vigorous research is ongoing for safer and more effective ovulation inducing agents. Long-acting recombinant follicle-stimulating hormone (FSH-CTP, corifollitropin alfa) is one such drug already described above that can help decrease daily gonadotropin injections in ART cycles to once in a week.[12] German research aimed at developing an orally effective FSH has started from 2013 December, which might pave way for injections free ART.

CONCLUSION

Ovulation induction in IUI cycles:

- CC 100 mg for 5 days from day 2/3 of cycle + follicular imaging + hCG trigger
- Letrozole 2.5 mg/anastrozole 1 mg/ tamoxifen 20 mg BD for 5 days from day 2/3 of cycle + follicular imaging + hCG rigger→in CC resistant cases
- CC for 5 days from day 2/3 of cycle + HMG/ FSH 75–150 IU SC/IM for 3–5 days from day 3 to day 5 of CC + hCG trigger → in CC resistant/failure.

OVULATION INDUCTION IN ART CYCLES

- Long agonist protocol
- Patient tailored FSH/HMG (150–450) IU SC/ IM daily from day 2 of period for 9–11 days

under coverage of GnRH agonist leuprolide 0.2–1 mg SC from day 21 of preceding cycle + follicular imaging + hCG trigger

- Antagonist protocol
- Patient tailored FSH/HMG (150–450) IU SC/IM daily from day 2 of period for 9–11 days with antagonist cetrorelix/ganirelix 0.25 mg SC coverage started on day 6 or when leading follicle more than 14 mm + follicular imaging + HCG trigger.
- Mild IVF
- CC for 5 days from day 2/3 of cycle + HMG/FSH 75–150 IU SC/IM from day 3 to day 5 of CC + follicular imaging + hCG trigger.

REFERENCES

1. Rowe PJ, Comhaire FH, Hargreave TB, et al. WHO manual for the standardized investigation and diagnosis of the infertile couple (Cambridge University Press, Cambridge, 1997).
2. Fritz MA, Speroff L. Assisted reproductive technologies. In: Clinical Gynecologic Endocrinology and Infertility, 8th edn, Philadelphia: Lippincott Williams and Wilkins; 2011.pp.1331-82.
3. Gardner DK, Weissman A, Howles CM, Shoham Z. Textbook of Assisted Reproductive Techniques Volume 1: Clinical Perspectives, 4th edn, pp. 99-157 CRC Press.
4. Gulekli B, Ozaksit G, Turhan NO, Senoz S, Oral H, Gokman O. Tamoxifen: An alternative approach in clomiphene resistant polycystic ovarian syndrome patients. J Pak Med Assoc. 1993;43:89-91.
5. Macklon NS, Stouffer RL, Giudice LL, Fauser Bart CJM. The Science behind 25 Years of Ovarian Stimulation for in vitro Fertilization, Endocrine Reviews. 2006;27(2):170-207.
6. Pavone ME, Bulun SE. The use of aromatase inhibitors for ovulation induction and superovulation. The Journal of Clinical Endocrinology & Metabolism. 2013;98(5):1838-44.
7. Ashraf M, Kiani K. The Role of Low-Dose hCG1 in the Late Follicular Phase of Controlled Ovarian Hyper Stimulation (COH) Protocols Shevach Friedler, editor, In Vitro Fertilization—Innovative Clinical and Laboratory Aspects, InTech, 2012.p.1-9.
8. Papanikolaou EG, Pados G, Grimbizis G, Bili E, et al. GnRH-agonist versus GnRH-antagonist IVF cycles: is the reproductive outcome affected by the incidence of progesterone elevation on the day of HCG triggering? A randomized prospective study Hum Reprod. 2012.doi: 10.1093/humrep/des066.
9. Youssef MA, Van der Veen F, Al-Inany HG, Mochtar MH, Griesinger G, Nagi Mohesen M, Aboulfoutouh I, van Wely M. Gonadotropin-releasing hormone agonist versus HCG for oocyte triggering in antagonist-assisted reproductive technology. Cochrane Database Syst Rev. 2014 Oct 31;10:CD008046.
10. Lin MH, Shao-Ying Wu F, Kuo-Kuang Lee R, Li SH, Lin SY, Hwu YM. Dual trigger with combination of gonadotropin-releasing hormone agonist and human chorionic gonadotropin significantly improves the live-birth rate for normal responders in GnRH-antagonist cycles. Fertil Steril. 2013 Aug 28. pii: S0015-0282(13)02762-3. doi: 10.1016/j.fertnstert.2013.07.1976.
11. Verberg MF, Macklon NS, Nargund G, et al. Mild ovarian stimulation for IVF. Hum Reprod Update. 2009;15:13-29.
12. Tarlatzis BC, Griesinger G, Leader A, Rombauts L, Ijzerman-Boon PC, Mannaerts BM. Comparative incidence of ovarian hyperstimulation syndrome following ovarian stimulation with corifollitropin alfa or recombinant FSH. Reprod Biomed Online. 2012 Apr;24(4):410-9. doi: 10.1016/j.rbmo.2012.01.005. Epub 2012 Jan 24.

CHAPTER 31

Postmenopausal Drug Therapy

Deepti Goswami

INTRODUCTION

Menopause occurs due to cessation of ovarian function and consequent decline in its hormonal secretion. The usual age for menopause is around 50-51 years. Thus, with growing life expectancy a woman is expected to spend about one third of her life in menopausal state.

Though menopause is a physiological event, a woman at this stage of life often manifests symptoms that occur due to cessation of ovarian hormone secretion particularly estrogen. The postmenopausal symptoms mainly comprise of vasomotor symptoms (hot flashes) and clinical manifestation of urogenital atrophy. The other important issue is that of osteoporosis which is not manifest clinically but makes the bones fragile and prone to fractures on minimal trauma. Aging related other problems also need to be dealt with in postmenopausal women.

Postmenopausal drug therapy mainly aims to address the menopausal symptoms and signs. Nearly 75% of menopausal women experience hot flashes that may continue to be bothersome for several years. These hot flashes occur due to vasomotor instability and are mediated at the level of hypothalamus. The most physiological and most effective means of controlling hot flashes involves estrogen replacement therapy. Progesterone is given along with estrogen to women with intact uterus. The nonhormonal alternatives for treating hot flashes include selective serotonin reuptake inhibitors (SSRIs) and gabapentin. The choice of drug depends on the clinical scenario and risk benefit assessment in a particular woman. Symptoms of vulvovaginal atrophy are managed with vaginal estrogens. Several drugs are available to manage postmenopausal osteoporosis, however, this treatment is usually provided in consultation with an endocrinologist.

POSTMENOPAUSAL HORMONE THERAPY

Postmenopausal hormone replacement therapy (HRT) involves use of estrogen either alone or along with progesterone. The use of systemic HRT has got restricted to managing vasomotor symptoms after the results of the Women's Health Initiative (WHI) study got published in 2002.[1] It is generally recommended that hormones should be used for shortest possible duration in lowest dose that is effective in curbing the menopausal symptoms. The risks versus benefits of hormone therapy should be assessed before prescribing it for symptomatic menopausal women. Presently, HRT is used for relief of bothersome vasomotor symptoms in women who have recently attained menopause. The duration of treatment is kept at less than 5 years. It is not indicated for the prevention of chronic disease in older women several years after menopause.[2]

Estrogen alone is sufficient for women who have undergone hysterectomy. Women with uterus *in situ* require progesterone in addition to estrogens to avoid endometrial hyperplasia. The use of combined treatment should be restricted to less than five years since a longer period of use may increase risk of breast cancer. In hysterectomized women receiving estrogens alone, the WHI study reported no increase in risk of breast cancer for up to 7 years of use. Thus postmenopausal hormone therapy needs to be individualized.

Different types of estrogen and progestogen are used to manage menopausal symptoms. The common preparations of estrogens include conjugated estrogens, estradiol and estriol. The progesterone preparations commonly used for HRT include medroxyprogesterone, norethisterone, dydrogesterone, and levonorgestrel.

Estrogens	Oral preparation: Conjugated equine estrogen Ethinyl estradiol
	Continuous release skin patch
	Low-dose preparations for local application
Progesterones	Medroxyprogesterone acetate Norethisterone acetate Micronized progesterone Dydrogesterone
Tibolane	Synthetic steroid hormone
Nonhormonal drugs for menopausal symptoms	Selective serotonin reuptake inhibitors (SSRIs)—Paroxetine Selective norepinephrine reuptake inhibitors (SNRIs)-Venlafaxine, Desvenlafaxine Gabapentin Clonidine
Medications to prevent or treat osteoporosis	Selective estrogen receptor modulator (SERM)-Raloxifen Biphosphonates Teriparatide Strontium ranelate Calcitonin Calcium Vitamin D

ESTROGENS

Systemic preparations of estrogens include oral (pills), transdermal (patches and gel) and subcutaneous (implants) preparations. Subcutaneous implants of estrogen are not available in India. Local preparations include cream, tablets and rings. Estrogen containing ring is not available in India.

- *Oral preparation:*
  - *Conjugated Equine Estrogen (CEE)*: This is a preparation containing natural estrogens and is considered to be safer to use in postmenopausal women as compared to the synthetic estrogens like ethinylestradiol. It contains conjugated estrogens which are sodium salts of the sulfate esters of natural estrogen. Sodium estrone sulfate is the main component of this preparation that gets converted to the active form—estrone (by action of enzyme estrone sulfatase) and estradiol.
  - *Ethinyl estradiol*: It is a derivative of estradiol
  - *Estardiol valerate*: It is the valeric-acid ester of estradiol and is chemically and biologically similar to endogenous human estradiol.
- *Continuous release skin patch* are available that contain estradiol as hemihydrate preparation.
- *Low-dose preparations for local application*: Vaginal estrogenic creams, rings and tablets are used for management of urogenital atrophy in postmenopausal women. These local preparations may contain estriol, estradiol or conjugated equine estrogen. Systemic absorption is very less so progesterone administration is not required.

Pharmacology

Estrogens are well absorbed by oral as well as transdermal route. They are present in circulation mainly in the bound form with plasma proteins like sex hormone binding globulin. Estrogens act through estrogen receptors that are of two types—alpha and beta with different sites of distribution. Alpha receptor is mainly sited in breast, ovarian stroma, endometrium, and vagina while the beta-receptor is located in the bone, coronary arteries (in endothelial cells), brain, kidneys and intestines. Oral estrogens are metabolized in liver and excretion is mainly in urine. Nonoral routes like dermal patches, gel, or implants are devoid of first pass effect on liver.

Indications (in menopausal women): Systemic estrogens are used mainly to treat vasomotor symptoms, i.e. hot flashes in postmenopausal women. Estrogens prevent postmenopausal osteoporosis, however, their use is not indicated solely for this purpose. Estrogen preparations for local application in vagina are used for managing urogenital atrophy.

Contraindications: The main contraindications to systemic estrogens include thromboembolic disease, active liver and gallbladder disease, cancer of breast and endometrium, abnormal uterine bleeding, porphyria.

Dosage

- *Oral preparations:*
  - *Conjugated equine estrogens (CEEs)*: The commonly used daily doses are 0.625 mg and 0.3 mg. The minimally effective daily dose for maintaining satisfactory bone density postmenopausally, is 0.625 mg of CEE.[3]
  - *Estradiol valerate*: 1–2 mg/day. Dose of 2 mg/day is needed for osteoporosis prevention.
  - *Ethinyl estradiol*: 10–20 μg/day.
- Transdermal patch containing estradiol is available in different strengths and accordingly release 25, 50 or 100 micrograms estradiol in 24 hours. The minimally effective daily dose for maintaining satisfactory bone density postmenopausally is 50 μg of transdermal estradiol. The patch is applied on the trunk area below waist. The skin at the site of application should be clean, dry and intact. The patch should not be applied near breasts. The site of application should be changed frequently to avoid local irritation. Initially, the patch is applied once a week. The dose can be subsequently adjusted to control symptoms.
- *Estrogen formulations for local application:*
  - Estriol cream (Evalon) is available in Indian markets which contains 1 mg of estriol per gram of the cream and the dose recommended is 1 applicator-ful applied intravaginally once or twice daily for 2 weeks, gradually reduced to 1/2-1 applicator-ful 2–3 times per week.
  - 17β-estradiol tablets each providing 25 μg of estradiol (Vagifem) are also marketed and are available with an applicator for vaginal use. The recommended dose is 1 tablet per day for 2 weeks after which 1 tablet twice per week is usually sufficient.
  - 17β-estradiol containing vaginal ring is not available in India.

Adverse drug reaction

- Side effects of systemic estrogens include nausea, mood swings, bloating and breast tenderness.
- Unopposed use of estrogens in women with uterus *in situ* can give rise to endometrial hyperplasia and endometrial cancer. Cyclical regimens of HRT involving sequential administration of estrogen and progesterone (10–14 days) also increase the risk after 5 years of use. Continuous combined regimen is not associated with this increased risk.
- Oral estrogen preparations undergo first-pass hepatic metabolism and lead to increased synthesis of various clotting factors, trigylcerides and vascular inflammatory marker like C-reactive protein.
- There is an increased risk of venous thromboembolism. Transdermal administration yields lower risk of this complication.[4]
- Long-term use of CEE with progesterone in postmenopausal women increases the risk of breast cancer (>5 years of continuous use) and stroke (WHI study).

- Multiple trials have thrown up conflicting data regarding effect of estrogens on cardiovascular system. WHI study showed that unopposed CEE does not affect the risk of cardiac events. Later studies like the Danish Osteoporosis Prevention Study concluded that early initiation of hormone therapy soon after menopause does not increased the risk of adverse cardiovascular events rather it reduces the risk of heart failure, myocardial infarction and overall mortality among the users.[5] The concept that hormone therapy may reduce cardiovascular diseases in recently postmenopausal women but potentially increase it in older women has been called the 'timing hypothesis'.[6]

Drug interaction: Patients receiving anti-coagulant treatment with warfarin need to be monitored for loss of anticoagulant effect if estrogen is co administered. Estrogens can inhibit the metabolism of cyclosporine. Estrogens may also interfere with action of some other drugs like-barbiturates, phenytoin, carbamazepine, phenylbutazone, and some antibiotics and anti-infective drugs—rifampicin, rifabutin, nevirapine, efavirenz, ritonavir and nelfinavir.

Preparations

- *Conjugated equine estrogen*: Premarin (Wyeth), Conjugase (Elder Pharmeceuticals)
- *Ethinyl estradiol*: Lynoral (Organon)
- *Estradiol valerate*: Progynova [Zydus Cadila Healthcare Ltd. (German Remedies)]
- *Transdermal patch*: Estraderm- MX 25, 50, 75, 100 patch (Novartis)
- Estriol Cream for vaginal application—Evalon (Infar India)
- *17β-estradiol vaginal tablets*: Vagifem (NovoNordisk)

Safety during pregnancy and lactation: Estrogens are contraindicated in pregnancy and are assigned category X by FDA for use in pregnancy.

PROGESTERONES

The rationale behind the use of progesterones in postmenopausal women is to prevent endometrial hyperplasia due to unopposed estrogen administration. Progesterones are prescribed in a cyclical or continuous manner with systemic estrogens. Cyclical regimen involves use of progesterones for at least 12 days per month to prevent endometrial hyperplasia.[7] Continuous-combined administration of estrogen and progesterones avoids the monthly bleeding associated with cyclical use of progesterones.

The two commonly used preparations are medroxyprogesterone acetate (a C-21 compound) and micronized progesterone. A French study has reported that use of micronized progesterone is associated with a lower relative risk of breast cancer than use of medroxyprogesterone acetate (1 versus 1.69).[8] The most common regimen is combined daily use of CEE 0.625 mg and medroxyprogesterone acetate 2.5 mg. There may be episodic unpredictable bleeding in the first few months of treatment, but by 6 months of use most of the women become amenorrheic.[9] Other progesterone preparations include dydrogesterone and C-19 nortestosterone derivatives like norethisterone acetate.

In women nontolerant to oral progesterones, levonorgestrel containing intrauterine device (MIRENA) has been used but this device is not approved by FDA for this indication. Use of vaginal gel containing micronized progesterone for managing menopausal symptoms is also not approved by the FDA.

Progesterones used for HRT

- *Medroxyprogesterone acetate (MPA)* is synthetic progesterone. The chemical compound in the drug is 17α-hydroxy-6α-methylprogesterone acetate.
- *Norethisterone acetate* is also synthetic progesterone. Norethisterone is a chemically 19-nor-17α-ethynyltestosterone.
- *Micronized progesterone*: Natural progesterone, chemically identical to the progesterone produced by the corpus luteum ($C_{12}H_{30}O_2$). Micronization improves its bioavailability.
- *Dydrogesterone*: The chemical compound is 9β, 10α-pregna-4, 6-diene-3, 20-dione.

This preparation has chemical structure and pharmacological action similar to that of endogenous progesterone. Unlike other synthetic progesterones, it does not have undesirable androgenic, anabolic and corticoid hormonal effects.

Pharmacology

All the above-mentioned progesterones are well absorbed orally. These are bound to plasma proteins in the blood and undergo first pass metabolism in liver where they are metabolized via hydroxylation and conjugation. Excretion is mainly in urine and also in feces.

Indications (in menopausal women): Post-menopausal HRT where it is used along with estrogens to prevent estrogen-induced endometrial hyperplasia.

Contraindications: Undiagnosed abnormal genital bleeding, breast cancer, estrogen- or progesterone-dependent neoplasia, history of thromboembolism, liver disease.

Dosage

- *MPA*: 2.5 mg for continuous and 5–10 mg/day for cyclical regimes of HRT
- *Norethisterone acetate*: 0.7 mg/day for continuous and 1 mg/day for cyclical regimes of HRT
- *Micronized progesterone*: 100–200 mg/day
- *Dydrogesterone*: 5 mg/day for continuous and 10 mg 1–2 times daily for cyclical regimes of HRT.

Preparations

- *MPA*: Deviry (Elder), Meprate (Serum Int), Modus (Glaxo-Smithkline), Orgamed (Infar)
- *Micronized progesterone*: Naturogest (German Remedies), Susten (Sun Pharma), Nidagen (Systopic), Endogest (Cipla)
- *Norethisterone acetate*: Primolut N [Zydus Cadila Healthcare Ltd. (German Remedies)] and Sysron N (Systopic) are available as 5 mg tablets. So ¼ tablet (1.25 mg) would be used for HRT.
- *Dydrogesterone*: Duphaston (Solvay).

Adverse drug reactions

- Breast tenderness is a common side effect. Nausea, bloating, headache, mood swings, blurred vision, and drowsiness are also reported.
- The use of combined estrogen and progesterone increases the risk for stroke, dementia and gallbladder disease.
- There is also an increased risk of venous thromboembolism and breast cancer (US Preventive Services Task Force 2013).[10] The risk of breast cancer is greater when estrogen-progesterone HRT is initiated close to the menopause.[11]

Drug interaction: Aminoglutethimide, drugs affecting liver enzymes such as, rifampin, antifungals such as itraconazole and certain antiseizure medicines, e.g. carbamazepine, phenobarbitone, phenytoin.

Safety during pregnancy and lactation: MPA and northeisterone acetate should not be used during pregnancy or lactation (Pregnancy Category X). Micronized progesterone and dydrogesterone are FDA category B.

TIBOLONE

Tibolone is a synthetic steroid hormone derived from the Mexican yam. It is an analog of norethynodrel which is a progesterone. Functionally, it is a gonadomimetic drug with estrogenic, progestogenic, and weak androgenic actions and is therefore used for postmenopausal hormone replacement therapy.

Pharmacology

The drug is administered orally. It is metabolized in intestine and liver into metabolites that yield estrogenic, progestogenic, and weak androgenic actions. It is as effective as estrogen-progesterones in relieving menopausal symptoms and preventing osteoporosis. It has a better effect than estrogens on sexual function due to its androgenic action. It has tissue-selective estrogenic effects. It has been called a selective tissue estrogenic activity regulator (STEAR). It has beneficial effect on bone (prevents osteoporosis), brain (controls hot flashes) and vagina (reduces vaginal dryness). However, unlike estrogen preparations, it does not have undesirable effects on breast and endometrium; rather it has progesterone like effect on endometrium.

Indications: Management of menopausal symptoms due to estrogen deficiency.[12]

Contraindications: Women treated for breast cancer, unexplained vaginal bleeding, liver or kidney disease. It should be used with caution in women with history of thromboembolism.

Dosage: A dose of 2.5 mg/day prevents postmenopausal osteoporosis. The risk for vertebral and non-vertebral fractures is reduced even with 1.25 mg/day.

Adverse drug reactions

- Side effects such as headache, nausea, abdominal pain, breast tenderness, swollen feet and itching may occur but are not common.
- Slight bleeding or spotting may commonly occur initially but amenorrhea is achieved by 1-3 months of use.[13]
- There is an increased risk of stroke in women more than 60 years of age (LIFT study).[14] A study has reported that tibolone may increase the risk of endometrial cancer, however, the data was not robust.[15] It decreases HDL cholesterol level but risk of atherosclerosis is not increased.[16] Observational studies do not show increased risk of venous thromboembolism with tibolone use.
- Discrepant results are reported for risk of breast cancer. While the Million woman year study reported increased risk, another case control study reported from the UK showed no increase in the risk of breast cancer with postmenopausal use of tibolone.[17,18]

Drug interaction: Tibolone may augment the effect of anticoagulants such as warfarin by increasing fibrinolytic activity in blood. It may also interact with cytochrome P450 3A4 substrates such as midazolam. Tibolone activity may be reduced in women taking liver enzyme-inducing drugs like rifampicin or anticonvulsants such as phenytoin, phenobarbitone, or carbamazepine. The requirement for insulin or other hypoglycemic agents may be increased in diabetics using tibolone.

Preparations: Livial (Organon), Tibofem (Cipla).

Drug approval: FDA does not approve tibolone for menopausal treatment in the USA. However, tibolone is widely available and marketed in countries outside the US, where it has been approved.

Safety during pregnancy and lactation: Tibolone is contraindicated in pregnancy-USFDA pregnancy category D.

NONHORMONAL DRUGS FOR MENOPAUSAL SYMPTOMS

There is currently only one FDA-approved non-hormonal pharmaceutical option for relief of hot flashes-Paroxetine which is a selective serotonin reuptake inhibitor (SSRI) compound primarily used as an antidepressant. The FDA approval for use in postmenopausal symptom was granted in June 2013.

However, for moderate-to-severe bothersome hot flashes, the other nonhormonal drugs used off label include: (a) clonidine; (b) other SSRIs (fluoxetine, sertraline); (c) norepinephrine reuptake inhibitors (SNRIs) like venlafaxine; and (d) gabapentin.[19-21] Serotonin and noradrenaline are the neurotransmitters that affect mood and also modulate thermoregulation and thereby have a role in management of postmenopausal hot flashes.

SELECTIVE SEROTONIN REUPTAKE INHIBITORS: PAROXETINE

Pharmacology

Serotonin primarily affects mood but may also impact thermoregulation. Paroxetine selectively inhibits the reuptake of serotonin. Oral paroxetine is well absorbed from the gastrointestinal tarct. The peak concentration in plasma is reached after 5 hours. More than 90% of the drug in circulation is protein-bound.

It undergoes extensive hepatic first-pass metabolism. It is metabolized by oxidation followed by methylation and formation of glucuronide and sulfate conjugates. It is excreted both in urine and feces.

Indications: It is approved by FDA for management of hot flashes associated with menopause. Otherwise the main use is as an antidepressant and for mood disorders. This drug may be particularly useful for women for whom estrogens are not safe and for those who require an antidepressant for mood disorder.

Contraindications: It should be used with caution in women suffering from liver and renal disease.

Dosage: The dosage for treatment of hot flashes is 10 mg once daily at bedtime. A higher is needed for treatment of depression.

Adverse drug reactions: Common side effects are nausea, vomiting, headache and fatigue. There may be an increased risk for abnormal bleeding and side effects due to serotonin syndrome, i.e. confusion, rapid heart rate, high blood pressure, etc. There may be visual disturbances and an increased risk of fractures.

Drug interaction: Paroxetine is a potent inhibitor of CYP2D6 and concomitant use with tamoxifen may reduce the efficacy of the latter. It should not be prescribed along with monoamine oxidase inhibitor, or antipsychotic medications like thioridazine or pimozide.

Preparations: Parotin (Cipla), Paxep (Intas).

Safety during pregnancy and lactation: Paroxetine should not be used in pregnant or breastfeeding women. It is FDA Category D drug implying that animal studies have shown adverse fetal effects.

SELECTIVE NOREPINEPHRINE REUPTAKE INHIBITORS

Selective norepinephrine reuptake inhibitors (SNRIs) include venlafaxine and desvenlafaxine, which is the succinate salt form of venlafaxine.

Pharmacology

Venlafaxine is a potent inhibitor of neuronal serotonin and norepinephrine reuptake and weak inhibitor of dopamine reuptake. Noradrenaline may impact thermoregulation. Venlafaxine is well absorbed orally. It is metabolized in liver and is excreted in mainly via the kidneys in urine.

Indications

Menopausal hot flashes.

Contraindications: Venlafaxine is contra-indicated in women suffering from heart disease, uncontrolled hypertension and dyselectrolytemia.

Dosage: Venlafaxine 75 mg SR and Desvenla-faxine 100 mg.

Adverse drug reactions: Insomnia or excite-ment, nausea, constipation, and anorexia. Blood pressure needs to be monitored with its use. It discontinuation is needed, the dose should be gradually tapered and not stopped abruptly. SSRIs and SNRIs can lead to hyponatremia in elderly women.

Drug interaction: Concomitant use of venla-faxine and ethanol can exacerbate the nervous system side effects such as dizziness and drowsiness, and make it difficult to concentrate. Using a non-steroidal anti-inflammatory drug (NSAID) with venlafaxine may cause easy bruising or bleeding.

Preparations: Flavix (Wockhart), Veniz XR (Sun).

Safety during pregnancy and lactation: FDA category C for pregnancy. It is secreted in breast milk.

GABAPENTIN

This drug is an analog of gamma-aminobutyric acid. The exact mechanism of action in controlling hot flashes is not known. Gabapentin binds to the voltage-gated calcium channels, which are present in the central nervous system and in periphery.[22] The benefit with gabapentin as compared to other nonhormonal preparations is its safety profile. There are no absolute contraindications to its use and the drug has no significant drug interactions.

Pharmacology

Gabapentin is not well absorbed after oral administration. It is distributed in the body in unbound form. It undergoes insignificant metabolism and is excreted mainly in urine.

Indications: It is used primarily for treating seizures, migraine and neuropathic pain. It also reduces hot flashes. This drug is useful in women where estrogen therapy is not safe or is not tolerated and in women who have migraines coexisting with menopausal symptoms.

Contraindications: Renal impairment.

Dosage: Gabapentin is started in a dose of 100 mg three times a day, gradually increased to 300 mg three times a day. Relief in hot flashes occurs within days.

Adverse drug reactions: Dizziness, headache, and somnolence (which improves over time), swelling of legs and weight gain. There is an increased risk of depression and suicidal thoughts. If the drug needs to be discontinued, its dose should be gradually reduced over a week's time.

Drug interaction: There are no significant interactions with other drugs.

Preparations: Gabator (Torrent), Gabastar (Lupin).

Safety during pregnancy and lactation: Effect of gabapentin on unborn fetus is not known. It belongs to FDA category C for use in pregnancy.

CLONIDINE

It is a centrally-acting alpha 2-adrenergic agonist. It reduces sympathetic signals from the central nervous system. It may control hot flashes by reducing the vascular reactivity.

Pharmacology

It is well absorbed orally and nearly 40% is bound to the plasma proteins. The drug is metabolized mainly in liver. Excretion is through urine and feces.

Indications: It is mainly used as an antihypertensive drug. It is also useful to prevent migraine and hot flashes.

Contraindications: It should be used with caution in patients with coronary artery disease, dysrhythmias, cerebrovascular disease or renal failure.

Dosage: The initial dose is 25 μg twice a day and is increased up to 75 μg twice a day. Sometimes a dose up to 150 μg twice a day may be needed. If there is no benefit after four weeks of use clonidine should be stopped. If reduction in dose is needed, it should be tapered gradually to avoid blood pressure related side-effects.

Adverse drug reactions: Sedation, dry mouth, and hypotension.

Drug interaction: Excessive drowsiness with concomitant use of hypnosedatives, antihistamines and alcohol. It may enhance digitalis, lithium toxicity and may antagonize oral hypoglycemic.

Preparations: Arkamine (Unichem), Catapres [Zydus Cadila Healthcare Ltd (German Remedies)].

Safety during pregnancy and lactation: It is FDA category C drug for use in pregnancy.

COMPLEMENTARY/ALTERNATIVE MEDICINES

Preparations like soy isoflavones, vitamin E, red clover and black cohosh show inconsistent effect on hot flashes and are not approved for this indication.

MEDICATIONS TO PREVENT OR TREAT OSTEOPOROSIS

Postmenopausal hypoestrogenemia leads to reduction in bone mineral density (BMD) leading to osteopenia, osteoporosis and increased risk of fragility fractures. There are several drugs that help reduce bone loss and risk of fractures in menopausal women. Most of these drugs are prescribed in consultation with an endocrinologist. These drugs are discussed in brief in the following section.

SELECTIVE ESTROGEN RECEPTOR MODULATOR

Selective estrogen receptor modulators (SERMs) are nonhormonal alternative to the HRT. These are used for preventing and managing osteoporosis in postmenopausal women. The most common preparation in this category of drugs is Raloxifene that reduce the risk of vertebral fracture in postmenopausal women.[23] These drugs have beneficial estrogen like effects on the skeletal and cardiovascular systems and there are no undesirable estrogenic effects on breast and uterus. However, the hot flashes may get worsened and there is risk of thromboembolism.

Preparations of raloxifene: Ralista 60 mg (Cipla).

Dosage: 1 tablet, i.e. 60 mg once a day.

Biphosphonates: Bisphosphonates increase the BMD in postmenopausal women and are effective in reducing the risk of vertebral and non-vertebral fractures. The calcium and vitamin D intake should be adequate for the beneficial effects of bisphosphonates.

Alendronate is the most common drug to be used from this category.

Dosage: 10 mg orally taken once a day; alternatively 70 mg can be taken orally once a week.

The tablet is taken on empty stomach in the morning with a full glass of plain water. Food intake should be delayed for at least 30 minutes after the drug intake. The woman should not lie down for at least 30 minutes after taking the medication to reduce the risk for esophageal irritation. Other medications should be taken at least 60 minutes after the bisphosphonate.

Preparations: Denfos (Dr Reddy Lab), Osteofos (Cipla).

Adverse drug reaction: Osteonecrosis is a serious, though rare, side effect of long-term treatment with high dose of bisphosphonate.

TERIPARATIDE

Teriparatide, an N-terminal analog of PTH, is a bone-forming agent that decreases resorption of bone. It is given as daily subcutaneous injection (20 µg). The drug is expensive and is recommended for selected patients who are at a high risk of fracture or in whom bisphosphonates are contraindicated.

Strontium Ranelate

Strontium ranelate 2 g/day prevents the loss of BMD in women in early menopause. Calcium reduces absorption of strontium. Strontium ranelate increases the risk of venous thromboembolism. It should not be used in women with severe renal impairment.

Calcitonin

It is a calcium-lowering hormone that inhibits osteoclastic activity. Salmon calcitonin is available as a nasal spray (100, 200, or 400 IU). It reduces the occurrence of vertebral fractures by one-third over five years of use. Side effects include nasal congestion or irritation. Calcitonin is safe, but long-term use may lead to resistance due to antibody formation.

Calcium

Postmenopausal women need a dietary intake of 1000–1500 mg of elemental calcium per day. The shortfall in dietary intake is compensated by giving oral calcium supplements. The two commonly used calcium preparations are calcium carbonate and calcium citrate. Calcium carbonate is 40% elemental calcium implying that 1000 mg of calcium carbonate will provide 400 mg of elemental calcium. It requires an acidic environment for absorption and is better absorbed when taken after meals. Calcium citrate does not depend on the presence of acid for calcium absorption. It contains about 21% elemental calcium implying that 1000 mg of calcium citrate will provide 210 mg of elemental calcium. It costs more than calcium carbonate. Calcium supplements can cause abdominal bloating and constipation. A large number of calcium preparations are available in the market.

Vitamin D

Vitamin D is needed for absorption of calcium in the gastrointestinal tract. The recommended daily dietary intake of vitamin D for postmenopausal women is 800–1000 IU. Vitamin D supplementation per se reduces the risk of fracture and of falling in elderly patients. Most of the urban Indian population has severe vitamin D deficiency.[24] The most commonly used vitamin D supplement is vitamin D_3 or cholecalciferol given in a dose of 60000 IU per week for 8 weeks. The treatment needs to be repeated after a few months to maintain adequate blood levels.[25] The drug is available in the form of granules and tablets, e.g. cholecalciferol granules are marketed as "Calcirol" (Cadila).

REFERENCES

1. Rossouw JE, Anderson GL, Prentice RL, LaCroix AZ, Kooperberg C, Stefanick ML, et al. Writing Group for the Women's Health Initiative Investigators. Risks and benefits of estrogen plus progestin in healthy postmenopausal women: Principal results from the Women's Health Initiative randomized controlled trial. JAMA. 2002;288(3):321-33.
2. Rossouw JE, Manson JE, Kaunitz AM, Anderson GL. Lessons learned from the Women's Health Initiative trials of menopausal hormone therapy. Obstet Gynecol. 2013;121(1):172-6.
3. Society of Obstetricians and Gynaecologists of Canada. The Canadian Consensus Conference on Menopause and Osteoporosis. J Soc Obstet Gynecol Can. 1998;20:26.
4. Canonico M, Oger E, Plu-Bureau G, Conard J, Meyer G, Lévesque H, et al. Hormone therapy and venous thromboembolism among postmenopausal women: Impact of the route of estrogen administration and progestogens: The ESTHER study. Circulation. 2007;115(7):840-5.
5. Schierbeck LL, Reynmark L, Tofteng CL, Stilgren L, Eiken P, Mosekilde L, et al. Effect of hormone replacement therapy on cardiovascular events in recently menopausal women: Randomized trial. BMJ. 2012;345:e6409.
6. Clarkson TB, Meléndez GC, Appt SE. Timing hypothesis for postmenopausal hormone therapy: Its origin, current status, and future. Menopause. 2013;20:342-53.
7. Whitehead MI, Townsend PT, Pryse-Davies J, Ryder T, Lane G, Siddle NC, et al. Effects of various types and dosages of progestogens on the postmenopausal endometrium. J Reprod Med. 1982;27(Suppl 8):539-48.
8. Fournier A, Berrino F, Clavel-Chapelon F. Unequal risks for breast cancer associated with different hormone replacement therapies: Results from the E3N cohort study. Breast Cancer Res Treat. 2008;107(1):103-11.
9. Archer DF, Pickar JH, Bottiglioni F. Bleeding patterns in postmenopausal women taking continuous combined or sequential regimens of conjugated estrogens with medroxyprogesterone acetate. Menopause Study Group. Obstet Gynecol. 1994;83:686-92.
10. Moyer VA. US Preventive Services Task Force. Menopausal hormone therapy for the primary prevention of chronic conditions: US Preventive Services Task Force Recommendation Statement. Ann Intern Med. 2013;158(1):47-54.
11. Chlebowski RT, Anderson GL. The influence of time from menopause and mammography on hormone therapy-related breast cancer risk assessment. J Natl Cancer Inst. 2011; 103(4): 284-5.
12. Huang KE, Baber R. Asia Pacific Tibolone Consensus Group. Updated clinical recommendations for the use of tibolone in Asian women. Climacteric. 2010;13(4):317-27.
13. Hammar M, Christau S, Nathorst-Böös J, Rud T, Garre K. A double-blind randomized trial comparing the effects of tibolone and continuous combined hormone replacement therapy in postmenopausal women with menopausal symptoms. Br J Obstet Gynecol. 1998;105:904-11.
14. Cummings SR, Ettinger B, Delmas PD, Kenemans P, Stathopoulos V, Verweij P, et al. LIFT Trial Investigators: The effects of tibolone in older postmenopausal women. New Eng J Med. 2008;359(7):697-708.

15. de Vries CS, Bromley SE, Thomas H, Farmer RDT. Tibolone and endometrial cancer: A cohort and nested case-control study in the UK. Drug Saf. 2005;28:241-9.
16. Morris EP, Denton ER, Robinson J, MacDonald LM, Rymer JM. High resolution ultrasound assessment of the carotid artery: Its relevance in postmenopausal women and the effects of tibolone on carotid artery ultrastructure. Climacteric. 1999;2:13-20.
17. Speroff L. The million women study and breast cancer. Editorial. Maturitas. 2003;46:1-6.
18. Allen DS, De Vries SS, Farmer RDT. Pharmaceutical content and regimen of hormone replacement therapy and risk of breast cancer. Pharmacoepidemiology and Drug Safety. 2002;11(Suppl 1):296.
19. Albertazzi P. A review of non-hormonal options for the relief of menopausal symptoms. Treat Endocrinol. 2006;5(2):101-13.
20. Sassarini J, Lumsden MA. Non-hormonal management of vasomotor symptoms. Climacteric. 2013;16(Suppl 1):31-6.
21. Rada G, Capurro D, Pantoja T, Corbalán J, Moreno G, Letelier LM, et al. Non-hormonal interventions for hot flushes in women with a history of breast cancer. Cochrane Database Syst Rev. 2010;(9):CD004923.
22. Yadav M, Volkar J. Potential role of gabapentin and extended-release gabapentin in the management of menopausal hot flashes. Int J Gen Med. 2013;6:657-64.
23. Ettinger B, Black DM, Mitlak BH, Knickerbocker RK, Nickelsen T, Genant HK, et al. Reduction of vertebral fracture risk in postmenopausal women with osteoporosis treated with raloxifene: Results from a 3-year randomized clinical trial. Multiple Outcomes of Raloxifene Evaluation (MORE) Investigators. JAMA. 1999;282(7):637-45.
24. Goswami R, Gupta N, Goswami D, Marwaha RK, Tandon N, Kochupillai N. Prevalence and significance of low 25-hydroxyvitamin D concentrations in healthy subjects in Delhi. Am J Clin Nutr. 2000;72:472-5.
25. Gupta A, Gupta N, Singh N, Goswami R. Presence of impaired intestinal calcium absorption in chronic hypovitaminosis D and its change after cholecalciferol supplementation: Assessment by the calcium load test. J Hum Nutr Diet. 2010;23: 54-60.

Section IX

ANTICANCER DRUGS

CHAPTER

CHAPTER 32

Chemotherapy in Gynecological Cancers

Gauri Gandhi, Shweta Tahlan, Snigdha Pathak

The various *antineoplastic drugs* used in gynecological cancers are classified as follows[1]:

Alkylating agents	Cyclophosphamide Ifosfamide Triethylenethiophosphoramide (TSPA, Thiotepa)
Alkylating like agents	Cisplatin Carboplatin
Antitumor antibiotics	Actinomycin D (Dactinomycin) Bleomycin Doxorubicin (Adriamycin) Liposomal doxorubicin
Antimetabolites	5-fluorouracil Methotrexate Hydroxyurea Gemcitabine
Plant alkaloids	Vincristine Vinblastine Etoposide Paclitaxel Docetaxel
Topoisomerase–1 inhibitors	Topotecan Irinotecan

ALKYLATING AGENTS

Pharmacology (Table 32.1)

Mechanism

They act primarily by chemically interacting with the DNA leading to inhibition of DNA, RNA and protein synthesis. These drugs are also called radiomimetic, as some effects are similar to irradiation.

Some alkylating agents used in gynecological cancers are tabulated in **Table 32.1**.

ALKYLATING-LIKE AGENTS

Precise mechanism less known. Tabulated in **Table 32.2**.

ANTITUMOR ANTIBIOTICS (TABLE 32.3)

Pharmacology

Mechanism

They are naturally occurring products that have complex chemical structures. They interact with DNA, often with intercalation, and the compound is inserted in between DNA base pairs. Also, they are believed to form free radicals that damage DNA, RNA and vital proteins. They are thought to be cell cycle—nonspecific.

Commonly used antitumor antibiotics are given in **Table 32.3**.

ANTIMETABOLITES (TABLE 32.4)

Pharmacology

Mechanism

These drugs interact with intracellular enzymes which leads to their inactivation or

Table 32.1: Alkylating agents

Drug	*Route*	*Dosage*	*Common toxicities*	*Gynecological cancers treated*
Cyclophosphamide (cytoxan)	PO, IV	• 10–50 mg/kg IV every 1–4 weeks; • 60–1000 mg/m^2 every 3–4 weeks	Myelosuppression, cystitis ± bladder fibrosis, alopecia, hepatitis, amenorrhea, azoospermia	Ovarian cancer
Ifosphamide	IV	1.0 or 1.2 g/m^2/day × 5 days with *mesna*: 200 mg/m^2 immediately before and 4h and 8 h after *ifosphamide*	Myelosuppression, bladder toxicity, central nervous system dysfunction, renal toxicity	Ovarian cancer Cervical cancer
Triethylenethiophosphoramide (TSPA, Thiotepa)	IV	IV: 0.8 mg/kg every 4–6 weeks	Myelosuppression, nausea and vomiting headaches fever (rare)	Ovarian, breast cancer
	Intracavitary	Intracavitary: 45–60 mg		For malignant effusions

Table 32.2: Alkylating-like agents

Cisplatin	IV	10–20 mg/m^2/day × 5 days; every 3 weeks (daily dosing) 40–75 mg/m^2 every 1–3 weeks (weekly dosing)	Nephrotoxicity, tinnitus and hearing loss, nausea or/and vomiting, myelosuppression, peripheral neuropathy	Epithelial ovarian cancer Germ cell tumors Cervical cancer Endometrial cancer
Carboplatin	IV	300–400 mg/m^2 × 6 every 3–4 weeks AUC 4–7.5	Less neuropathy, ototoxicity, and nephrotoxicity but more hematopoietic toxicity, especially thrombocytopenia, than *cisplatin*	Epithelial ovarian cancers Germ cell tumors Endometrial cancer

Table 32.3: Anti-tumor antibiotics

Drugs	*Route*	*Dosage*	*Toxicity*	*Gynecological cancers treated*
Actinomycin D (Dactinomycin)	IV	0.3–0.5 mg/m^2 IV × 5 days every 3–4 weeks	• GI Toxicity—Nausea and vomiting, mucosal ulceration • Skin necrosis • Myelosuppression	Germ cell ovarian tumors, choriocarcinoma

Contd...

Contd...

Drugs	*Route*	*Dosage*	*Toxicity*	*Gynecological cancers treated*
Bleomycin	IV, SC, IM, IP	10–20 units/m^2 1–2 times/week to total dose of 400 units; for effusions, 60–120 units	Fever, dermatologic reactions, pulmonary toxicity, anaphylactic reactions	Cervical, germ cell ovarian tumors, malignant effusions
Doxorubicin (Adriamycin)	IV	60–90 mg/m^2; 3 weekly; or 20–35 mg/m^2/day for 3 days; 3 weekly	Myelosuppression, alopecia, cardiotoxicity, local vesicant, nausea and vomiting, mucosal ulcerations	Ovarian cancer endometrial cancer
Liposomal doxorubicin	IV	40–50 mg/m^2; every 4 weeks	Palmar-plantar erythrodysesthesia, myelosuppression, stomatitis	Ovarian and endometrial cancers

Table 32.4: Anti-metabolites				
5-fluorouracil (fluorouracil, 5-FU)	IV	10–15 mg/kg/week	Myelosuppression, nausea and vomiting, anorexia, alopecia	Ovarian cancer
Methotrexate (MTX, amethopterin	PO, IV, intrathecal	PO: 15–40 mg/day × 5 days; IV: 240 mg/m^2 with leucovorin rescue; intrathecal: 12–15 mg/m^2/week	Mucosal ulceration, myelosuppression, hepatotoxicity, allergic pneumonitis; with intrathecal: meningeal irritation	Choriocarcinoma, ovarian cancer
Hydroxyurea (Hydrea)	PO, IV	1–2 g/m^2/day for 2–6 weeks	Myelosuppression, nausea and vomiting, anorexia	Cervical cancer
Gemcitabine (Gemzar)	IV	800–1000 mg/m^2/week for 3 weeks, then 1 week rest, then repeated	Myelosuppression, fever	Ovarian cancer, leiomyosarcoma

formation of products which are incapable of normal intracellular function. Structurally they resemble normal purines and pyrimidines analogs. These drugs are usually act more on actively proliferating cells. Therefore, they are classed in general as cell cycle specific agents. Usually, they are used in combinations because of their cell cycle specificity.

PLANT ALKALOIDS (TABLE 32.5)

Pharmacology

Mechanism

Derived from plants, these natural compounds are large and complex molecules. Vincristine and vinblastine act primarily by binding to vital intracellular micotubular proteins, particularly tubulin. This produces inhibition of microtubule assembly and destruction of the mitotic spindle and the cells are arrested in mitosis. These are cell cycle specific drugs.

Paclitaxel's mechanism of action is unique as it preferentially binds to microtubules and causes their polymerization and stabilization.

TOPOISOMERASE-1 INHIBITORS

Topotecan, Irinotecan

These drugs act through inhibition of the enzyme topoisomerase-1. This enzyme is a very important enzyme in DNA replication, transcription and DNA repair. The inhibition leads to permanent strand breaking. Topotecan is used in Platinum refractory ovarian cancer and cervical cancer. Its main toxicity is bone marrow suppression. Irinotecan is the second drug of the class, active in ovarian and cervical cancers.

COMPLICATIONS AND SIDE EFFECTS OF CHEMOTHERAPY

Hematological Toxicity

The precursor cells in bone marrow are very susceptible. Granulocytopenia and thrombocytopenia are common with most of the agents. The severity and duration depends upon the drug used, its dosage, schedule and previous exposures to chemotherapy or radiotherapy. Usually, granulocytopenia occurs 6–12 days

Table 32.5: Plant alkaloids

Vincristine (Oncovin)	IV	0.01–0.03 mg/kg/week	Neurotoxicity, alopecia, myelosuppression, cranial nerve palsies, gastrointestinal	Germ cell tumors, sarcomas, cervical cancer
Vinblastine (Velban)	IV	5–6 mg/m^2 every 1–2 weeks	Myelosuppression, alopecia, nausea and vomiting, neurotoxicity	Germ cell tumors, choriocarcinoma
Etoposide	IV	300–600 mg/m^2 divided over 3–4 days every 3–4 weeks	Myelosuppression, alopecia, hypotension	Germ cell tumors. choriocarcinoma
	PO	50 mg/m^2/day × 21 days, then 1 week rest, then repeat		Ovarian cancer
Paclitaxel (Taxol)	IV	135–250 mg/m^2 as a 3- to 24-hour infusion every 3 weeks	Myelosuppression and peripheral sensory neuropathy (Dose limiting toxicities) alopecia, allergic reactions, cardiac arrhythmias	Ovarian cancer Endometrial cancer Cervical cancer
Docetaxel (Taxotere)	IV	60–100 mg/m^2 every 3–4 weeks	Myelosuppression (Dose limiting toxicity), alopecia, hypersensitivity reactions	Ovarian cancer

after the chemotherapeutic drugs are given. The recovery of granulocytopenia usually occurs in 21–24 days. Thrombocytopenia occurs 4–5 days later and its recovery also follows the WBC recovery. Drugs like mitomycin C and nitrosoureas cause delayed suppression of marrow, at 28–42 days. The recovery is also delayed up to 2 months.

Neutropenia

Neutropenia is defined as absolute neutrophil count (ANC) of less than 1500/μL. Based on the level of ANC, it is categorized as mild, moderate or severe. It is called mild neutropenia when ANC is between 1000 microL and 1500/microL, moderate neutropenia when ANC is between 500 and 1000/microL, and it is called severe when ANC is less than 500/microL. Below an ANC of 1000/microL, the risk of infection begins to increase. The risk of clinically important infection increases when the ANC goes below 500 cells/microL and the risk is higher when the duration of neutropenia is prolonged (>7 days).[2]

Evaluation and Treatment

In a neutropenic patient, fever might be the only and earliest sign of infection. Fever in these patients is defined as a single oral temperature of >38.3°C (101°F) or a temperature of >38.0°C (100.4°F) sustained for more than one hour.[2] Fever should be monitored 4 hourly in a neutropenic patient and should be taken as a medical emergency. Mortality rates of up to 70% have been documented in earlier studies if initiation of antibiotics was delayed.[3]

Therefore, initial evaluation should be done promptly by taking detailed history and doing a complete physical examination to identify the focus of infection. Common sites are—skin, catheter sites, biopsy and bone marrow aspirate sites, oral cavity, mucosal membranes, perianal and genital areas. Blood cultures and cultures from other relevant sites should be sent.

Neutropenia is treated with broad spectrum antibiotics and colony stimulating factors.

a. *Broad spectrum antibiotics* which cover both the gram-positive and gram-negative organisms should be started within 60 minutes of presentation and at full doses. The recommended initial empiric oral antibacterial regimen for low-risk patients (neutropenia <7 days, no comorbidities) involves a combination of a fluoroquinolone (*Ciprofloxacin* 750 mg orally BD or *levofloxacin* 750 mg orally OD) and a beta-lactam agent, such as amoxicillin (500 mg)—clavulanic acid (125 mg) (orally three times daily).[2,4] For patients who have a history of penicillin hypersensitivity, *clindamycin* (300 mg four times daily) may be given in place of amoxicillin—clavulanic acid or, if a cephalosporin is deemed to be safe, *cefixime* (400 mg once daily) may be given.[2] Antibiotic therapy may be changed according to patient's condition and culture reports. The duration of antibacterial therapy in low-risk patients with negative blood cultures is for at least two afebrile days after the ANC has recovered (more than 500/microL). Among patients in whom the ANC has not recovered to >500 cells/microL, antibacterial therapy should be continued until the patient has been afebrile for 5–7 days.[2,5] Antifungal drug is added after 7 days of fever despite antibiotics. For high-risk patients (neutropenia >7 days, other comorbidities) with neutropenic fever, empiric monotherapy with a beta-lactam agent which has antipseudomonas activity, like *Cefepime, Meropenem, Imipenem,* or *Piperacillin-Tazobactam* are recommended.
b. *Colony stimulating factors*: There are two colony stimulating factors available—recombinant human granulocyte colony-stimulating factor (G-CSF, filgrastim and pegylated filgrastim, trade name—neupogen) and granulocyte-macrophage colony-stimulating factor (GM-CSF, sargramostim). Usually, G-CSF's are used; however, none is recommended over the other.

Primary prophylaxis[2]: G-CSF is given as primary prophylaxis when anticipated incidence of neutropenic fever is 20% or higher in dose-intense chemotherapy regimens.

Secondary prophylaxis[2]: G-CSF may be given as secondary prophylaxis when neutropenic fever has occurred in a prior cycle.

Dosage and timing of G-CSF: 5 microgram/kg/day is recommended.

Therapy is usually begun 24–72 hours after cessation of chemotherapy and continues twice weekly with monitoring of blood counts, until the absolute neutrophil count reaches 5000–10000/microL.[6] Growth factors should be stopped several days before the next cycle of chemotherapy and they should not be given on the same day as chemotherapy as rapidly dividing myeloid cells can be sensitive to cytotoxic chemotherapy.[7] Also, they should not be given with concurrent radiotherapy.

Therapeutic use in neutropenia without fever: Role of CSF's in this condition is not established.[8] However, in prolonged neutropenia, neupogen can be given in the same dose as above.

Therapeutic use in neutropenic fever: Though the role is controversial, ASCO guidelines[9] recommend its use in high risk patients (age > 65 years, pneumonitis, sepsis, prolonged and severe neutropenia). NCCN[10] guidelines recommend CSF to be continued in patients who receive prophylactic CSF and even in patients with high risk factors who did not receive prophylactic CSF.

Gastrointestinal Toxicity

Mucositis in upper GI tract leads to painful ulceration in mouth and pharynx, esophagitis, oral candidiasis. Mucositis in lower GI tract causes diarrhea. It can also cause bowel perforation, hemorrhage and necrotizing enterocolitis. Mucositis usually occurs 3–5 days earlier than myelosuppression.

Dermatologic Reactions

Extravasation can cause erythema, skin necrosis and skin sloughing and chronic ulceration. Alopecia is also common.

Genitourinary Toxicity

Cisplatin, methotrexate, nitrosoureas, mitomycin C are all nephrotoxic and can cause *renal failure*. Treatment includes discontinuation of the offending drug, increase glomerular filtration by increasing blood volume and treatment of specific metabolic abnormalities. Short-term dialysis may also be required. The dose of cisplatin and carboplatin should be adjusted according to renal function of the patient.

Dose (mg) = Target AUC × (Creatinine clearance + 25)

The desired target AUC (area under curve) is 4–5 mg/mL for previously treated patients and 5–7 mg/mL for untreated patients.

The use of nephrotoxic antibiotics will enhance the renal toxicity of platins and this important drug interaction should be kept in mind.

High dose cyclophosphamide and ifosfamide can cause bladder irritation and hemorrhagic cystitis. This can be prevented by the use of mesna (sodium mercaptoethanesulfonate). Mesna acts by deactivating acrolein, which is the toxic metabolite.

Neurotoxicity

Vinca alkaloids, mainly vincristine, can cause peripheral motor, sensory and autonomic neuropathies. Cisplatin and paclitaxel are also neurotoxic.

Cisplatin causes a progressive and delayed peripheral neuropathy when used in high doses. It involves sensory and proprioceptory functions but motor function is usually saved.

Paclitaxel causes peripheral sensory neuropathy and the severity and incidence of neuropathy symptoms is associated with peak levels of drug in the plasma.

Also, combination of platins + paclitaxel is more neurotoxic than each agent alone.

Hepatotoxicity

Slight elevations in bilirubin, ALT, AST, ALP are commonly seen with many drugs.

This usually resolves after treatment. Long-term methotrexate therapy can cause hepatic fibrosis leading to cirrhosis. Patients with pre-existing liver disease increases the risk of toxicity. Drug induced hepatitis and cirrhosis require removal of the toxic drug and supportive treatment.

Pulmonary Complications

Interstitial pneumonitis with pulmonary fibrosis is the usual insult. Bleomycin, alkylating agents, gemcitabine and nitrosoureas cause this damage. Management includes discontinuation of the offending agent and supportive care.

Cardiac Toxicity

Doxorubicin and daunomycin can cause severe cardiomyopathy. Cardiotoxicity increases with total cumulative dose. Therefore, a cumulative dose of 500 mg/m^2 is used as maximum tolerable dose of doxorubicin. Early detection of LV dysfunction before CHF occurs is important and discontinuation of the drug at earliest indication. Bevacizumab can cause the development of hypertension. In cardiac patients, this effect can cause deterioration in cardiac function.

Vascular and Hypersensitivity Reactions

The hypersensitivity reactions can be reduced by giving intravenous dexamethasone infusion (20 mg) along with tablet diphenhydramine (50 mg), 30 minutes before administration of drug.

Secondary Malignancies

Etoposide's prolonged use has been associated with development of leukemia. Combined chemotherapy with extensive radiotherapy is high risk for second malignancy.

Gonadal Dysfunction

Many drugs, especially alkylating agents, can cause amenorrhea. Secondary sexual characters are usually not disturbed. Short-term intensive chemotherapy, like that given in germ cell tumors and gestational trophoblastic disease, with the use of antimetabolites, vinca alkaloids and antitumor antibiotics, causes less injury to reproductive system. These patients usually recover their reproductive capacity after treatment.

Metabolic Abnormalities

Rapid tumor lysis can cause hyperuricemia, hyperkalemia, hyperphosphatemia, hypocalcemia, and can be life threatening.

Chemotherapy in Pregnancy

Use of chemotherapy in the first trimester, especially antimetabolites, can cause congenital abnormalities. The anomalies are usually not seen with chemotherapy in second and third trimester, but very few studies have been done.

CASE SCENARIOS

Case 1: A 45-year-old lady, P4 L4, with chief complaints of postcoital bleeding since past 3 months. On examination, there was a large growth of size 5 × 6 cm replacing the cervix, involving medial half of parametrium. What is the treatment of choice?

The patient is having *cancer cervix stage IIB*. This is a locally advanced cancer cervix.

[Locally advanced cancer cervix includes - Stages 1B2, IIA2, IIB, IIIA, IIIB, IVA].

The preferred treatment for locally advanced cervical cancer is *concurrent chemoradiation*. (NCCN guidelines 2015).[11] This involves external pelvic irradiation + concurrent cisplatin containing chemotherapy + brachytherapy (Category 1). Concurrent cisplatin containing chemotherapy has single agent cisplatin or cisplatin + 5-flurouracil. The regimens used are given below:

Different Regimes[12] for Concurrent Chemoradiation

- Cisplatin 40 mg/m^2 IV once weekly (not to exceed 70 mg/wk) *plus* radiation therapy

1.8–2 Gy per fraction (minimum 4 cycles; maximum 6 cycles) or

- Cisplatin 50–75 mg/m² IV on day 1 *plus* 5-fluorouracil (5-FU) 1000 mg/m² continuous IV infusion on days 2–5 and days 30–33 (total dose 4000 mg/m² each course)
- Cisplatin 50–75 mg/m² IV on day 1 *plus* 5-FU 1000 mg/m² continuous IV infusion over 24 hours on days 1–4 (total dose 4000 mg/m² each cycle) every 3 weeks for a total of 3–4 cycles.

Single agent cisplatin used with RT has similar outcomes but reduced toxicity as compared to cisplatin plus 5 FU,[13] therefore, it is generally preferred.

Neoadjuvant Chemotherapy in Locally Advanced Cancer Cervix

In areas where radiotherapy facilities are limited, such as our country, NACT followed by Radical surgery is an option for patients with stage IB2, IIA2 and IIB. Two phase III trials are ongoing to study NACT in this group—EORTC 55994 and NCT00193739. Tata Memorial Hospital, Mumbai is conducting the randomnized controlled trial NCT00193739 to compare NACT (3 courses of paclitaxel-carboplatin) followed by surgery to concurrent chemoradiation in stages IB2 to IIB squamous cell cancer cervix. The final results are awaited.

Case 2: A 47-year-old patient is diagnosed with metastatic cancer cervix-stage IVB. What is the preferred treatment?

Metastatic and recurrent cancer cervix is primarily treated with chemotherapy. If the disease is amenable to local treatment, resection and radiotherapy is considered.[11]

NCCN recommends following drugs for recurrent or metastatic cervical cancer.

First Line Combinations[11,14,15]

- Cisplatin/paclitaxel/bevacizumab (category 1): Bevacizumab 15 mg/kg IV over 30–90 minutes *plus* cisplatin 50 mg/m² IV over 30–90 minutes on days 1 or 2 *plus* paclitaxel 135 or 175 mg/m² IV over 3 or 24 hours on day 1 every 3 weeks.
- Cisplatin/paclitaxel (category 1): Paclitaxel 135 mg/m² IV over 24 hours (dosing at 175 mg/m² IV over 3 hours is also acceptable) *plus* cisplatin 50 mg/m² IV on day 1 every 3 weeks.
- Topotecan/paclitaxel/bevacizumab (category 1): Bevacizumab 15 mg/kg IV over 30–90 minutes *plus* paclitaxel 175 mg/m² IV over 3 hours on day 1 *plus* topotecan 0.75 mg/m² IV over 30 minutes on days 1–3 every 3 weeks.
- Carboplatin/paclitaxel
- Cisplatin/topotecan: Topotecan 0.75 mg/m² IV (or 0.6 mg/m² IV if prior radiation therapy) on days 1–3 *plus* cisplatin 50 mg/m² IV on day 1 every 3 weeks.
- Topotecan/paclitaxel: Topotecan 0.75 mg/m² IV (or 0.6 mg/m² IV if prior radiation therapy) on days 1–3 *plus* paclitaxel 175 mg/m² IV over 3 hours on day 1 every 3 weeks.
- Cisplatin/gemcitabine (category 3).

Case 3: A 55-year-old female presents with ascites and abdominopelvic mass. CA-125 is 3400. Imaging shows bilateral solid cystic adenexal masses of size 10 × 10 cm, likely malignant, with peritoneal nodules. Cytology from ascitic fluid shows malignant cells. What is the management?

The case is one of *advanced stage ovarian cancer*, likely Stage IIC. The preferred treatment is primary surgical cytoreduction followed by adjuvant systemic chemotherapy.

Indications for adjuvant chemotherapy in ovarian cancer: (NCCN Guidelines 2015)

- Stage IA and IB—Grade 2
- Stage IA and IB—clear cell types (any grade)
- Stage IC—any grade
- Stage II, III, IV

Cases that don't require chemotherapy—Stage IA and IB—Grade 1.

Cases that can be either observed/given chemotherapy—Stage IA and IB Grade 2.

Number of cycles—Stage I—3–6 cycles; stage II/III/IV—6–8 cycles.

Recommended therapy:

- IV platin + taxane or

- Combination intraperitoneal + IV chemotherapy—for optimally debulked stage II and III patients.

Patients who are not poor candidates for surgery due to the site and volume of disease involvement or medical comorbidities at the time of diagnosis may be considered for *neoadjuvant chemotherapy*.

Recommended regimes[16] are:

- Paclitaxel 175 mg/m² IV over 3 hours followed by carboplatin AUC 5-6 IV over 1 hour—Day 1. Repeat every 3 weeks for 6 cycles (category 1).
- Dose dense paclitaxel 80 mg/m² IV over 1 hour—days 1, 8, 15 followed by carboplatin AUC 5-6 over 1 hour on day 1. Repeat every 3 weeks for 6 cycles (category 1).
- Paclitaxel 60 mg/m² IV over 1 hour followed by carboplatin AUC 2 IV over 30 minutes. Weekly for 18 weeks (category 1).
- Docetaxel 60-75 mg/m² IV over 1 hour followed by carboplatin AUC 5-6 IV over 1 hour—day 1. Repeat every 3 weeks for 6 cycles (category 1).
- Cisplatin (75 mg/m²) plus paclitaxel (135 mg/m² over 24 hours) every three weeks for six cycles[17]
- *Combined IP/IV regimen*: Paclitaxel 135 mg/m² IV continuous infusion over 3 or 24 hours on day 1; cisplatin 75-100 mg/m² IP, day 2 after IV paclitaxel; paclitaxel 60 mg/m² IP on day 8. Repeat every 3 weeks for 6 cycles (category 1).

Carboplatin is the preferred platin as it produces equivalent response rates and survival outcomes as cisplatin but causes less toxicity as shown by phase III studies.[18,19] Carboplatin plus docetaxel is equivalent to carboplatin with paclitaxel, although docetaxel causes a lower incidence of neuropathy, myalgias, and weakness, but it increases the risk of neutropenia, hypersensitivity reactions, and severe nausea and vomiting, as shown by the scotroc study.[20]

Role of bevacizumab[16]: NCCN does not recommend the use of bevacizumab as initial adjuvant chemotherapy or as maintenance therapy. It is recommended to be given with carboplatin and paclitaxel (category 3).

Maintenance chemotherapy: The impact of maintenance chemotherapy for epithelial ovarian cancer was reviewed by a meta-analysis of 6 randomized trials (n = 902)[21]. The 5 years survival rate showed no significant improvement and the study concluded that the administration of maintenance therapy was not justifiable.

Monitoring of patients on chemotherapy[16] as follows:

- Pelvic examination at least every 2-3 cycles
- Complete hemogram as indicated
- Liver and kidney function tests, blood sugar; as and when required
- CA-125 levels or other tumor markers, prior to each cycle of chemotherapy
- Radiographic imaging if indicated.

CHEMOTHERAPY FOR GERM CELL TUMORS

NCCN[16] recommends adjuvant chemotherapy in the following cases:

- Embryonal tumor—any stage
- Endodermal sinus tumor (yolk sac tumor)-any stage
- Dysgerminoma—stage II-IV
- Immature teratoma—Stage I, grade 2, 3 or stage II-IV.

Recommended chemotherapy is 3-4 cycles of bleomycin/etoposide/cisplatin, given as follows:[22]

- Bleomycin 30 units/week IV on days 1, 8, and 15 *plus*
- Etoposide 100 mg/m ²/day IV *and*
- Cisplatin 20 mg/m ²/day IV on days 1-5
- BEP is given every 21 days for three cycles (4 cycles if the patient had bulky residual disease after surgery).

Pulmonary function tests are recommended if bleomycin is considered.[16]

In selected patients, where minimizing toxicity is critical, 3 courses of etoposide/carboplatin can be used.[16]

CHEMOTHERAPY IN ENDOMETRIAL CANCERS

Indications for adjuvant chemotherapy (alongwith radiotherapy) in endometrial cancers:

- Stage IB and II—Grade 3 (Category 2B)[23]
- Stage III and IV—all grades (Category 2A)
- Serous adenocarcinoma, clear cell adenocarcinoma, carcinosarcoma—all stages[23]

Recommended chemotherapeutic agents for endometrial cancer[23] are as follows:

Multiagent chemotherapy regimens preferred, if tolerated:

- Carboplatin/paclitaxel
- Carboplatin/docetaxel
- Cisplatin/doxorubicin
- Cisplatin/doxorubicin/paclitaxel
- Ifosfamide/paclitaxel (category 1 for carcinosarcoma)
- Cisplatin/ifosfamide (for carcinosarcoma)

UTERINE SARCOMA

Chemotherapy is recommended in high grade (undifferentiated) endometrial sarcoma and uterine leiomyosarcoma, stages II, III, IV; with radiotherapy (category 2A recommendation). In stage I, chemotherapy can be given vs observation (category 2B recommendation).[23]

Chemotherapeutic agents have no role in endometrial stromal sarcoma (ESS), where hormone therapy (progesterones, aromatase inhibitors, GnRH analogs), is given as adjuvant therapy with radiotherapy.[23]

GESTATIONAL TROPHOBLASTIC NEOPLASIA

These tumors are highly chemosensitive and curable cancers, even when metastatic. Chemotherapy is the main line of treatment for GTN.

Chemotherapy for Low-risk GTN

Single agent chemotherapy[24,25]: It is given in low-risk GTN. Methotrexate (MTX) and dactinomycin (Actinomycin-D) are the two commonly drugs used in this setting. MTX is preferred, as the side effects and toxicity of MTX is less than that of dactinomycin. Etoposide and 5-FU have also been used. Various regimes are as follows.

- *8-day alternating MTX regimen*: MTX-1 mg/kg IM days (1, 3, 5, and 7) *plus* leucovorin calcium—0.1 mg/kg, given once, 24 hours after each MTX dose (on days 2, 4, 6, and 8). Repeat cycle every 14 days. This regime is most widely used as it is easy to administer and well tolerated. Overall response rates are 74–90% and stage I remission rates are more than 90%.
- *Infusional MTX therapy*: MTX 100 mg/m^2 as IV bolus over 30 minutes, *then* 200 mg/m^2 in 500 mL D5W infused over 12 hours on day 1 *plus* folinic acid 15 mg IM/PO every 12 hours for 4 doses. Initiate folinic acid 24 hours after start of MTX. Repeat cycle every 18 days or as needed.
- *5-day MTX regimen*: MTX 0.4 mg/kg/day IV or IM for 5 days, not to exceed 25 mg/day. Repeat cycle every 14 days.
- *Weekly MTX*: MTX 30–50 mg/m^2 IM weekly. Treatment is repeated until the serum beta-hCG concentration falls to normal (less than 5 mIU/mL) for three consecutive weeks.

  Significant toxicity with MTX usually not seen, but hematologic values should be carefully monitored during therapy. Prior to every treatment, normal renal and liver function should be checked, as MTX is excreted entirely by kidneys and it may cause liver damage. Sometimes, MTX has been associated with idiopathic interstitial pneumonitis.
- *Dactinomycin 5 day regime*: Act-D 0.5 mg IV/day for 5 days, repeat cycle after every 14 days.
- *Pulsed Act-D regime*: 1.25 mg/m^2 IV every 2 weeks.

Chemotherapy for High-risk GTN

Multi agent therapy: It is used for high risk GTN—stage IV disease or stage II/III disease with high prognostic score, disease that is resistant to single agent therapy, and for PSTT.

Etoposide, methotrexate, actinomycin-D followed by cyclophosphamide and vincristine (EMA/CO) is the most preferred regimen for initial treatment of highrisk GTD.[26-28]

- Etoposide—100 mg/m² IV over 30 minutes on days 1 and 2 +
- Methotrexate—100 mg/m² IV push followed by 200 mg/m² IV over 12 hours on day 1 +
- Dactinomycin—0.5 mg IV bolus on days 1 and 2 +
- Leucovorin calcium—15 mg orally every 12 hours for four doses, starting 24 hours after start of MTX +
- Cyclophosphamide—600 mg/m² IV on day 8
- Vincristine (Oncovin®)—1.0 mg/m² IV on day 8.

The regimen is repeated every two weeks until remission (remission is normalization of beta-hCG and disappearance of all radiographically evident disease), and usually continued for an additional three cycles (six weeks).

Some other regimes which are used are:

- *EMA*: The EMA regimen uses the same doses as for the EMA/CO regimen, but without the cyclophosphamide and vincristine.
- *MAC*: Methotrexate, actinomycin-D, cyclophosphamide.

VULVAR CANCER

Chemotherapy in vulvar cancer has little role. Chemoradiation is an alternative to radical surgery in selected patients with locally advanced vulvar cancer. Patients with anorectal or bladder involvement (to avoid colostomy and urostomy) and patients with disease fixed to the bone can be offered chemoradiation over surgery. Surgical resection can be done if residual disease remains.[29] A gynecologic oncology group (GOG) trial[30] used *cisplatin* (50 mg/m² on day 1 of each course of RT) and 5-FU (1000 mg/m² per day as a 24 hours continuous infusion for the first four days of each course of RT). Palliative chemotherapy can be given for metastatic stage IV B patients or frail inoperable patients.

REFERENCES

1. Berek and Hacker's Gynaecologic Oncology 5th edition. 2010. Chapter 3: Chemotherapy
2. Freifeld AG, Bow EJ, Sepkowitz KA, et al. Clinical practice guideline for the use of antimicrobial agents in neutropenic patients with cancer: 2010 update by the infectious diseases society of america. Clin Infect Dis. 2011; 52:e56.
3. Schimpff S, Satterlee W, Young VM, Serpick A. Empiric therapy with carbenicillin and gentamicin for febrile patients with cancer and granulocytopenia. N Engl J Med. 1971;284:1061.
4. Flowers CR, Seidenfeld J, Bow EJ, et al. Antimicrobial prophylaxis and outpatient management of fever and neutropenia in adults treated for malignancy: American Society of Clinical Oncology clinical practice guideline. J Clin Oncol. 2013;31:794.
5. de Naurois J, Novitzky-Basso I, Gill MJ, et al. Management of febrile neutropenia: ESMO Clinical Practice Guidelines. Ann Oncol. 2010;21 (Suppl 5):v252.
6. Ozer H, Armitage JO, Bennett CL, et al. 2000 update of recommendations for the use of hematopoietic colony-stimulating factors: evidence-based, clinical practice guidelines. American Society of Clinical Oncology Growth Factors Expert Panel. J Clin Oncol. 2000;18:3558.
7. Skarlos DV, Timotheadou E, Galani E, et al. Pegfilgrastim administered on the same day with dose-dense adjuvant chemotherapy for breast cancer is associated with a higher incidence of febrile neutropenia as compared to conventional growth factor support: matched case-control study of the Hellenic Cooperative Oncology Group. Oncology. 2009;77:107.
8. Hartmann LC, Tschetter LK, Habermann TM, et al. Granulocyte colony-stimulating factor in severe chemotherapy-induced afebrile neutropenia. N Engl J Med. 1997;336:1776.
9. Smith TJ, Khatcheressian J, Lyman GH, et al. 2006 update of recommendations for the use of white blood cell growth factors: an evidence-based clinical practice guideline. J Clin Oncol. 2006;24:3187.
10. National Comprehensive Cancer Network (NCCN) guidelines. Available at: www.nccn.org (Accessed on May 15, 2012).
11. NCCN guidelines Version 2. 2015—Cervical Cancer.
12. Chemoradiotherapy for Cervical Cancer Meta-Analysis Collaboration. Reducing uncertainties

about the effects of chemoradiotherapy for cervical cancer: a systematic review and meta-analysis of individual patient data from 18 randomized trials. J Clin Oncol. 2008;26(35): 5802-12.
13. Chemoradiotherapy for Cervical Cancer Meta-Analysis Collaboration. Reducing uncertainties about the effects of chemoradiotherapy for cervical cancer: a systematic review and meta-analysis of individual patient data from 18 randomized trials. J Clin Oncol. 2008;26(35): 5802-12.
14. Monk BJ, Sill MW, McMeekin DS, et al. Phase III trial of four cisplatin-containing doublet combinations in stage IVB, recurrent, or persistent cervical carcinoma: a Gynecologic Oncology Group study. J Clin Oncol. 2009;27(28): 4649-55.
15. Tewari KS, Monk BJ. Recent achievements and future developments in advanced and recurrent cervical cancer: trials of the Gynecologic Oncology Group. Semin Oncol. 2009;36(2):170-80.
16. NCCN Guidelines version 1. 2015—Epithelial ovarian cancer/fallopian tube cancer/primary peritoneal cancer.
17. McGuire WP, Hoskins WJ, Brady MF, et al. Cyclophosphamide and cisplatin compared with paclitaxel and cisplatin in patients with stage III and stage IV ovarian cancer. N Engl J Med. 1996; 334:1.
18. Aabo K, Adams M, Adnitt P, et al. Chemotherapy in advanced ovarian cancer: four systematic meta-analyses of individual patient data from 37 randomized trials. Advanced Ovarian Cancer Trialists' Group. Br J Cancer. 1998;78:1479.
19. Chemotherapy for advanced ovarian cancer. Advanced Ovarian Cancer Trialists Group. Cochrane Database Syst Rev. 2000;CD001418.
20. Vasey PA, Jayson GC, Gordon A, et al. Phase III randomized trial of docetaxel-carboplatin versus paclitaxel-carboplatin as first-line chemotherapy for ovarian carcinoma. J Natl Cancer Inst. 2004;96:1682.
21. Mei L, Chen H, Wei DM, et al. Maintenance chemotherapy for ovarian cancer. Cochrane Database Syst Rev 2010;CD007414.
22. Williams S, Blessing JA, Liao SY, Ball H, Hanjani P. Adjuvant therapy of ovarian germ cell tumors with cisplatin, etoposide, and bleomycin: a trial of the Gynecologic Oncology Group. J Clin Oncol. 1994;12(4):701-6.
23. NCCN guidelines version 2. 2015—Endometrial Carcinoma.
24. Aghajanian C. Treatment of low-risk gestational trophoblastic neoplasia. J Clin Oncol. 2011;29(7): 786-8. [Medline].
25. Lurain JR. Gestational trophoblastic disease II: classification and management of gestational trophoblastic neoplasia. Am J Obstet Gynecol. 2011;204(1):11-8. [Medline].
26. Lurain JR, Singh DK, Schink JC. Primary treatment of metastatic high-risk gestational trophoblastic neoplasia with EMA-CO chemotherapy. J Reprod Med. 2006;51:767.
27. Escobar PF, Lurain JR, Singh DK, et al. Treatment of high-risk gestational trophoblastic neoplasia with etoposide, methotrexate, actinomycin D, cyclophosphamide, and vincristine chemotherapy. Gynecol Oncol. 2003;91:552.
28. Deng L, Zhang J, Wu T, Lawrie TA. Combination chemotherapy for primary treatment of high-risk gestational trophoblastic tumour. Cochrane Database Syst Rev. 2013;1:CD005196.
29. Elkas JC, Berek JS. Vulvar cancer; staging, treatment and prognosis. Uptodate 2013.
30. Montana GS, Thomas GM, Moore DH, et al. Preoperative chemo-radiation for carcinoma of the vulva with N2/N3 nodes: a gynecologic oncology group study. Int J Radiat Oncol Biol Phys. 2000;48:1007.

Section X

MISCELLANEOUS

CHAPTERS

CHAPTER 33

Fetal Therapy

Krishna Agarwal, Anoosha K Ravi

A therapeutic intervention for the sick fetus or anomalous fetus *in utero* has been made possible by the advances in the diagnostic modalities in fetal medicine. These therapeutic interventions include medical and surgical interventions. Some of the fetal conditions could be treated by giving drugs to the mother which are transferred transplacentally to the fetus. Here we will discuss few fetal conditions amenable to pharmacological treatment **(Table 33.1)**.

Table 33.1: Medical treatment of fetal disorders

Fetal disorder	*Drug(s)*
Cardiac arrhythmias	Digoxin
	Flecainide
	Amiodarone
	Sotalol
Thyroid disorders	Propylthiouracil
	Methimazole
	Carbimazole
	Intra-amniotic T4
	Intra-amniotic T3
	Triac
Adrenal disorders	Dexamethasone

CARDIAC ARRHYTHMIAS

Normal cardiac rhythm is regular and range from 110 to 160 beats per minute. Any irregularity in this is termed dysrhythmia. It can be benign extrasystoles or sustained arrhythmias resulting in fetal hydrops, congestive heart failure or even fetal demise. The most common causes of fetal tachycardia are atrioventricular re-entry supraventricular tachycardia (5%), atrial flutter (1.5%) and sinus tachycardia (0.5%).[1] The most common cause of fetal bradycardia is complete AV block (2.8%).[1] Arrhythmias are mostly diagnosed and monitored by echocardiography.

Fetal Tachycardia

Various drugs used for treatment of fetal tachycardia are digoxin, flecainide, amiodarone and sotalol. Drugs are usually administered to the mother. If fetus is hydropic or mother is at risk of arrhythmias or placental transfer is unsatisfactory, direct administration of intramuscular injection can be considered.

Digoxin

Pharmacology: Acts by slowing ventricular rate by partial blockage of AV node. It gets metabolized in liver and excreted by kidney. Half-life is 36–48 hour.[1]

Indications: Short ventriculoatrial tachycardia, atrial flutter, atrial fibrillation.

Contraindications: Liver and renal disease.

Dosage: Loading dose: 1200–1500 mcg IV. The required dose is added to 50–100 mL sodium chloride 0.9% or glucose 5%. Given as single infusion over at least 2 hours or given in divided doses as IV infusions over 20 minutes.

Maintenance 375 to 875 mcg orally in 2 divided doses.

Adverse effects: Nausea, vomiting, diarrhea, visual disturbances, dizziness, extrasystoles, bradycardia, dysrhythmias, first degree or second degree AV block.

Drug interaction: Verapamil and amiodarone increases plasma concentration by reducing clearance of digoxin.

Monitoring: Therapeutic plasma level of 1–2 ng/mL to be maintained.

Preparations

- *Digoxin*: 0.5 mg per 2 mL vial as injection
- *Lanoxin*: 0.25 tablet
- *Digox*: 0.25 tablet
- *Digitran*: 0.25 tablet.

Safety during pregnancy and lactation: It is FDA Category C drug.

Flecainide

Pharmacology: Inhibits sodium channels and slows down conduction velocity by increasing action potential duration. Given orally, metabolizes in liver and excreted by kidney. Half-life is 20 hours.

Indications: Short ventriculoatrial tachycardia, long ventriculoatrial tachycardia, atrial ectopic tachycardia.

Contraindications: Liver and renal disease, congestive heart failure.

Dosage: 100–400 mg/day orally in 2–4 divided doses.

Adverse effects: QT interval prolongation, torsades de pointes, proarrhythmia, fetal death, drug-induced interstitial lung disease.

Drug interaction: Blood levels are increased by amiodarone. Flecainide decreases levels of digoxin.

Monitoring: Therapeutic level is 0.2–10 mcg/mL.

Preparations

Tambocor: 100 mg tablet.

Safety during pregnancy and lactation: It is FDA category C drug.

Amiodarone

Pharmacology: It is a class III antiarrhythmic drug with action on K channels, Na channels and has beta blocker effect. It is given orally, metabolized in liver and excretion is hepatic and biliary.[1]

Indications: Short ventriculoatrial tachycardia, junctional ectopic tachycardia, ventricular tachycardia.

Contraindications: AV block, bradycardia, liver disease.

Dosage: Loading dose 1200 mg orally 6 hourly. Maintenance dose is 600–900 mg/day.

Adverse effects: Interstitial lung disease, QT interval prolongation, hypothyroidism/hyperthyroidism, visual disturbance, thrombocytopenia, etc.

Drug interaction: It also inhibits cytochrome P450 isozyme and thus, reduces clearance of digoxin, flecainide and warfarin.

Monitoring: Used with great caution with monitoring for maternal ECG and other side effects.

Preparations

- *Cordarone tablet*: 200 mg
- *Pacerone tablet*: 200 mg.

Safety during pregnancy and lactation: FDA category D drug.

Sotalol

Pharmacology: Mechanism of action is nonselective beta blockade and K channel blockade. It is only excreted by kidney and not metabolized. Half-life is 12 hours.[2]

Indications: Short ventriculoatrial tachycardia, long ventriculoatrial tachycardia, atrial flutter, junctional ectopic tachycardia, ventricular tachycardia.

Contraindications: Long QT syndrome, asthma, kidney disease.

Dosage: 80–160 mg orally in 2–4 divided doses.[2]

Adverse effects: QT interval prolongation, torsades de pointes (polymorphic ventricular tachycardia), dizziness, nausea, headache.

Drug Interaction

Monitoring: ECG, echocardiography and serum electrolytes.

Preparations

- *Solet*: 40 mg tablets
- *Sotagard*: 40, 80 mg tablets
- *Sotalar*: 40, 80 mg tablets.

Safety during pregnancy and lactation: FDA category C drug.

Monitoring for Antiarrhythmic Drugs

1. Maternal ECG
2. Fetal echocardiography
3. Fetal hydrops
4. Maternal serum electrolytes (potassium levels in digoxin and flecainide-hypokalemia predisposes to arrhythmias).

Fetal Bradycardia

1. If heart rate is below 55, salbutamol/terbutaline may be considered but it is deleterious if given in long QT syndrome.
2. Complete heart block is mostly due to anti-Ro/La antibodies. But the effect of immunoglobulins is doubtful.
3. Dexamethasone 4 mg orally daily may reverse first degree heart block but is ineffective for second and third degree heart block.

THYROID DISORDERS

Fetal thyroid starts functioning at 10–12 weeks but appreciable amounts of thyroid hormones are released only from 14–16 weeks. So, early fetus is dependent on maternal thyroid secretions. Moreover, maternal thyroid hormones contribute to the fetal thyroid hormone levels till birth as evident from neonates with complete thyroid agenesis. The placenta is permeable to T3 and T4, TRH, iodide substrates, thyroid stimulating hormone receptor antibodies (TRAbs) but is impermeable to TSH. Fetal thyroid status is assessed indirectly by maternal thyroid function and antibody tests: TSH, FT4, TSAb (TSH receptor stimulating antibodies), TBAb (TSH receptor blocking antibodies), TBII (TSH binding inhibitory immunoglobulin) and directly by fetal imaging by ultrasound or MRI and fetal thyroid function tests.[3]

Fetal Hyperthyroidism

Causes of fetal hyperthyroidism are maternal autoimmune disorders like Graves' disease and Hashimoto's thyroiditis.

Drugs: Thioamides like propylthiouracil (PTU), methimazole, carbimazole are used in treatment of fetal hyperthyroidism.

Dosage: PTU 100 mg 8 hourly later reduced to 50 mg 8 hourly. Carbimazole 20 mg 12 hourly. Dose titrated according to the response.[2]

Monitoring

- Maternal thyroid function tests 4–6 weekly
- Ultrasound for fetal thyroid size and color Doppler for thyroid vascularization

- Fetal bone maturation
- Fetal heart rate
- Fetal thyroid function tests by fetal blood sampling in fetuses with goiter and persistent tachycardia
- Complete blood counts, liver function tests and prothrombin time for PTU.

Fetal Hypothyroidism

Cause of fetal hypothyroidism are thyroid dysgenesis (aplasia, hypoplasia, ectopic thyroid)— most common, hypothalamic or pituitary deficiency, defects in thyroid hormone synthesis, thyroid hormone resistance, Graves' disease (TSH receptor blocking antibodies), iodine deficiency or excessive iodine, antithyroid drugs, radioiodine, etc.

Drugs used in fetal hypothyroidism are intra-amniotic T4, intra-amniotic T3, 3'-triiodothyroacetic acid (Triac).

Intra-amniotic T4, Intra-amniotic T3 and 3,3', 5-triiodothyroacetic Acid (Triac)

Pharmacology: Intra-amniotic T3 is absorbed faster than intra-amniotic T4 (90% in 24 hours) and effects are evident in 4–8 hours. But it has a shorter half-life of 1-2 days compared to 6–7 days with intra-amniotic T4. Intra-amniotic is the route of administration as the doses required for fetal therapy result in maternal thyrotoxicity if administered to the mother.

Triac is T3 derived analog: Crosses placenta and binds to thyroid hormone receptors (TR beta 1) with higher affinity than T3. Triprop or 3,5,3'-triiodothyropropionic acid is also a T3 analog with higher affinity than T3.[4]

Intra-amniotic T4 is the drug of choice.

Indications: Fetal hypothyroidism.

Triac is given in 2 conditions. One for PTU-induced hypothyroidism and the other mutation of TR-beta gene leading to resistance of thyroid hormones.

Dosage: Intra-amniotic T4 250 mcg weekly to 500–600 mcg every 14 days. intra-amniotic T3 60–120 mcg.[5]

Triac-oral 2.1–2.8 mg/day for PTU-induced hypothyroidism and 2.1–3.5 mg/day for reducing TSH in TR-beta gene mutation.[4]

Adverse effects: Fetal hyperthyroidism.

Monitoring

- Fetal movements (reduced) and fetal heart rate (both tachycardia and bradycardia may occur)
- Fetal skeletal maturity
- Ultrasound for polyhydramnios, cardiomegaly and goiter. Color Doppler for vascularization.
- Fetal TSH and FT4 after 1–2 weeks of starting therapy. Repeat sampling required if there is worsening of hypothyroidism.

Preparation

- Triacana
- Teatrois

ADRENAL DISORDERS

Congenital Adrenal Hyperplasia

It is an autosomal recessive disorder. Deficiency of any of the 5 enzymes in steroidogenic pathway, can result in deficiency of cortisol and increase in ACTH. Thus, the precursors are now available for excess androgen synthesis. This results in virilization of female fetuses (pseudohermaphroditism). Most common is 21 hydroxylase deficiency. Differentiation of external genitalia occurs at around 7 weeks of gestation. So, intervention is needed before 7 weeks gestation.[6]

Dexamethasone

Pharmacology: Maternal administration of dexamethasone can suppress fetal adrenal gland.[6] It is given oral, IV or IM. Half-life is about 3 hours.

Indications: In a suspected congenital adrenal hyperplasia (CAH) fetus (couples that are carrier of classic CAH, previously affected sibling or first-degree relative, genetic analysis), dexamethasone should be started as early as 5 weeks. Sex determination is done by PCR (DYS14- Y chromosome specific sequence). If 2 separate samples of DYS14 PCR is positive (indicative of male fetus), dexamethasone is stopped. If negative, continue treatment till diagnostic chorionic villus sampling at 11 weeks to detect affected female fetus. Dexamethasone can be discontinued in unaffected fetus. In affected female, dexamethasone is continued and stress dose should be given during labor.

Contraindications: Hypersensitivity, uncontrolled infections.

Dosage: 20 mcg/kg pre-pregnancy weight per day in 2–3 divided doses maximum up to 1.5 mg/day.

Adverse effects: Edema, cutaneous striae, excessive weight gain, mood swings in the mother.[7]

Possible adverse effects in fetus include hydrocephalus, mental retardation, and failure to thrive, corpus callosum agenesis.[8,9]

Monitoring

- Maternal serum estriol and cortisol every 6–8 weeks.
- Ultrasound for external genitalia. If virilization suspected, dose of dexamethasone titrated according to amniotic fluid 17-hydroxyprogesterone.
- Maternal side effects like weight gain.

Drug interaction: Phenytoin induces its metabolism and hence, dose should be increased if given along with it.

Preparations

- *Dexamethasone*: 0.5 mg tablets, 4 mg/2 mL injection
- *Dexona*: 0.5 mg tablets, 4 mg/2 mL injection
- *Wymesone*: 0.5 mg tablets, 4 mg/2 mL injection

Safety during pregnancy and lactation: It is a FDA Category A/C drug.

REFERENCES

1. Tripathi KD (Ed). Essentials of Medical Pharmacology (7th Edn). Jaypee Publishers, 2007.
2. James, et al. High risk pregnancy management options (4th Edn). Fetal cardiac arrhythmias. Fetal thyroid and adrenal disease, 2011.
3. Haddow JE, et al. Maternal thyroid deficiency during pregnancy and subsequent neuropsychological development of the child. New Eng J Med. 1999;341:549-55.
4. Kawaguchi H, Pilbeam CC, Woodiel FN, Raisz LG. Comparison of the effects of 3, 5, 3'-triiodothyroacetic acid and triiodothyronine on bone resorption in cultured fetal rat long bones and neonatal mouse calvariae. J Bone Miner Res. 1994;9(2):247-53.
5. Bruinse HW, et al. Fetal treatment for thyrotoxicosis in non-thyrotoxic pregnant women. Fetal Ther. 1988;3(3):152-7.
6. Concalves J, Friaes A, Maura L. Congenital adrenal hyperplasia: focus on the molecular basis of 21-hydroxylase deficiency. Expert Rev Mol Med. 2007;9:1-23.
7. New MI, et al. Prenatal diagnosis for congenital adrenal hyperplasia in 532 pregnancies. Clin Endocrinol Metab. 2001;86:5651-7.
8. Forest MG, Dorr HG. Prenatal treatment of congenital adrenal hyperplasia (CAH) due to 21-hydroxylase deficiency: European experience in 223 pregnancies at risk. Pediatr Res. 1993;33:S3.
9. Lajic S, et al. Long-term somatic follow-up of prenatally treated children with congenital adrenal hyperplasia; 1998.pp.3872-80.

CHAPTER 34

Vaccines

Devender Kumar, Asmita Patil

INTRODUCTION

Adolescent girls and women should be vaccinated against vaccine preventable diseases, ideally before the conception. However in few conditions, it may be required to give vaccine even during pregnancy, if it is safe and it is going to protect mother as well as her fetus. In some conditions, the immunization has to be completed after child birth.[1]

Vaccines in Adolescent Girls and During Pregnancy

Table 34.1 enumerates the vaccines which should be given to adolescent girls and during pregnancy. Most international organizations (ACOG, SOGC) and Indian Academy of Pediatrics recommend these vaccinations.[2-4] However, Government of India recommends only tetanus toxoid (TT) vaccine during pregnancy under the National Immunization Program.[5]

Human Papilloma Virus Vaccine

Human papilloma virus (HPV) vaccine has emerged as one of the effective way of preventing cervical cancer.

HPV is a DNA virus. There are more than 100 types of HPVs and out of these 40 different types of HPV spread through sexual or direct contact. These types can be grouped under low risk (type 6 and 11) and high risk (type 16 and 18) depending on their carcinogenic potential.[6,7]

Pharmacology: Viruses like particles (VLP) are made from HPV surface components using recombinant technique. VLPs have outer L1 protein coat of HPV but no genetic material. These VLPs are very immunogenic and antibodies produced are effective against HPV. Vaccines use this property and if this person is exposed to HPV, antibodies against L1 protein will coat the virus and would prevent it from causing infection.

Two vaccines are prepared by recombinant DNA technology that produce VLPs comprising L1 proteins of HPV. These vaccines protect only against the HPV serotypes against which VLPs are present in the vaccine and the subject has not been infected earlier with that serotype. The vaccines are only prophylactic and not curative. It does not provide 100% protection against cancer and routine screening is recommended.[6,7]

The quadrivalent vaccine contains L1 protein of HPV 6, 11, 16 and 18 and aluminum based adjuvant. Clinical studies with 0, 2 and 6 months schedule is found to be 100% efficacious. Bivalent vaccine contains L1 proteins of HPV serotypes 16 and 18 and AS04

Table 34.1: Vaccines recommended during adolescence and pregnancy

Vaccine	*Age/time of vaccination*	*Type of vaccine*	*Recommendation*
HPV	Given between 9 and 26 years, contraindicated during pregnancy, given at 0,1,6 month for quadrivalent 0,2,6 month for bivalent	Live	ACOG, IAP
MMR	Given at 15 month of age, if not given at that time should be given during adolescence, should delay pregnancy for one month, contraindicated during pregnancy, if not received earlier then to be given after delivery	Live	SOGC, ACOG
Varicella*	Given at 1 year of age, if not given can be given during adolescence, contraindicated during pregnancy, pregnancy should be avoided for 1 month, if not received earlier then to be given after delivery	Live	SOGC, ACOG
TT	Given in childhood, booster dose given in second trimester, 2 doses 4 weeks apart, then every 10 years	Tetanus toxoid	UIP (Government of India), SOGC, ACOG
Td	TT can be combined with diphtheria vaccine and can be given in pregnancy in the same schedule as TT, it provides protection of new born against tetanus as well as diphtheria	Toxoid of tetanus and diphtheria	SOGC, ACOG, IAP
Tdap	TT can be combined with diphtheria and pertussis and can be given during pregnancy, it has benefit of providing protection to the newborn against tetanus, diphtheria and pertussis	Tetanus toxoid, reduced diphtheria toxin and acellular pertussis vaccine	Not yet well studied so as of now only given if risk of having pertussis SOGC, ACOG, IAP
H1N1 influenza	Can be given during pregnancy if mother is at risk, preferably to be given in second trimester, but if needed can be given in first trimester. Pregnant women are at increased risk of serious complications due to changes in respiratory, cardiovascular and immune systems. Single dose of vaccine provides protection to mother as well as the newborn and actually it is the only way to provide protection to the baby till 6 months of age because up to 6 months baby cannot be given this vaccine	Killed vaccine, administered by SC injection	SOGC, ACOG
Rabies	Can be given during pregnancy if mother is at risk of rabies	Killed vaccine	SOGC, ACOG, RCOG

*Inadvertent administration is not an indication for termination of pregnancy

as adjuvant. Clinical trials with 0, 1 and 6 month schedule is found to be 90% effective.[8-10]

Indications

IAP recommendations: Though vaccine is not part of National Immunization Program but Indian Academy of Pediatrics on immunization recommends HPV vaccine to all girls who can afford the vaccine. It should be given before the sexual debut. It recommends vaccine in girls at 11–12 years with 3 doses of vaccine. It can be given as early as 9 years and to those between 13 and 26 years if vaccination is not complete. As cervical cancer is the leading cause of cancer related morbidity and mortality, Indian Academy of Pediatrics recommends that all adolescent girls should be offered HPV vaccine at age 9–13 years.[1,2,7]

ACOG recommendations: HPV to all female patients between 9 and 26 years of age and recommends continued regular screening.

American Cancer Society warns against routine vaccination in women older than 18 years of age.

Contraindication: Vaccine is contraindicated in individuals with hypersensitivity to yeast or any other component in the vaccine.

Adverse effects: Common adverse effects are pain, swelling and erythema at the injection site. In 4% patients there may be fever.

Monitoring: Patient should be observed for 15 minutes after the injection for any syncope or other effects.

Dosage and preparation: Two types of vaccines are licensed by Food and Drug Administration (FDA) and are also available in India.[7,8] These are quadrivalent vaccine available by trade name Gardasil and a bivalent vaccine available as cervarix. Gardasil is quadrivalent as it provides protection against type 6, 11, 16 and 18 of HPV. Cervarix is very effective against 16 and 18 types only so know as bivalent vaccine. A third vaccine named as Gardasil 9 is approved by FDA and it provides protection against HPV types 6, 11,16, 18, 31, 33, 45, 52 and 58.

Vaccine is available as injection in a single dose vial or prefilled syringe and given as 0.5 mL intramuscular injection in the deltoid muscle or in the anterolateral thigh. Total of 3 doses are recommended. Quadrivalent vaccine is given at 0, 2, 6 months interval and bivalent vaccine is given at 0,1,6 months interval.

First dose is given at 9–14 years of age and booster doses can be given up to 26 years of age. If the schedule of HPV vaccine is interrupted, it need not be restarted. If a second dose is missed, it should be administered as soon as possible and interval between 2nd and 3rd dose should be at least 12 weeks. If third dose is missed, give it as soon as possible.

Vaccine is stored at 2–8°C in refrigerator and should not be frozen. It can be kept at higher temperature up to 25°C for 72 hours.

Food and Drug Administrations (FDA)/ Drugs Controller General of India (DCGI) approval: Both quadrivalent and bivalent vaccines are approved by FDA and DCGI. However, in India cost is the major concern.

Tetanus Toxoid

Tetanus is caused by a toxin produced by bacteria known as *Clostridium tetani.* The spores of this *Bacterium* are ubiquitous in the environment. Broken skin and dead tissue such as wounds provide a perfect anaerobic condition for the growth of the spores of this *Bacterium.* Infection of the cut end of umbilical cord can lead to neonatal tetanus.

Tetanus vaccination is given during pregnancy so as to prevent the mother and the newborn from tetanus. Tetanus vaccination produces protective antibodies and these antibodies are passed on to fetus. At birth both the mother and the newborn are at high risk of developing tetanus and these circulating protective antibodies protect both the mother and her fetus from neonatal tetanus. These antibodies provide protection to mother at the time of delivery and to the newborn.

Tetanus vaccine is safe during pregnancy. Two doses of TT provide protection for 1-3 years.

Pharmacology: The tetanus toxin is purified and inactivated by treatment with formaldehyde to produce the toxoid antigen. After purification and sterilization, tetanus toxoid is formulated with aluminum or calcium salts and available as single or multiple dose ampules as a single antigen vaccine (TT). It is also available in combination with diphtheria toxoid (DT and Td), and in combination with diphtheria and whole-cell or acellular pertussis (Tdap) (mentioned later in this chapter).

TT is stored at 2–8°C in refrigerator and should not be frozen.

Dosage and schedule: Primary immunization is performed under universal immunization program (Government of India) and includes 7 doses. Three doses are given as DPT followed by 2 booster doses at

18–24 months and at 5 years (as DT). Two booster doses are given at 10 and 15 years of age and then booster doses are recommended every 10 years. If a person encounters injury then may require booster at that time. According to Government of India (national immunization program), a pregnant woman is given 2 doses of TT, in second trimester and the second dose is given 4 weeks later. If the woman becomes pregnant again and has received TT within 3 years then she needs just one dose in the second trimester. Pregnant woman if undergoes abortion should receive TT vaccine and if undergoes unsafe abortion may even need tetanus immunoglobulin.[11-13]

However, WHO recommends 3 doses of TT during pregnancy, first dose is given at the first visit in the first trimester; second dose is given after 4 weeks and the third dose after 6 months. According to WHO, if a woman of child bearing age or a pregnant woman has not been immunized or the status is unknown then 5 doses of TT should be given according to schedule given in **Table 34.2.**[11,12]

Td and Tdap

ACOG and SOGC recommend use of Td instead of TT during pregnancy because Td provides protection to the newborn against diphtheria till the time the child gets vaccination. Recently Center for Disease Control and Prevention Advisory Committee on immunization Practice (ACOG 2013) has updated their guidelines and advised to use Tdap instead of TT or DT. Tdap contains tetanus toxoid, reduced diphtheria toxin and acellular pertussis vaccine. During pregnancy, this recommendation is based on the strong assumption that it protects newborn from pertussis in addition to tetanus and diphtheria and it is safe in pregnancy.

ACOG recommends booster injection during pregnancy. In a woman who had completed her immunization schedule before pregnancy, it recommends that Tdap should be administered between 27 and 36 weeks of gestation so that maximum benefit is achieved in terms of newborn protection against three diseases. Tdap at 27–36 weeks would provide better protection. It is repeated if already given. If booster is to be given, it can be given between 27 and 36 weeks.[3]

However if pregnant woman's vaccination status is unknown, ACOG recommends 3 doses of vaccine containing tetanus and diphtheria toxoid at 0, 4 weeks and 6–12 months. Recently it recommends that last dose should be Tdap instead of Td and should be given between 27 and 36 weeks of gestation.

REFERENCES

1. Indian Academy of Pediatrics Committee on Immunization (IAPCOI). Consensus recommendations on immunization and IAP immunization timetable. Indian Pediatr. 2012;49:549-64.
2. Vashishtha VM, Choudhury P, Bansal CP, Yewale VN, Agarwal R (eds). IAP Guidebook on

Table 34.2: Tetanus toxoid immunization schedule for women of childbearing age and pregnant women without previous exposure to TT, Td or Tdap

Dose of TT or Td	*When to give*	*Expected duration of protection*
TT 1	At first contact or as early as possible	None
TT 2	At least 4 weeks after TT 1	1–3 years
TT 3	At least 6 months after TT 2 or during subsequent pregnancy	At least 5 years
TT 4	At least 1 year after TT 3 or during subsequent pregnancy	At least 10 years
TT 5	At least 1 year after TT4 or during subsequent pregnancy	For all childbearing age years and possibly longer

Immunization 2013-2014. National Publication House, Indian Academy of Pediatrics, Gwalior, 2014.

3. American College of Obstetricians and Gynecologists. Committee opinion: update on immunization and pregnancy. June 2013, No. 566. Available at: http://www.acog.org/-/media/Committee-Opinions/Committee-on-Obstetric-Practice/co566.pdf?dmc=1andts=20150901T1130519590.
4. SOGC clinical practice guidelines. Immunization in pregnancy. No. 220, December 2008. Available at: http://sogc.org/wp-content uploads /2013/01/gui220CPG0812.pdf
5. MOHFW. Universal immunization program. Available at: http://mohfw.nic.in/WriteReadData/l892s/Immunization_UIP.pdf
6. World health Organization. Evidence Based Recommendations on Human Papilloma Virus (HPV) Vaccines Schedules. Background paper for SAGE discussions, March 11, 2014. Available from: http://www.who.int/immunization/sage/meetings/2014/april/1_HPV_Evidence_based_recommendationsWHO_with_Appendices2_3.pdf?ua=1. Accessed June 15, 2014.
7. Centers for Disease Control and Prevention. Advisory Committee on Immunization Practices (ACIP) recommended immunization schedule for persons aged 0 through 18 Years—United States, 2013. Atlanta (GA): CDC; 2013. Available at: http://www.cdc.gov/vaccines/schedules/down loads/child/mmwr-0-18yrs-catchup schedule.pdf
8. Sankaranarayanan R. Two vs three doses HPV vaccine schedule: low- and middle-income countries, in Eurogin 2013 International Multidisciplinary Congress. 2013: Florence, Italy.
9. Sankaranarayanan R. Trial of two versus three doses of Human Papillomavirus (HPV) vaccine in India. 2013 [cited 2013 Nov 15]; Available from: http://clinicaltrials.gov/show/NCT00923702. Accessed July 4, 2014.
10. Sankaranarayanan R. Evaluation of fewer than three doses of HPV vaccination in India, in WHO Consultation Meeting. 2013: WHO, Geneva.
11. Galazka AM. The immunological basis for immunization series. Module 3: tetanus. Geneva, World Health Organization, 1993. Available at: http://www.who.int/vaccines-documents/DocsPDF-IBI-e/mod3_e.pdf
12. The immunological basis for immunization series. Module 3: Tetanus update 2006. Geneva, World Health Organization, 2007 (http://wholibdoc.who.int/publications/2007/9789241595551_eng.pdf, accessed 24 June 2013).
13. Transplacental immunisation of the human foetus to tetanus by immunisation of the mother. J Clin Invest. 1983;72:987.

CHAPTER 35

Analgesics

Krishna Agarwal, Shailja Verma

INTRODUCTION

Commonly used analgesics in obstetrics and gynecology are given in **Table 35.1**. Ibuprofen, naproxen, tramadol, morphine, pethidine and fentanyl have been discussed in detail elsewhere. The remaining will be described here.

Non-opioid Analgesics

Paracetamol (Acetaminophen)

Pharmacology: It is a unique analgesic and is different from other ones. It has only weak anti-inflammatory action unlike NSAIDs. It has a weak analgesic action in therapeutic doses but it is a good and promptly acting antipyretic.

Table 35.1: Analgesics used commonly in obstetrics and gynecology

Class	*Drug (s)*
Nonopioid analgesics	Paracetamol
	Nonselective NSAIDs:* Diclofenac, mefanamic acid, ibuprofen, naproxane
Opioids analgesics	Tramadol, morphine, pethidine, pentazocine, fentanyl

* NSAIDs—nonsteroidal anti-inflammatory drugs

Unlike opioid analgesics it has no effect on acid-base balance, cardiovascular system and no respiratory depression.

It is well absorbed orally, only about 1/3rd is protein bound in plasma and it is uniformly distributed in the body. It is conjugated with glucuronic acid and sulfate and is excreted rapidly in urine. Plasma half-life is 2–3 hours. Effect of an oral dose lasts in 3–5 hours. It is metabolized in liver and is hepatotoxic in heavy doses and on prolonged use.

Its exact mechanism of action is not known. Recent experimental work has suggested that its analgesic action is by indirect activation of cannabinoid receptors. It has been proposed that it acts by inhibiting cyclooxygenase and it specifically acts on COX 2 receptors. It does not inhibit thromboxane and thus does not affect coagulation unlike aspirin.[1,2]

Indication of use: It is one of the most commonly used 'over the counter' analgesic for headache and musculoskeletal pain. It provides more effective analgesia when combined with opioids than with either drug alone.

It is one of the best drugs to be used as antipyretic.

It is a safest analgesic and antipyretic during pregnancy.

IV infusion is found to be effective in providing postoperative analgesia.

Contraindications: Hypersensitivity reactions though it is rare.

Dosage
- 325–650 mg orally every 4—6 hourly or 1000 mg three times a day
- *Rectal*: 650 mg every 6 hourly
- IV paracetamol
  - Less than 50 kg body weight—12.5 mg/kg every 4 hourly or 15 mg/kg 6 hourly
  - When weight is 50 kg or more—650 mg every 4 hours or 1000 mg every 6 hours.

Recently due to risk of hepatotoxicity, the maximum daily dose of paracetamol has been brought down to 3 g daily.

Adverse effects: Nausea and rashes occur occasionally, leukopenia rarely.

Acute liver failure is the most serious side effect of paracetamol toxicity. Acute paracetamol poisoning occurs specially in small children with low hepatic glutathione conjugating ability and can even be fatal beyond certain level. In case of overdose activated charcoal can be used. It prevents further absorption. Acetyl cysteine is an antidote in cases of paracetamol poisoning and it acts as a precursor of glutathione and enhances nontoxic metabolism of paracetamol.

Analgesic nephropathy can occur after years of heavy ingestion of analgesic and causes personality defects along with renal fibrosis.

Drug interactions: It interacts with warfarin (prolong INR), isoniazid and CYP450—inducing drugs.

Monitoring: No specific monitoring is required for short term use required.

Preparations
- Crocin—500 mg and 1 g tablets.
- Calpol, Metacin, Paracin—500 mg tablets, 125 mg/5 mL syrup.
- Neomol 2 mL injection—300 mg/2 mL.
- Mol—150 mg per 2 mL injection.
- Perfalgan—1 g/100 mL solution in infusion vial.

Safety during pregnancy and lactation: FDA category C drug. It does not increase the risk of congenital malformations and does not cause closure of ductus arteriosus in fetus as happens with opioid analgesics and this is the recommended drug for pain and fever during pregnancy.

Diclofenac Sodium

Pharmacology: It is a nonsteroidal anti-inflammatory drug. It is the most potent NSAIDs.

It causes inhibition of cyclooxygenase (COX) which leads to inhibition of prostaglandin synthesis. It inhibits lipoxygenase pathway and therefore decreased synthesis of leukotrienes. It may also inhibits phospholipase A2.[3,4]

Indications of use
- Postoperative pain relief
- Dysmenorrhea
- Endometriosis
- Inflammatory disorders.

Contraindications: Hypersensitivity, third trimester of pregnancy (can cause closure of ductus arteriosus) peptic ulcer, inflammatory bowel disease, dengue fever (it may induce capillary leak and heart failure), skin reaction.

Dosage: 50 mg orally or per rectally every 8 hourly maximum dose 150 mg daily.

50 mg IM or IV 8 hourly, maximum dose of 150 mg daily.

Adverse effects: This is a better tolerated NSAID.

Most common side effects is development of peptic ulcer and gastrointestinal bleeding. Rarely it can cause hepatitis. Prolonged use can cause kidney damage by inhibition of synthesis of prostaglandins in kidney. Rarely it can lead to marrow depression. There is increased risk of cardiac failure.

Drug interactions: Aspirin, paracetamol, vitamin D3, antidepressants, anticoagulants, etc.

Monitoring: CBC, liver enzymes, electrolytes, serum creatinine are monitored. Monitor urine output and blood pressure.

Preparations
- Voveran—75 mg CR capsule and tablets
- Diclofenac—50 mg dispersible tablets, 25 mg/mL injection

- Diclomove—100 mg tablet and capsule
- Jonac—100 mg suppository, 25 mg/mL injection
- Nac-75 mg tablet and capsule and 75 mg injection.

Safety during pregnancy and lactation: It is category C drug. It should be avoided in late pregnancy as may cause closure of ductus arteriosus. Prolonged use should be avoided during lactation.

Mefenamic Acid

Pharmacology: It is a nonselective COX inhibitor, which exerts both a peripheral as well as central analgesic action. It also antagonizes certain actions of prostaglandins (PGs). Its oral absorption is slow but almost complete. As it is highly plasma protein bound, displacement interactions with other drugs can occur. It is partly metabolized and excreted in urine and rest in bile. Plasma half-life is 2–4 hours, also excreted in human breast milk.

Indication of use: It is used primarily for analgesia of muscle, joints and soft tissue pain.

It is also pretty effective in primary dysmenorrhea and to some extent in rheumatoid osteoarthritis.

Contraindications: Known hypersensitivity to mefenamic acid, asthmatics, history of urticarial or type 1 allergic reactions after taking aspirin or other NSAIDs, acute active ulceration or chronic inflammation of either upper or lower GIT.

Adjustments of dose required in renal or hepatic dysfunction patients.

Dosage: 250–500 mg TDS.

Adverse effects: Diarrhea is the most important dose related side effect. There may be epigastric distress but gut bleeding is not significant with it. Skin rashes, dizziness and other CNS manifestations are rare complications. Hemolytic anemia is also a rare yet serious complication.

It can also cause new onset hypertension or worsening of preexisting one and so can contribute to increased incidence of CV events.

Drug interactions: Concomitant ingestion of antacids containing magnesium hydroxide has been shown to significantly decrease the rate and extent of mefenamic acid absorption.

Reports suggest it may diminish the antihypertensive effect of ACE inhibitors.

Avoid its use with aspirin as it increases adverse effects.

With lithium careful signs of lithium toxicity to be observed.

It may prolong prothrombin time and give false lab values.

Monitoring: Blood pressure should be monitored closely during initiation and throughout the course of treatment.

Preparations: Meftal 250, 500 mg tablet; 100 mg/5 mL susp.

Medol 250, 500 mg capsule.

Safety during pregnancy and lactation: It is FDA category C drug.

Pentazocine

Used in moderate to severe pain before minor surgical procedures.

Pharmacology: It is agonist of kappa opiate receptors and partial agonist of Mu opiate receptors in CNS.

Indications of use

- As analgesic for preoperative pain relief
- In labor pain relief.

Contraindications: Allergy, diarrhea.

Dosage: Analgesia—30–60 mg IM or IV every 4 hourly maximum 360 mg per day.

Labor pain—30 mg IM once or 20 mg IV every 3 hours, maximum total dose of 60 mg.

Adverse effects: Drowsiness, nausea, vomiting, lightheadedness, swelling or irritation at injection site. Severe allergic reaction—rash, difficulty in breathing, tightness of chest, swelling of face, lips or tongue, blurred vision, fainting, hallucinations, seizures, etc.

Interactions: Diuretics, doxylamine, magnesium sulfate, etc.

Monitoring: Mental status, blood pressure and respiratory system monitoring.

Preparations

- Fortwin—25, 30 mg tablets; 30 mg injection
- Pentazocine lactate, Forstar—30 mg injection
- Zocin—30 mg/mL.

Safety in pregnancy and lactation: FDA category C. It is FDA approved for labor analgesia. Though it may temporarily affect fetal heart rate.

REFERENCES

1. Bertolini A, Ferrari A, Ottani A, Guerzoni S, Tacchi R, Leone S. Paracetamol: New vistas of an old drug. CNS Drug Rev. 2006 Fall-Winter;12(3-4):250-75. Review.
2. McNicol ED, Tzortzopoulou A, Cepeda MS, Francia MB, Farhat T, Schumann R. Single-dose intravenous paracetamol or propacetamol for prevention or treatment of postoperative pain: A systematic review and meta-analysis. Br J Anaesth. 2011;106:764-75.
3. Dahl V, Hagen IE, Sveen AM, Norseng H, Koss KS, Steen T. High-dose diclofenac for postoperative analgesia after elective caesarean section in regional anaesthesia. Int J Obstet Anesth. 2002;11(2):91-4.
4. Al-Waili NS. Efficacy and safety of repeated postoperative administration of intramuscular diclofenac sodium in the treatment of post-cesarean section pain: A double-blind study. Arch Med Res. 2001;32:148-54.

Index

Page numbers followed by *f* refer to figure and *t* refer table

D

E

F